Rural Mental Health

K. Bryant Smalley, PhD, PsyD, is a licensed clinical psychologist with experience in research and practice in rural areas. He is the founding Co-Executive Director of the Rural Health Research Institute, an innovative, interdisciplinary hub of research and outreach dedicated to improving health outcomes and reducing health disparities in rural populations. He is also the Associate Director of Clinical Training for the PsyD program at Georgia Southern University, a clinical psychology program focused on preparing mental health practitioners for rural practice. Dr. Smalley currently serves on the Georgia Psychological Association board as the Rural Health Committee Chair. His research has appeared in numerous journals and texts, including *Health and Technology, Psychology of Men and Masculinity, The International Journal of Men's Health*, and *Journal of Clinical Psychology: In Session*, and has been funded by organizations such as the Office of Rural Health Policy within the Health Resources and Services Administration (HRSA).

Jacob C. Warren, PhD, is a behavioral epidemiologist specializing in health disparities research. He has been a Principal Investigator or Co-Investigator on numerous federally funded research and service grants, including funding from the Centers for Disease Control and Prevention, the National Institutes of Health, and the Federal Office of Rural Health Policy within the Health Resources and Services Administration (HRSA). He is the founding Co-Executive Director of the Rural Health Research Institute and has presented his research at numerous national and international conferences. He has published in journals including *Health and Technology, Drug and Alcohol Dependence, Journal of Ethnicity and Substance Abuse, Pan American Journal of Public Health, AIDS and Behavior*, and *AIDS Education and Prevention*.

Jackson P. Rainer, PhD, is a nationally known and respected psychotherapist, teacher, and supervisor. In rural and urban settings, he has directed community mental health institutions and agencies, practiced psychotherapy with children, adults, couples and families, and taught in universities and professional settings for more than 25 years. In addition to being the Department Head of the Department of Psychology and Counseling at Valdosta State University, he serves as a national consultant for psychotherapy and supervision. His research appears in journals such as *Innovations in Clinical Practice* and the *Journal of Clinical Psychology: In Session,* and his most recent book is *Crisis Counseling and Therapy,* coauthored with Frieda Brown.

Rural Mental Health
Issues, Policies, and Best Practices

K. Bryant Smalley, PhD, PsyD
Jacob C. Warren, PhD
Jackson P. Rainer, PhD
Editors

SPRINGER PUBLISHING COMPANY
NEW YORK

Springer Publishing Company, LLC
11 West 42nd Street
New York, NY 10036
www.springerpub.com

Acquisitions Editor: Margaret Zuccarini
Production Editor: Michael O'Connor
Composition: Techset

ISBN: 978-0-8261-0799-2
E-book ISBN: 978-0-8261-0800-5

12 13 14 15 / 5 4 3 2 1

The author and the publisher of this Work have made every effort to use sources believed to be reliable to provide information that is accurate and compatible with the standards generally accepted at the time of publication. Because medical science is continually advancing, our knowledge base continues to expand. Therefore, as new information becomes available, changes in procedures become necessary. We recommend that the reader always consult current research and specific institutional policies before performing any clinical procedure. The author and publisher shall not be liable for any special, consequential, or exemplary damages resulting, in whole or in part, from the readers' use of, or reliance on, the information contained in this book. The publisher has no responsibility for the persistence or accuracy of URLs for external or third-party Internet Web sites referred to in this publication and does not guarantee that any content on such Web sites is, or will remain, accurate or appropriate.

Library of Congress Cataloging-in-Publication Data

Rural mental health : issues, policies, and best practices/K. Bryant Smalley, Jacob C. Warren, Jackson P. Rainer, editors.
  p. ; cm.
  Includes bibliographical references and index.
  ISBN 978-0-8261-0799-2 -- ISBN 978-0-8261-0800-5 (e-book)
  1. Smalley, K. Bryant. II. Warren, Jacob C. III. Rainer, Jackson P.
  [DNLM: 1. Mental Health Services--United States. 2. Rural Health Services--United States. 3. Health Policy--United States. 4. Mental Health--United States. 5. Rural Health--United States. WA 390]
  LC classification not assigned
  362.1968900973--dc23
                                                                    2012015887

Special discounts on bulk quantities of our books are available to corporations, professional associations, pharmaceutical companies, health care organizations, and other qualifying groups.

If you are interested in a custom book, including chapters from more than one of our titles, we can provide that service as well.

For details, please contact:
Special Sales Department, Springer Publishing Company, LLC
11 West 42nd Street, 15th Floor, New York, NY 10036-8002s
Phone: 877-687-7476 or 212-431-4370; Fax: 212-941-7842
Email: sales@springerpub.com

Printed in the United States of America by Gasch printing

To my parents, Becky and Terry - Bryant

To my parents, Rita and Mark - Jacob

To my wife, Karen - Jack

Contents

Contributors

Jamie Aten, PhD, Associate Professor, Psychology Department, Wheaton College, Wheaton, Illinois

Audrey L. Austin, MPH, MA, Department of Psychology, The University of Alabama, Tuscaloosa, Alabama

Jaedon P. Avey, MS, Department of Psychology, University of Alaska—Anchorage, Anchorage, Alaska

Carmen Broussard, PhD, Associate Professor, Department of Psychology and Counselor Education, Nicholls State University, Thibodaux, Louisiana

Frieda Farfour Brown, PhD, Professor of Psychology and Counseling, School of Psychology and Counseling, Gardner-Webb University, Boiling Springs, North Carolina

Clark Campbell, PhD, ABPP, Dean, Rosemead School of Psychology, Biola University, La Mirada, California

Courtney Cantrell, MS, Center for Psychological Studies, Nova Southeastern University, Fort Lauderdale, Florida

Ralph E. Cash, PhD, NCSP, Professor, Center for Psychological Studies, Nova Southeastern University, Fort Lauderdale, Florida

Patrick W. Corrigan, PsyD, Associate Dean of Psychology Research, College of Psychology, Illinois Institute of Technology, Chicago, Illinois

Thomas P. Cothran, College of Psychology, Illinois Institute of Technology, Chicago, Illinois

Martha R. Crowther, PhD, MPH, Associate Professor, Department of Psychology, The University of Alabama, Tuscaloosa, Alabama

Lisa Curtin, PhD, Professor of Psychology, Department of Psychology, Appalachian State University, Boone, North Carolina

Tamara L. DeHay, PhD, Behavioral Health Research Associate, Mental Health Program, Western Interstate Commission for Higher Education (WICHE), Boulder, Colorado

Patrick H. DeLeon, PhD, JD, MPH, Former President, American Psychological Association, Washington, District of Columbia

Angela Banitt Duncan, PhD, Senior Research Associate, Center for Telemedicine and Telehealth, University of Kansas, Kansas City, Kansas

Robert Eley, PhD, Senior Research Fellow, Centre for Rural and Remote Area Health, University of Southern Queensland, Toowoomba, Queensland, Australia

John A. Gale, MS, Research Associate, Maine Rural Health Research Center, University of Southern Maine, Portland, Maine

Don Gorman, RN, DipNEd, BEd, MEd, EdD, FRCNA, Director, Centre for Rural and Remote Area Health, University of Southern Queensland, Toowoomba, Queensland, Australia

Kristin Guilfou, Department of Psychology and Counselor Education, Nicholls State University, Thibodaux, Louisiana

Patrick Hall, MDiv, Psychology Department, Wheaton College, Wheaton, Illinois

David S. Hargrove, PhD, ABPP, Georgetown Family Center, Washington, District of Columbia

David Hartley, PhD, MHA, Research Professor and Director, Maine Rural Health Research Center, University of Southern Maine, Portland, Maine

Delwar Hossain, PhD, Research Fellow, Centre for Rural and Remote Area Health, University of Southern Queensland, Toowoomba, Queensland, Australia

John Paul Jameson, PhD, Assistant Professor, Department of Psychology, Appalachian State University, Boone, North Carolina

Mary Beth Kenkel, PhD, Dean and Professor, College of Psychology and Liberal Arts, Florida Institute of Technology, Melbourne, Florida

Amanda Brown Kotis, MA, DMD, Private Practice, Huntersville, North Carolina

David Lambert, PhD, Research Associate Professor, Maine Rural Health Research Center, University of Southern Maine, Portland, Maine

Jonathon E. Larson, EdD, MS, LCPC, CRC, Assistant Professor, College of Psychology, Illinois Institute of Technology, Chicago, Illinois

Jennifer D. Lenardson, MHS, Research Associate, Maine Rural Health Research Center, University of Southern Maine, Portland, Maine

Michael Mangis, PhD, Professor of Psychology, Psychology Department, Wheaton College, Wheaton, Illinois

Johnathan C. Martin, EdS, Psychology Department, Georgia Southern University, Statesboro, Georgia

Mimi McFaul, PsyD, Associate Director, Mental Health Program, Western Interstate Commission for Higher Education (WICHE), Boulder, Colorado

Dennis Mohatt, MA, Vice President for Behavioral Health, Western Interstate Commission for Higher Education (WICHE), Boulder, Colorado

Eve-Lynn Nelson, PhD, Associate Professor, Pediatrics and Telemedicine, University of Kansas Medical Center, Kansas City, Kansas

Karen B. Pearson, MLIS, MA, Policy Analyst, Maine Rural Health Research Center, University of Southern Maine, Portland, Maine

Amanda Pellegrino, PsyS, Educational Specialist, Regents Center for Learning Disorders, Georgia Southern University, Statesboro, Georgia

Heidi Liss Radunovich, PhD, Assistant Professor, Department of Family, Youth, and Community Sciences, University of Florida, Gainesville, Florida

Jackson P. Rainer, PhD, ABPP, Department Head, Psychology and Counseling, Valdosta State University, Valdosta, Georgia

Forrest Scogin, PhD, Coordinator, Clinical Geropsychology, Department of Psychology, The University of Alabama, Tuscaloosa, Alabama

Diana V. Shaw, PhD, MPH, MBA, FACMPE, Lanai Community Health Center, Lanai City, Hawaii

K. Bryant Smalley, PhD, PsyD, Co-Executive Director, Rural Health Research Institute, Georgia Southern University, Statesboro, Georgia

Sarah Valley-Gray, PsyD, Associate Professor, Center for Psychological Studies, Nova Southeastern University, Fort Lauderdale, Florida

Sarah E. Velasquez, MAB, MS, Senior Coordinator, Center for Telemedicine and Telehealth, University of Kansas, Kansas City, Kansas

Angela M. Waguespack, PhD, Associate Professor, Center for Psychological Studies, Nova Southeastern University, Fort Lauderdale, Florida

Shannon P. Warden, PhD, LPC, NCC, Mental Health Counseling Coordinator, Boiling Springs Campus, School of Psychology and Counseling, Gardner-Webb University, Boiling Springs, North Carolina

Jacob C. Warren, PhD, Co-Executive Director, Rural Health Research Institute, Georgia Southern University, Statesboro, Georgia

Ernest Wayde, MA, Department of Psychology, The University of Alabama, Tuscaloosa, Alabama

Isaac Weaver, Psychology Department, Wheaton College, Wheaton, Illinois

James L. Werth, Jr., PhD, ABPP, Director, PsyD Program in Counseling Psychology, Department of Psychology, Radford University, Radford, Virginia

Brenda A. Wiens, PhD, Clinical Assistant Professor, Department of Clinical and Health Psychology, University of Florida, Gainesville, Florida

Derick Williams, PhD, Assistant Professor, Curry School of Education, University of Virginia, Charlottesville, Virginia

Ishan Williams, PhD, Assistant Professor, School of Nursing, University of Virginia, Charlottesville, Virginia.

Preface

Rural residents, accounting for 20% of the United States population, represent one of the largest population groups with recognized challenges in receipt of mental health services. For decades, there has been national recognition that individuals and families in rural areas face barriers to health and wellness beyond those faced by urban residents. In addition to being more likely than individuals in urban areas to be without a regular source of health care, without health insurance, and to be coping with a chronic or serious illness, rural residents face stark burdens of mental illness and barriers to receipt of quality mental health services. In addition, mental health clinicians practicing in rural areas face additional challenges not as frequently encountered by their urban counterparts.

The repeating themes of rural mental health involve mounting needs, restricted or limited resources, and widespread provider shortages; unique geographic and cultural challenges to service delivery for which clinicians receive little to no training; service providers struggling to operate under urban models and assumptions imposed by funding sources and regulators; consistent and pervasive misunderstandings of rural realities; and the tendency to not take "rural" into account in public policy or the tendency to want a single policy solution to rural issues. Despite many years of attention, there remain innumerable examples of challenges rural residents face in maintaining and improving their mental health that are widespread and require consideration of multiple unique features of rural living.

In our roles ranging from rural-based clinicians to university-based researchers, we have seen daily the impact that rural residence has on mental health—both in mental health stressors and in ability to receive care. These ongoing observations provided the impetus for this book. While much attention has been paid to rural mental health, there was a lack of a cohesive, up-to-date resource focusing on all areas of need within rural mental health (ranging from cultural factors to specific evidence-based best practices for particular rural groups). We have written *Rural Mental Health* in the hope of bringing much-needed attention to the distinct mental health needs of rural populations. The book first offers a summary and background of the current state of rural mental health and special consideration in working with rural populations, followed by discussion on some of the major models of service delivery that have been developed to address specific challenges faced in the delivery of quality mental health services. The book then examines specific considerations and best practices for working with distinct subgroups in rural areas, ranging from minority groups to veterans. It concludes with a discussion on the next steps in advancing the mental health of rural groups.

The book has been written for practitioners, researchers, and students seeking recommendations, a guide to best practices and new models of service delivery, and as a useful reference for current issues and concerns in rural mental health. The text examines the intricacies of improving mental health in rural practice and offers clear, research-driven recommendations for clinicians and scholars, able to be adopted into current practice or training programs. In preparing the text, we assembled a group of seasoned researchers and clinicians from Georgia to Alaska to Australia who speak from their direct experience as to the current state of rural mental health, new models for service delivery, and the best practices for working with specific rural populations.

We hope that this text serves as both a resource and a call-to-action for rural mental health. Together, we can help bridge the gap between rural and urban areas and improve the mental health of the 60 million people who live in rural America.

K. Bryant Smalley, PhD, PsyD
Co-Executive Director, Rural Health Research Institute
Associate Director of Clinical Training, Department of Psychology
Georgia Southern University

Jacob C. Warren, PhD
Co-Executive Director, Rural Health Research Institute
Georgia Southern University

Jackson P. Rainer, PhD
Department Head, Psychology and Counseling
Valdosta State University

Rural Mental Health

I

Introduction and Special Considerations

1

The Current State of Rural Mental Health

K. BRYANT SMALLEY AND JACOB C. WARREN

INTRODUCTION

*R*ural Americans comprise an estimated 20% of the U.S. population (U.S. Census Bureau, 2010) and represent a larger subgroup of Americans than any racial or ethnic minority. Unfortunately, persistent disparities in rates, severity, and outcomes of mental illness in rural America have remained relatively unchanged over the past several decades, and federal funding for rural mental health research lags behind funding received for other disparity groups. Practitioners and researchers have long recognized the unique mental health challenges faced by rural Americans, but organized movements toward improving mental health in rural areas did not come to the forefront until the 1970s. At the time, the most pressing mental health concerns in rural areas were the lack of doctoral-level psychologists available at community mental health centers in rural areas, the lack of training of mental health professionals in the particular needs of rural residents, and the high rate of turnover in rural mental health positions (Hollingsworth & Hendrix, 1977)—concerns that unfortunately continue today. The federal response to rural mental health has heightened in recent years; one of the most significant advancements was the establishment of the Office of Rural Health Policy and the National Rural Health Advisory Committee in 1987 within the Health Resources and Services Administration (HRSA; DeLeon, Wakefield, Schultz, Williams, & VandenBos, 1989). Many other federal steps have been taken to improve rural mental health (and are discussed in detail in Chapter 2); however, despite nearly 30 years of intensified focus on rural mental health, rural populations continue to face increased mental health burden and distinct challenges in receiving mental health services.

Portions of this chapter are adapted from material that previously appeared in the Journal of Clinical Psychology.

The goal of this book is to summarize the current status of rural mental health and to individually examine the many complex subcomponents of improving mental health throughout rural regions. This chapter provides a broad introduction to the current state of rural mental health, briefly touching on many of the issues that are examined in depth in later chapters.

WHAT IS RURAL?

Throughout the psychological literature, inconsistent findings with respect to rural residence abound in mental health diagnoses and outcomes. This is due in large part to the fact that unlike many other underserved populations (such as racial or ethnic minorities), there is no single, consistent definition of what *rural* actually is (HRSA, 2005). Definitions of rurality are frequently based on population size, population density, and/or economic factors—each of which have distinct limitations in their application. For instance, a common definition of "rural" is a county with less than 50,000 residents. This definition, however, does not take into account population *density*. As a result, counties with more geographic area may not be labeled as rural, even if they have fewer residents per square mile than a geographically smaller county with proportionately more residents.

Similar complications arise with nearly every definition of rural, leading to a vast array of inconsistent definitions applied across the rural health literature. The lack of consistency in the definition of rurality has unfortunately clouded what can definitively be stated about rural mental health prevalence and outcomes. Despite this, some differences have been repeatedly demonstrated, and the impact of the unique culture of rural living on mental health is evident; in fact, being from a rural background can have such strong influence on an individual's perceptions of mental health that "rurality" can be viewed by mental health practitioners as a diversity issue similar to being from a racial, ethnic, or other minority background (see Chapter 3).

Even within the somewhat nebulous concept of "rural," there are well-recognized degrees of rurality. Traditionally, rurality has been divided into two main categories, rural and frontier, with frontier communities representing the extreme of rurality (sometimes with "neighbors" separated from each other by miles). As with "rural," defining "frontier" is difficult; definitions range from having a population density less than or equal to six people per square mile (Hewitt 1989) to complex scoring methods that take into account travel time to market centers and medical care (Center for Rural Health, 2006; Frontier Education Center, 2007). Most frontier communities are concentrated in the Western United States and Alaska. Many of the differences presented below and throughout this book are even more amplified in frontier areas because of their extreme geographic isolation; challenges with geographical barriers, poverty, travel distance, and lack of mental health care providers are particularly acute in frontier settings (see Chapter 20).

Regardless of the definition used or the degree of rurality of a given community, rural areas have unique health problems, resource shortages, demographic characteristics, cultural behaviors, and economic concerns that combine to impact on the mental health of its residents. While cultural factors and demographic characteristics vary across rural regions, two consistent characteristics across most rural populations are poverty and inability to access affordable mental health services. An estimated 17% of adult rural residents live below the federal poverty line, as compared with 14% of urban residents (Economic Research Service [ERS], 2011). Poverty rates are even higher for minority rural residents: 32% of rural African Americans and 28% of rural Hispanics live below the poverty line (ERS, 2011). Rural residents have been shown to go longer periods of time without health insurance, and are less likely to seek care when they cannot pay because of pride and the lack of reduced-price medical care services in rural areas (Mueller, Patil, & Ullrich, 1997). Even if an individual decides to seek care, rural areas are plagued by shortages in mental health care professionals (Murray & Keller, 1991). These cultural, economic, and provider shortage challenges combine to sustain mental health problems in rural areas that unfortunately are not easily addressed.

MENTAL HEALTH IN RURAL AREAS

The impact of mental health disorders in rural areas is greater than in urban areas due to a three-part problem of accessibility, availability, and acceptability of mental health services (HRSA, 2005; Human & Wasem, 1991). Key challenges with accessibility of mental health services in rural areas include transportation to and from services and ability to pay for services. Availability of services is impacted upon mainly by health professional shortages; more than 85% of Mental Health Professional Shortage Areas (MHPSAs) are in rural areas (Bird, Dempsey, & Hartley, 2001), and more than one half of all the counties in the United States do not have a single psychologist, psychiatrist, or social worker (American Psychological Association, 2001; National Advisory Committee on Rural Health, 1993). Practitioner shortages have been attributed to challenges in recruiting and retaining professionals because of lower salaries, limited social/cultural outlets, and increased risk of professional burnout (HRSA, 2005; see Chapter 8). Rural providers also face additional ethical dilemmas in their practice (see Chapter 7) that may serve as a deterrent to establishing and maintaining a practice in rural areas.

Acceptability of receiving psychological services in rural areas is lowered due to increased stigma and decreased anonymity in seeking psychological services (HRSA, 2005). The impact of stigma is well recognized in rural areas (see Chapter 4), mainly related to traditional cultural beliefs and a lack of understanding of mental health issues (Letvak, 2002). The level of stigma toward mental health services has been shown to be stronger the smaller the community is (Hoyt, Conger, Valde, & Weihs, 1997). In addition, because of the interconnected nature of rural communities, there is less anonymity when seeking mental health services (Helbok, 2003). For instance, by parking at a psychologist's office, clients face the possibility of word spreading of their use of services. The increased stigma and decreased anonymity likely make rural residents less likely to seek care than their urban counterparts (Wagenfeld & Buffum, 1983), and may contribute to rural residents' perceptions that psychological services are less available and accessible to them (Rost, Fortney, Zhang, Smith, & Smith, 1999). Ironically, despite the tight-knit nature of rural communities, rural residents face increased burdens of isolation and loneliness (see Chapter 5) not only because of their often extended geographic separations from friends and family, but because of the high levels of stigma regarding mental illness that can leave those seeking psychological services feeling even more detached from their communities.

Because of lowered accessibility, availability, and acceptability, rural residents suffering from mental health disorders tend to enter mental health care later, enter with more serious symptoms, and as a result require more intensive treatment (Rost, Fortney, Fischer, & Smith, 2002; Wagenfeld, Murray, Mohatt, & DeBruyn, 1994). Not all cultural aspects of rural living have negative impacts on mental health, however. Religiosity, highly prevalent in rural areas, can have a protective and therapeutic effect. Emerging evidence suggests that incorporating religious themes into therapy with rural populations can be particularly effective (see Chapter 6 for more details).

While large-scale, systematic differences are not routinely found in mental health prevalence in rural areas, some relatively consistent differences have emerged. Rural residents have been shown to have higher levels of depression, domestic violence, and child abuse (Bushy, 1998; Cellucci & Vik, 2001) and demonstrate higher involvement in behavioral health risk factors such as sedentary lifestyle and smoking (Eberhardt, Ingram, & Makuc, 2001; Eberhardt & Pamuk, 2004).

Disproportionate burdens of substance use and suicide are among the most robust differences found between rural and urban areas, and the reasons for these differences are complex and often intertwined with the physical and cultural realities of rural living (see Chapter 12). While illegal drugs have traditionally been thought of as an "urban" problem, methamphetamine use in particular is becoming an increasing problem in rural settings (Gfroerer, Larson, & Colliver, 2008). Rural youth face particular drug use disparities, having higher rates of substance use than their urban counterparts, including alcohol, tobacco, methamphetamines, prescription drugs, inhalants, marijuana, and cocaine (Lambert, Gale, & Hartley, 2008; National Center on Addiction and Substance Abuse, 2000; Substance Abuse and Mental Health Services Administration [SAMHSA], 2001). Unfortunately, access to appropriate inpatient and outpatient substance use care is lower in rural areas and prevents rural populations from accessing evidence-based care for substance use (American Society of Addiction Medicine, 2001, 2005; Center for Substance Abuse Treatment [CSAT], 2000; Sowers & Rohland, 2004). Compounding difficulties in treatment of substance use disorders is the fact that up to 40% of mentally ill individuals in rural areas have a comorbid substance use disorder (Gogek, 1992), complicating the receipt of appropriate services even more.

Rural residents also have higher rates of suicide than their nonrural counterparts. Rural areas have consistently demonstrated more suicide deaths and a higher rate of suicide completion than urban areas (Center for Disease Control and Prevention [CDC] 2007; Goldsmith, Pellmar, Kleinman, & Bunney, 2002; Institute of Medicine, 2002; New Freedom Commission Subcommittee on Rural Issues, 2003); in some areas, the rural–urban differences are as much as 300% (Mulder et al., 2001). The differences in suicide attempts are even more striking among adolescents, sometimes demonstrated to be 15 times higher among rural adolescents when compared to urban (Forrest, 1988). Many factors have been identified as driving these disparities in suicide rates (and are discussed in detail in Chapter 13), including access to lethal means, geographic and social isolation, and mental health stigma.

Although rural populations share many characteristics, there is tremendous diversity within rural populations, and different subgroups of rural populations face varying mental health stressors and experience different mental health burdens. Minority groups face disparate burdens of many mental health conditions (see Chapter 14). Rural minority groups face a disproportionate burden of poverty and an underutilization of mental health services that lead rural minorities to have an increased utilization of mental health emergency services due to delays in receipt of treatment (Snowden, Masland, Libby, Wallace, & Fawley, 2008). When examining nonemergency care, African Americans and Hispanic populations receive less mental health treatment even when age, gender, and insurance status are controlled for (Goodwin, Koenen, Hellman, Guardino, & Struening, 2002; Han & Lui, 2005; Padgett, Patrick, Burns, & Schlesinger, 1994; Zito, Safer, Zuckerman, Gardner, & Soeken, 2005). As with all rural populations, rural minorities face challenges in accessibility, availability, and acceptability of services; however, rural minorities are even more impacted upon by reduced acceptability of services. For instance, rural African Americans have been shown to be less likely to seek mental health care services (even when needed and available) due to distrust of professionals and even more pronounced stigmatization of mental health problems (Corbie-Smith, Thomas, & St. George, 2001; Fox, Blank, Rovnyak, & Barnett, 2001; Fox, Merwin, & Blank, 1995; Menke & Flynn, 2009; Ward, Clark, & Hendrich, 2009).

Rural lesbian, gay, bisexual, and questioning (LGBQ) residents also face unique mental health challenges due to increased prevalence of mental health risk factors including vicitimization and discrimination, internalized heterosexism, minimal social opportunities with other LGBQ individuals, lack of family and social support, and decreased comfort in disclosing their sexual identity to others (Kennedy, 2010; Leedy & Connolly, 2007; McCarthy, 2000; Preston, D'Augelli, Kassab, & Starks, 2007; Willging, Salvador, & Kano, 2006a). These risk factors lead to increased concerns regarding substance abuse and suicidality (Waldo, Hesson-McInnis, & D'Augelli, 1998; Willging et al., 2006a) in a setting where mental health providers often have little or no experience or training in the mental health needs of rural LGBQ clients (Willging et al., 2006b; see Chapter 14 for further discussion).

There are also differences by gender in rural mental health (see Chapters 15 and 16). Rural men report poorer levels of overall mental health and higher rates of suicide (Alston, 2010; Dresang, 2001; Hauenstein et al., 2006). Because of gender-based norms of stoicism and self-reliance that are particularly strong in rural areas (Kosberg & Fei Sun, 2010), rural men are more likely to avoid treatment and present at later stages in the course of their mental health diagnosis (Francis, Boyd, Aisbett, Newnham, & Newnham, 2006; Murray et al., 2008). Rural women face mental health concerns in a context with limited mental health services specific for them (Thorndyke, 2005). They face increased risk of hospitalization for depression (Badger, Robinson, & Farley, 1999) and as with their urban counterparts, struggle with eating disorders and loneliness (Birmingham, Su, Hlynsky, Goldner, & Gao 2005). Rural women's mental health is affected by a number of sociocultural factors including increased risk for abuse, increased isolation, economic instability, and a lack of childcare support that have each been linked with mood disorders (Boyd & Mackey, 2000; Bushy, 1993; Dimmitt & Davila, 1995; Hauenstein & Boyd, 1994).

Other groups that require special consideration in provision of mental health services in rural areas include the elderly, as well as children/adolescents and their families. While the overall U.S. population is increasingly older, rural populations have higher numbers of older adults than nonrural areas (National Advisory Committee on Rural Health and Human Services [NACRHHS], 2004; U.S. Census Bureau, 2000), leading to unique mental health needs in a context with typically poorer mental health status among the elderly (Guralnick, Kemele, Stamm, & Greving, 2003). Older adults in rural areas face many challenges (see Chapter 18), including depression, higher burden of medical care, and lack of specialized elderly mental health expertise (Buckwalter, Smith, Zevenbergen, & Russell, 1991; Unutzer et al., 1997). Rural children and adolescents also face significant barriers to maintaining mental health (see Chapter 17), including increased incidence of poverty, obesity, physical abuse, and substance use often coupled with inferior educational, transportation, health care, and mental health care services (Slovak & Singer, 2002; Welsh, Domitrovich, Bierman, & Lang, 2003). Rural children have been shown to be at increased risk of many mental and behavioral health issues including substance use, depression, and anxiety (Peden, Reed, & Rayens, 2005; Sears, 2004; Spoth, Goldberg, Neppl, Trudeau, & Ramisetty-Mikler, 2001), but a low proportion of rural children actually receive care for diagnosed conditions (Angold et al., 2002).

An additional group within rural settings with particular mental health needs is rural veterans (see Chapter 19). With rural recruits overrepresented in the military (Richardson & Waldrop, 2003) and the increased likelihood of rural veterans experiencing combat casualties in recent armed conflicts (O'Hare & Bishop, 2006), there will be an increased demand for mental health services in rural areas for veterans in the coming years. Unfortunately, this increased need occurs in a context that is already recognized as having broad shortages in mental health care. With high rates of posttraumatic stress disorder (PTSD), other anxiety disorders, depression, substance use, and traumatic brain injuries (Fontana & Rosenheck, 2008; Hoge et al., 2008; Petrakis, Rosenheck, & Desai, 2011; Wallace, Weeks, Wang, Lee, & Kazis, 2006; Zatzick et al., 1997), rural veterans have very specific psychological needs that frequently cannot be addressed in rural settings. Unfortunately, the Veterans Affairs (VA) system—the safety net for physical and mental health care of veterans—often does not operate in rural areas and rural veterans frequently find themselves having difficulty securing transportation to distant VA service locations (Weeks, Wallace, West, Heady, & Hawthorne, 2008).

ADDRESSING CORE PROBLEMS IN RURAL MENTAL HEALTH

A number of strategies have been developed to address the problems faced by rural populations in achieving a healthy mental status and are discussed throughout this book. Many of these approaches directly counteract some of the barriers to maintaining mental health or receiving mental health services that rural residents face. Three of the most promising approaches are integrated care services, telehealth technologies, and school- and home-based interventions.

The concept of integrated care (provision of physical and mental health services within the same context) addresses several concerns, including increasing access to services and decreasing stigma in receipt of services. It also addresses the high degree of comorbidity between physical and mental health conditions; an estimated 34% to 41% of patients in primary care in rural areas have a diagnosable mental health disorder (Sears, Evans, & Kuper, 2003), and more than 40% of individuals with mental health needs originally seek treatment in a primary care setting (Chapa, 2004). This high overlap led the President's New Freedom Commission on Mental Health (2003) to highlight the need of increasing access to and quality of mental health care in rural areas through integrated care, specifically stating that there is a need to "screen for mental disorders in primary health care, across the life span, and connect to treatment and supports" (p. 11). Additional details on integrated care, including best practices and evidence base, can be found in Chapter 9.

Telehealth (the provision of clinical care or consultation via technology-enhanced means) also holds tremendous promise in addressing the core problems rural residents face in receiving mental health services. Such approaches improve accessibility because they can be deployed in almost any setting, improve availability because they increase the reach of providers into rural settings without requiring providers to actually be within the rural area, and improve acceptability because of their ability to be deployed within trusted settings including doctors' offices and the home. Chapter 10 presents a comprehensive review of telehealth technologies and the impact they have on rural mental health.

The school is also a natural place for mental health intervention (see Chapter 11) given that nearly all children in rural areas attend school, and transportation to schools is already required (Owens & Murphy, 2004; Stein et al., 2002; Weist & Evans, 2005). Provision of services within the school setting automatically minimizes stigma and accessibility concerns, and centralizes resources in a setting with maximum reach. Telehealth has broadened the possibilities of providing school-based care, connecting students at school with mental health care located in other areas (Myers, Valentine, & Melzer, 2008; Myers et al., 2010; Nelson & Bui, 2010). Many other evidence-based school programs have emerged, including those that involve family–school partnerships and interagency collaborations (Minke, 2006).

CONCLUSION

While there are many challenges in providing for the mental health needs of rural populations, there are also many emerging opportunities for addressing the needs of this highly underserved population. By becoming familiar with the unique needs, mental health burdens, and cultural influences of rural populations and combining that knowledge with the latest information on evidence-based approaches to address barriers to care in rural areas, mental health professionals can begin to make a difference in the lives of rural populations and address the disproportionate mental health burden they face. We hope this book can serve as a guide to this process.

REFERENCES

Alston, M. (2010). Rural male suicide in Australia. *Social Science & Medicine*, 74(4), 515–522.

American Psychological Association. (2001). *Caring for the rural community: 2000–2001 report*. Retrieved from http://www.apa.org/rural/APAforWeb72.pdf

American Society of Addiction Medicine. (2001). Preface. In D. Mee-Lee (Ed.), *ASAM patient placement criteria for the treatment of substance-related disorders* (2nd ed. Revised). Chevy Chase, MD: American Society of Addiction Medicine, Inc.

American Society of Addiction Medicine. (2005). *Public policy statement on treatment for alcoholism and other drug dependencies*. Chevy Chase, MD: Author.

Angold, A., Erkanli, A., Farmer, E. M. Z., Fairbank, J. A., Burns, B. J., Keeler, G., & ... Costello, E. J. (2002). Psychiatric disorder, impairment, and service use in rural African American and White youth. *Archives of General Psychiatry, 59*, 893-901. doi: 10.1001/archpsyc.59.10.893

Badger, L., Robinson, H., & Farley, T. (1999). Management of mental disorders in rural primary care. *The Journal of Family Practice, 2*(2), 15-22.

Bird, D. C., Dempsey, P., & Hartley, D. (2001). *Addressing mental health workforce needs in underserved rural areas: Accomplishments and challenges.* Portland, ME: Maine Rural Health Research Center.

Birmingham, C. L., Su, J., Hlynsky, J., Goldner, E. M., & Gao, M. (2005). The mortality rate from anorexia nervosa. *International Journal of Eating Disorders, 38*(2), 143-146.

Boyd, M. R., & Mackey, M. C. (2000). Running away to nowhere: Rural women's experiences of becoming alcohol dependent. *Archives of Psychiatric Nursing, 14*(3), 142-149.

Buckwalter, K. C., Smith, M., Zevenbergen, P., & Russell, D. (1991). Mental health services of the rural elderly outreach program. *The Gerontologist, 31*(3), 408-412.

Bushy, A. (1993). Rural women: Lifestyles and health status. *Nursing Clinics of North America, 28*(1), 187-197.

Bushy, A. (1998). Health issues of women in rural environments: An overview. *Journal of the American Medical Women's Association, 53*(2), 53-56.

Cellucci, T., & Vik, P. (2001). Training for substance abuse treatment among psychologists in a rural state. *Professional Psychology: Research and Practice, 32*(3), 248-252.

Center for Rural Health. (2006). *Defining the term "frontier area" for programs implemented through the Office for the Advancement of Telehealth.* Bismark, ND: Univeristy of North Dakota.

Center for Substance Abuse Treatment. (2000). *Changing the conversation: Improving substance abuse treatment* (SMA 00-3480). Rockville, MD: U.S. Department of Health and Human Services, The National Treatment Plan Initiative.

Centers for Disease Control and Prevention. (2007). *Preventing suicide.* Retrieved from http://www.cdc.gov/violenceprevention/pdf/PreventingSuicide-a.pdf

Chapa, T. (2004). *Mental health services in primary care settings for racial and ethnic minority populations* (Issue Brief draft). Rockville, MD: Office of Minority Health.

Corbie-Smith, G., Thomas, S. B., & St. George, M. (2002). Distrust, race, and research. *Archives of Internal Medicine, 162*(21), 2458-2463.

DeLeon, P. H., Wakefield, M., Schultz, A. J., Williams, J., & VandenBos, G. R. (1989). Rural America: Unique opportunities for health care delivery and health services research. *American Psychologist, 44*(10), 1298-1306.

Dimmitt, J., & Davila, Y. (1995). Group psychotherapy for abused women: A survivor group prototype. *Applied Nursing Research, 8*, 3-8.

Dresang, L. (2001). Gun deaths in rural and urban settings: Recommendations for prevention. *Guns and Violence Prevention, 14*(2), 107-115.

Eberhardt, M. S., & Pamuk, E. R. (2004). The importance of place of residence: Examining health in rural and nonrural areas. *American Journal of Public Health, 94*, 1682-1686.

Eberhardt, M. S., Ingram, D. D., & Makuc, D. M. (2001). *Urban and rural health chartbook: Health United States 2001.* Hyattsville, MD: National Center for Health Statistics.

Economic Research Service. (2004). *Rural poverty at a glance.* Washington, DC: United States Department of Agriculture.

Economic Research Service. (2011). *Rural income, poverty, and welfare: Summary of conditions and trends.* Retrieved from http://www.ers.usda.gov/Briefing/IncomePovertyWelfare/Overview.htm

Fontana, A., & Rosenheck, R. (2008). Treatment-seeking veterans of Iraq and Afghanistan: Comparison with veterans of previous wars. *Journal of Nervous & Mental Disease, 196,* 513–521.

Forrest, S. (1988). Suicide and the rural adolescent. *Adolescence, 23*(90), 341–346.

Fox, J. C., Blank, M., Rovnyak, V. G., & Barnett, R. Y. (2001). Barriers to help seeking for mental disorders in a rural impoverished population. *Community Mental Health Journal, 37*(5), 421–436.

Fox, J., Merwin, E., & Blank, M. (1995). DeFacto mental health services in the rural south. *Journal of Health Care for the Poor and Underserved, 6*(4), 434–468.

Francis, K., Boyd, C. P., Aisbett, D. L., & Newnham, K. (2006). Rural adolescents' perceptions of barriers to seeking help for mental health problems. *Youth Studies Australia, 25*(4), 42–49.

Frontier Education Center. (2007). *Frontier: A new definition.* Retrieved from http://www.frontierus.org/documents/consensus_paper.htm

Gfroerer, J. C., Larson, S. L., & Colliver, J. D. (2008). Drug use patterns and trends in rural communities. *The Journal of Rural Health, 23*(s1), 10–15.

Gogek, L. B. (1992). Letters to the editor. *American Journal of Psychiatry, 149,* 1286.

Goldsmith, S., Pellmar, T., Kleinman, A., & Bunney, W. (Eds.). (2002). *Reducing suicide: A national imperative.* Washington, DC: The National Academies Press.

Goodwin, R., Koenen, K. C., Hellman, F., Guardino, M., & Struening, E. (2002). Helpseeking and access to mental health treatment for obsessive–compulsive disorder. *Acta Psychiatrica Scandinavica, 106*(2), 143–149.

Guralnick, S., Kemele, K., Stamm, B. H., & Greving, A. M. (2003). Rural geriatrics and gerontology. In B. H. Stamm (Ed.), *Rural behavioral health care: An interdisciplinary guide* (pp. 193–202). Washington, DC: American Psychological Association.

Han, E., & Liu, G. G. (2005). Racial disparities in prescription drug use for mental illness among population in U.S. *Journal of Mental Health Policy Economics, 8*(3), 131–143.

Hauenstein, E. J., & Boyd, M. R. (1994). Depressive symptoms in young women of the Piedmont: Prevalence in rural women. *Women and Health, 21,* 105–123.

Hauenstein, E. J., Petterson, S., Merwin, E., Rovnyak, V., Heise, B., & Wagner, D. (2006). Rurality, gender, and mental health treatment. *Community Health, 29*(3), 169–185.

Health Resources and Services Administration. (2005). *Mental health and rural America*: 1994–2005. Rockville, MD: Author.

Helbok, C. M. (2003). The practice of psychology in rural communities: Potential ethical dilemmas. *Ethics & Behavior, 13,* 367–384.

Hewitt, M. E. (1989). *Defining "rural" areas: Impact on health care policy and research.* Darby, PA: Diane Publishing.

Hoge, C. W., McGurk, D., Thomas, J. L., Cox, A. L., Engel, C. C., & Castro, C. A. (2008). Mild traumatic brain injury in U.S. soldiers returning from Iraq. *New England Journal of Medicine, 358*, 453–463.

Hollingsworth, R., & Hendrix, E. M. (1977). Community mental health in rural settings. *Professional Psychology, 8*, 232–238.

Hoyt, D. R., Conger, R. D., Valde, J. G., & Weihs, K. (1997). Psychological distress and help seeking in rural America. *American Journal of Community Psychology, 25*(4), 449–470.

Human, J., & Wasem, C. (1991). Rural mental health in America. *American Psychologist, 46*(3), 232–239.

Institute of Medicine. (2002). *Reducing suicide: A national imperative.* Retrieved from http://www.nimh.nih.gov/health/topics/suicide-prevention/reducing-suicide-a-national-imperative.shtml

Kennedy, M. (2010). Rural men, sexual identity and community. *Journal of Homosexuality, 57*(8), 1051–1091. doi:10.1080/00918369.2010.507421

Kosberg, J. I., & Fei Sun, M. S. W. (2010). Meeting the mental health needs of rural men. *Rural Mental Health, 34*(1), 5–22.

Lambert, D., Gale, J. A., & Hartley, D. (2008). Substance abuse by youth and young adults in rural America. *Journal of Rural Health, 24*(3), 221–228.

Leedy, G., & Connolly, C. (2007). Out of the cowboy state: A look at lesbian and gay lives in Wyoming. *Journal of Gay & Lesbian Social Services: Issues in Practice, Policy & Research, 19*(1), 17–34. doi:10.1300/J041v19n01_02

Letvak, S. (2002). The importance of social support for rural mental health. *Issues in Mental Health Nursing, 23*, 249–261.

McCarthy, L. (2000). Poppies in a wheat field: Exploring the lives of rural lesbians. *Journal of Homosexuality, 39*(1), 75–94. doi:10.1300/J082v39n01_05

Menke, R., & Flynn, H. (2009). Relationships between stigma, depression, and treatment in white and African American primary care patients. *Journal of Nervous and Mental Disease, 197*(6). Retrieved from http://www.ncbi.nlm.nih.gov/pubmed/19525740

Minke, K. M. (2006). Parent–teacher relationships. In G. G. Bear, & K. M. Minke (Eds.), *Children's needs III: Development, prevention, and intervention* (pp. 73–85). Washington, DC: National Association of School Psychologists.

Mueller, K., Patil, K., & Ullrich, F. (1997). Lengthening spells of uninsurance and their consequences. *The Journal of Rural Health, 13*(1), 29–37.

Mulder, P. L., Kenken, M. B., Shellenberger, S., Constantine, M. G., Streigel, R., Sears, S. F., Jumper-Thurman, P., Kalodner, M., Danda, C. E., & Hager, A. (2001). *The behavioral health care needs of rural women.* Retrieved from American Psychological Association website: http://www.apa.org /rural/ruralwomen.pdf

Murray, G., Judd, F., Jackson, H., Fraser, C., Komiti, A., Pattison, P., & ...Robins, G. (2008). Big boys don't cry: An investigation of stoicism and its mental health outcomes. *Personality and Individual Differences, 44*(6), 1369–1381. doi: 10.1016/j.paid.2007.12.005

Murray, J. D., & Keller, P. A. (1991). Psychology and rural America: Current status and future directions. *American Psychologist, 46*, 220–231.

Myers, K. M., Valentine, J. M., & Melzer, S. M. (2008). Child and adolescent telepsychiatry: Utilization and satisfaction. *Telemedicine and e-Health, 14*(2), 131–137.

Myers, K. M., Vander Stoep, A., McCarty, C. A., Klein, J. B., Palmer, N. B., Geyer, J. R., & Melzer, S. M. (2010). Child and adolescent telepsychiatry: Variations in utilization, referral patterns and practice trends. *Journal of Telemedicine and Telecare, 16*, 128-133. doi: 10.1258/jtt.2009.090712

National Advisory Committee on Rural Health and Human Services. (2004). The 2004 Report to the Secretary. *Rural Health and Human Services Issues, April*, 35-43.

National Advisory Committee on Rural Health. (1993). *Sixth annual report on rural health*. Rockville, MD: Office of Rural Health Policy, Health Resources and Services Administration.

National Center on Addiction and Substance Abuse. (2000). *No place to hide: Substance abuse in mid-size cities and rural America*. New York: Author.

Nelson, E., & Bui, T. (2010). Rural telepsychology services for children and adolescents. *Journal of Clinical Psychology, 66*(5), 490-501.

New Freedom Commission Subcommittee on Rural Issues. (2003). Retrieved from http://govinfo.library.unt.edu/mentalhealthcommission/subcommittee/Sub_Chairs.htm

O'Hare, W., & Bishop, B. (2006). *U.S. rural soldiers account for a disproportionately high share of casualties in Iraq and Afghanistan* (Fact Sheet No. 3). Retrieved from the Carsey Institute, University of New Hampshire website: http://www.carseyinstitute.unh.edu/publications/FS_ruralsoldiers_06.pdf

Owens, J. S., & Murphy, C. E. (2004). Effectiveness research in the context of school-based mental health. *Clinical Child and Family Psychology Review, 7*, 195-209. doi:10.1007/s10567-004-6085-x

Padgett, D. K., Patrick, C., Burns, B. J., & Schlesinger, H. J. (1994). Ethnicity and use of outpatient mental health services in a national insured population. *American Journal of Public Health, 84*(2), 222-226.

Peden, A. R., Reed, D. B., & Rayens, M. K. (2005). Depressive symptoms in adolescents living in rural America. *The Journal of Rural Health, 21*(4), 310-316. doi:10.1111/j.1748-0361.2005.tb00100.x

Petrakis, I. L., Rosenheck, R., & Desai, R. (2011). Substance use comorbidity among Veterans with posttraumatic stress disorder and other psychiatric illness. *The American Journal on Addictions, 20*, 185-189.

President's New Freedom Commission on Mental Health. (2003). *Achieving the promise: Transforming mental health care in America*. Final report (DHHS Pub. No SMA-03-3832). Rockville, MD: U.S. Department of Health and Human Services.

Preston, D., D'Augelli, A. R., Kassab, C. D., & Starks, M. T. (2007). The relationship of stigma to the sexual risk behavior of rural men who have sex with men. *AIDS Education and Prevention, 19*(3), 218-230. doi:10.1521/aeap.2007.19.3.218

Richardson, C., & Waldrop, J. (2003). *Veterans: 2000* (Report No. C2KBR-22). Retrieved from United States Census Bureau website: http://www.census.gov/prod/2003pubs/c2kbr-22.pdf

Rost, K. J., Fortney, M., Zhang, M., Smith, J., & Smith, G. R. (1999). Treatment of depression in rural Arkansas: Policy implications for improving care. *Journal of Rural Health, 15*(3), 308-315.

Rost, K., Fortney, J., Fischer, E., & Smith, J. (2002). Use, quality, and outcomes of care for mental health: The rural perspective. *Medical Care and Review, 59*(3), 231-265.

Sears, H. A. (2004). Adolescents in rural communities seeking help: Who reports problems and who sees professionals? *Journal of Child Psychology & Psychiatry, 45*(2), 396–404. doi:10.1111/j.1469-7610.2004.00230.x

Sears, S. F., Evans, G. D., & Kuper, B. D. (2003). Rural social services systems as behavioral health delivery systems. In B. H. Stamm (Ed.), *Rural behavioral health care: An interdisciplinary guide* (pp. 109–120). Washington, DC: American Psychological Association.

Slovak, K., & Singer, M. I. (2002). Children and violence: Findings and implications from a rural community. *Child and Adolescent Social Work Journal, 19*, 35–56. doi:10.1023/A:1014003306441

Snowden, L. R., Masland, M. C., Libby, A. M., Wallace, N., & Fawley, K. (2008). Racial/ethnic minority children's use of psychiatric emergency care in California's public mental health system. *American Journal of Public Health, 98*(1), 118–124.

Sowers, W. E., & Rohland, B. (2004). American Association of Community Psychiatrists' principles for managing transitions in behavioral health services. *Psychiatric Services, 55*(11), 1271–1275.

Spoth, R., Goldberg, C., Neppl, T., Trudeau, L., & Ramisetty-Mikler, S. (2001). Rural-urban differences in the distribution of parent-reported risk factors for substance use among young adolescents. *Journal of Substance Abuse, 13*, 609–623. doi:10.1016/S0899-3289(01)00091-8

Stein, B. D., Kataoka, S., Jaycox, L. H., Wong, M., Fink, A., Escudero, P., & Zaragoza, C. (2002). Theoretical basis and program design of a school-based mental health intervention for traumatized immigrant children: A collaborative research partnership. *Journal of Behavioral Health Services & Research, 29*, 318–326. doi:10.1007/BF02287371

Substance Abuse and Mental Health Services Administration. (2001). *Summary of findings from the 2001 National Household Survey on Drug Abuse.* Rockville, MD: Office of Applied Studies.

Thorndyke, L. E. (2005). Rural women's health: A research agenda for the future. *Women's Health Issues, 15*, 200–203.

U.S. Census Bureau. (2000). *Projections of the total resident population by 5-year age groups, race, and Hispanic origin with special age categories: Middle series, 1999–2000 and 2050–2070.* Retrieved from http://www.census.gov/population/projections/nation/summary/np-t4.a-g.txt.

U.S. Census Bureau. (2010). *American FactFinder.* Retrieved from http://factfinder.census.gov/servlet/DCGeoSelectServlet?ds_name=DEC_2000_SF1_U

Unutzer, J., Patrick, D. L., Simon, G., Grembowski, D., Walker, E., Rutter, C., & Katon, W. (1997). Depressive symptoms and the cost of health services in HMO patients aged 65 years and older: A 4-year prospective study. *Journal of the American Medical Association, 277*, 1618–1623.

Wagenfeld, M. O., & Buffum, W. E. (1983). Problems in, and prospects for, rural mental health services in the United States. *International Journal of Rural Health, 12*, 89–107.

Wagenfeld, M. O., Murray, J. D., Mohatt, J. D., & DeBruyn, J. C. (1994). *Mental health and rural America 1980–1993: An overview and annotated bibliography.* Rockville, MD: Department of Health and Human Services.

Waldo, C. R., Hesson-McInnis, M. S., & D'Augelli, A. R. (1998). Antecedents and consequences of victimization of lesbian, gay, and bisexual young people: A structural model comparing rural university and urban samples. *American Journal of Community Psychology, 26*(2), 307-334. doi:10.1023/A:1022184704174

Wallace, A. E., Weeks, W. B., Wang, S., Lee, A., & Kazis, L. E. (2006). Rural and urban disparities in health-related quality of life among veterans with psychiatric disorders. *Psychiatric Services, 57*, 851-856.

Ward, E. C., Clark, L. O., & Heidrich, S. (2009). African American women's beliefs, coping behaviors, and barriers to seeking mental health services. *Qualitative Health Research, 19*(11). Retrieved from http://www.ncbi.nlm.nih.gov/pubmed/19843967

Weeks, W. B., Wallace, A. E., West, A. N., Heady, H. R., & Hawthorne, K. (2008). Research on rural veterans: An analysis of the literature. *The Journal of Rural Health, 24*, 337-344.

Weist, M. D., & Evans, S. W. (2005). Expanded school mental health: Challenges and opportunities in an emerging field. *Journal of Youth and Adolescence, 34*, 3-6. doi:10.1007/s10964-005-1330-2

Welsh, J., Domitrovich, C. E., Bierman, K., & Lang, J. (2003). Promoting safe schools and healthy students in rural Pennsylvania. *Psychology in the Schools, 40*, 457-472. doi:10.1002/pits.10103

Willging, C. E., Salvador, M., & Kano, M. (2006a). Pragmatic help seeking: How sexual and gender minority groups access mental health care in a rural state. *Psychiatric Services, 57*(6), 871-874. doi:10.1176/appi.ps.57.6.871

Willging, C. E., Salvador, M., & Kano, M. (2006b). Unequal treatment: Mental health care for sexual and gender minority groups in a rural state. *Psychiatric Services, 57*(6), 867-870. doi:10.1176/appi.ps.57.6.867

Zatzick, D. F., Marmar, C. R., Weiss, D. S., Browner, W. S., Metzler, T. J., Golding, J. M., . . . Wells, K. B. (1997). Posttraumatic stress disorder and functioning and quality of life in a nationally representative sample of Vietnam veterans. *American Journal of Psychiatry, 154*, 1690-1695.

Zito, J. M., Safer, D. J., Zuckerman, I. H., Gardner, J. F., & Soeken, K. (2005). Effect of Medicaid eligibility category on racial disparities in the use of psychotropic medications among youths. *Psychiatric Services, 56*(2), 157-163.

2

Advancing Federal Policies in Rural Mental Health

PATRICK H. DELEON, MARY BETH KENKEL, AND DIANA V. SHAW

INTRODUCTION

*D*uring the summer of 2011, President Obama by Executive Order # 13575 established the White House Rural Council naming access to affordable health care among the Council's top priorities. Excerpts from the order, presented below, highlight the need for the Council and lay out its current charge:

> Sixteen percent of the American population lives in rural counties. Strong, sustainable rural communities are essential to winning the future and ensuring American competitiveness in the years ahead. These communities supply our food, fiber, and energy, safeguard our natural resources, and are essential in the development of science and innovation. Though rural communities face numerous challenges, they also present enormous economic potential. The Federal Government has an important role to play in order to expand access to the capital necessary for economic growth, promote innovation, improve access to health care and education, and expand outdoor recreational activities on public lands. To enhance the Federal Government's efforts to address the needs of rural America, this order establishes a council to better coordinate Federal programs and maximize the impact of Federal investment to promote economic prosperity and quality of life in our rural communities . . . . The Council shall . . . coordinate and increase the effectiveness of Federal engagement with rural stakeholders, including agricultural organizations, small businesses, education and training institutions, health-care providers, telecommunications services providers, research and land grant institutions, law enforcement, State, local,

and tribal governments, and nongovernmental organizations regarding the needs of rural America . . . .

—Obama, 2011, pp. 34841–34842

The broad, sweeping nature of the President's charge reflects the natural interdependency of rural America. The National Rural Health Association, in particular, expressed its enthusiastic support for the President's vision, highlighting that the 62 million Americans who live in rural America have continually had difficulty in accessing health care providers of all disciplines, including mental health.

THREE HISTORICAL VIEWS OF RURAL MENTAL HEALTH THAT SHAPED POLICY DIRECTIONS

At the request of the Congressional rural caucuses, in 1990 the then-Office of Technology Assessment (OTA) issued a comprehensive report titled *Health Care in Rural America* (DeLeon, Wakefield, & Hagglund, 2003; OTA, 1990). At that time, America's rural population was becoming an increasingly smaller proportion of the total population, with 23% to 27% of the nation being considered "rural." The elderly, with their chronic health impairments, made up a greater proportion of rural America than urban America. Rural residents were characterized by relatively low mortality (with the exception of injury-related causes), but relatively high rates of chronic disease. Prolonged distances, adverse weather, and other physical obstacles were viewed as common and significant barriers to receipt of care. Economic barriers, including lack of access to health insurance, were significant. Rural hospitals were frequently described as "going broke" and health care providers of all disciplines were insignificant in number. Clinicians' and health policy experts' ability to access relevant scientific and clinical advances was deemed "questionable" at best. The OTA found that rural residents appeared to use preventive screening services less often than urban residents did; they had lesser contact with health care providers than individuals in urban areas, with rural areas having less than one-half as many physicians per capita as urban areas. Throughout the report, OTA emphasized that the federal government had a distinct role in protecting the well-being of rural America, noting that the federal government was already providing nearly one-half of the resources for rural health activities. Stressing the importance of a centralized focus for rural health policy, the Congressional rural caucuses were instrumental in the establishment of the Office of Rural Health Policy within the Department of Health and Human Service (HHS) in 1987 (subsequently codified by P.L. 100-203 in the Omnibus Budget Reconciliation Act of 1987).

The key to access throughout rural America has historically been the network of federally qualified community health centers (FQHCs) and rural health clinics. In describing her FY 2012 budget request, HHS Secretary Kathleen Sebelius noted that her budget includes $3.3 billion for the Health Centers Program, including $1.2 billion in mandatory funding provided through the Affordable Care Act Community Health Center Fund, to expand the capacity of existing health center services and create new access points. This level of funding would enable health centers to serve 900,000 new patients and increase access to medical, oral, and behavioral health services to a total of 24 million patients. Within HHS, the Health Resources and Services Administration (HRSA) has been the central health agency for rural activities and strategic planning. Rural America, and particularly our nation's federally qualified community health centers with their emphasis upon providing integrated health care, provides psychology with an extraordinary opportunity to broaden its scope of practice and expertise beyond that of being exclusively a mental health discipline. It provides the opportunity to become one of our nation's bona fide *health care* professions, including fostering a maturing focus on the behavioral and psychosocial aspects of chronic care treatments (DeLeon, Giesting, & Kenkel, 2003; Puente, in press).

The 1990 OTA report included a chapter focusing upon rural mental health care. Most interesting was the extent to which verifiable data on the prevalence of mental disorders and the availability of mental health services were scarce and difficult to obtain. It was felt that the differences in mental health status between rural and urban residents were probably slight, but that alcohol dependence (unlike drug abuse) was apparently higher among rural than urban residents. At that time, little data were required to be reported to the various federal agencies; however, dramatic differences between rural and urban areas in the availability of local inpatient mental health services were found. Two-thirds of metropolitan counties possessed some kind of inpatient services in 1983, while only 13% of nonmetropolitan counties had such facilities. Although, as we indicated, objective data were scarce, OTA felt that rural areas were not only less likely to have comprehensive mental health services available, where such services did exist they were also narrower in scope. Emergency mental health services were seen as particularly crucial, but unavailable, in rural areas. There was an apparent lack of awareness among the potential beneficiary population in rural areas that mental health services existed and that they could actually be helpful. Transportation availability, confidentiality concerns, and difficulty in recruiting and retaining mental health professionals were noted as continuing problems. Health care providers, including mental health specialists, must often become generalists and part of the local community in order to be effective. As discussed in Chapter 8, this potential overlap between personal and professional roles can lead to burnout and conflicts between professional impartiality and personal values. The mental and physical health care systems were seen as interdependent, but specialist knowledge in the nuances of mental health care was often simply unavailable. For example, nonpsychiatrist physicians provided almost one half of the patient visits resulting in a diagnosis of a mental disorder and approximately 85% of all psychoactive drug prescriptions.

In 1996, the Agency for Healthcare Research and Quality (AHRQ) high-lighted its Research in Action efforts and came to similar conclusions as those of the OTA. One quarter of America's population lived in rural areas and compared with urban Americans, rural residents had higher poverty rates, a larger percentage of elderly, tended to be in poorer health; they had fewer doctors, hospitals, and other health resources; and faced more difficulty getting to both physical and mental health services. Hospital closures and other market changes had adversely affected rural areas. Considerable changes in the health care delivery system over the prior decade had intensified the need for new approaches to health care in rural areas. AHRQ's primary mission is research and its efforts to develop a viable rural research agenda focused upon several specific issues:

- Access to care. Many small rural hospitals had closed, while other health care facilities were in financial straits. Unavailability of resources and transportation problems were barriers to access for rural populations.
- Supply of primary care physicians and other health care providers. The supply of primary care practitioners and other health care providers in rural areas had been decreasing. Some were leaving rural areas to join managed care organizations elsewhere.
- Health promotion and disease prevention. Goals for improving the Nation's health over the next decade, as outlined in *Healthy People 2000 (US DHHS, 1991)*, could be achieved only if rural populations were specifically included in efforts to remove barriers to access and use of clinical preventive services.
- Health care technology. Technologies including telemedicine offered promise of improved access to health care, but their most efficient and effective applications needed further evaluation.
- Organization of services for vulnerable rural populations. Low population density in rural areas made it inherently difficult to deliver services that targeted persons with special health needs. Groups at particular risk included: the elderly, the poor, people with HIV or AIDS, the homeless; mothers, children, and adolescents; racial or ethnic minorities; and persons with disability.
- Consumer choice and the rural hospital. Factors that drove changes in rural hospitals had a critical effect on consumer choice and access.
- Almost one in three adults living in rural America was in "poor to fair health." Nearly half had at least one major chronic illness. Yet, rural residents averaged fewer physician contacts per year than those in urban communities.
- Traumatic injuries were more common in rural areas, and residents faced worse outcomes and higher risks of death than urban patients, partly because of transportation problems and lack of advanced life support training for emergency medical personnel.
- Rural hospitals showed a greater shift toward outpatient services and greater declines in admissions and lengths of stay than urban hospitals. Economic pressures had driven rural hospitals to shift rapidly to outpatient care.

- Alcoholism and drug abuse were growing problems in rural areas. With a scarcity of mental health professions in rural areas, less than one in five rural hospitals had treatment services for these conditions.
- Rural and urban residents were equally likely to lack health insurance. Under-insurance was as much of a problem for rural residents as being uninsured.
- Analytic geographic mapping techniques were valuable for rural health policy and health services research.
- Different solutions are required to keep primary care providers in rural areas than are needed to attract them there initially.

The HHS Office of Rural Health subsequently commissioned an OTA follow-up report, which was released in 1999. "Almost 10 years have passed since the report's release and much of the data and information it contained have changed. The same decade witnessed the development of several policy initiatives including legislation to assist rural hospitals, strengthen efforts to place professionals in rural areas, and modify payment systems to be more equitable to rural citizens that were supported by that report. Despite these efforts, many of the same problems that confronted rural America in the 1980s remain in the 1990s, despite the best efforts of interested policy makers and their supporters" (Ricketts, 1999, p. vii). There remained a significant shortage of health professionals of all disciplines. Rural residents saw doctors less often and usually later in the course of an illness than their urban counterparts; specialty services (such as mental health care) were also utilized less often. Technological advances may have resulted in new clinical tools for rural practitioners (i.e., telehealth); however, their high costs led to a concentration into fewer, more urban areas.

In this later report, there was once again a specific focus upon rural mental health, this time including substance abuse. The report found that evolving national trends (such as parity legislation) may be breaking down some of the historic barriers between the mental and physical health care delivery systems. However, the concerns of rural mental health and substance abuse service providers and consumers were seen as often still overlooked at the national level. Although primary care providers demonstrate some success in treating a number of mental health problems, rural residents whose mental health problems are so persistent that they require ongoing professional care must often move to urban areas to obtain the necessary care. "Rural mental health professionals may require special training above and beyond that appropriate to their disciplines if they are to be successful at their work. Such training should emphasize the realities of the rural *environment*, such as physical distance, cultural factors, and resource limitations and of the rural practice—for example, the need to establish a relationship with the whole community, to assume the role of a generalist, to accept the lack of anonymity and the accompanying ethical dilemmas, and to cope with professional isolation and the potential for burnout" (Ricketts, 1999, p. 170). Fortunately, there was the clear notion that the authors of the follow-up study had access to considerably more comparative data than the original OTA study authors did, and that there was also a significantly enhanced appreciation for the clinical importance of addressing the psychosocial–economic–cultural gradient of health care (Anderson & Anderson, 2003).

THE IMPORTANCE OF PERSONAL INVOLVEMENT IN ADVOCACY AND LONG-TERM VISION FOR MENTAL HEALTH PROVIDERS IN RURAL AREAS

As discussed in more detail later in this chapter and throughout this text, the advent of telehealth and telepsychology has opened up an entirely new chapter in the delivery of mental health and behavioral health care in rural America. Significant change, however, always takes considerable time and often more than one would initially expect, even if unquestioningly beneficial (DeLeon, Kenkel, Oliveira Gray, & Sammons, 2011). For example, the far-reaching mental health parity legislation (The Paul Wellstone and Pete Domenici Mental Health Parity and Addiction Equity Act of 2008; P.L. 110-343) took over a decade to come to fruition. Back in April 1996, Senator Domenici told his Senate colleagues that "Now is the time" to pass legislation requiring insurance companies to cover mental illness just like any other medical condition; yet it took until 2008 for the political forces and societal issues to come together to develop broad support for his legislation. Those who have been personally involved in the public policy process over the years have learned the critical importance of five key mediators of success: patience, persistence, partnerships, personal relationships, and a long-term perspective for the field.

During its consideration of the Balanced Budget Act of 1997 (P.L. 105-33), the Congress noted, more than a decade ago, that the then-Health Care Financing Administration (HCFA) (currently the Centers for Medicare and Medicaid Services (CMS)) was conducting a 3-year demonstration project under which Medicare would pay for telemedicine services at 57 Medicare-Certified facilities. The demonstration was to focus on medical consultations between medical specialists located at medical center facilities and primary care providers treating Medicare patients at remote rural sites. At that time, five telemedicine centers were participating in the project. The Senate proposed that the Secretary submit a report to Congress no later than January 1, 1998, which would analyze in detail: (1) how telemedicine and telehealth systems are expanding access to health care services; (2) the clinical efficacy and cost-effectiveness of telemedicine and telehealth applications; (3) the quality of telemedicine and telehealth services delivered; and (4) the reasonable cost of telecommunication charges incurred in practicing telemedicine and telehealth in rural, frontier, and underserved areas. The conferees included the Senate provision with several amendments and required the Secretary to make Part B payments for telehealth services by January 1, 1999. In determining the amount of payments for telehealth services, the payments would be subject to Medicare coinsurance and deductible requirements. Beneficiaries could not be billed for any telephone line charges or any facility fees. A demonstration project was authorized in order to explore improving patient access to, and compliance with, appropriate care guidelines for individuals with diabetes mellitus through a direct telecommunication link with information networks, in order to improve patient quality-of-life and reduce overall health care costs. This latter project was also directed to develop a curriculum to train health professionals (particularly primary care health professionals) in the use of medical informatics and telecommunications.

Opportunities for Involvement in Rural Mental Health Advocacy

One of APA's continuing, yet unheralded "diamonds in the rough" is the APA Congressional Fellowship program whose 2010–2011 Fellowship class marked its 37th year. As of that time, APA had sponsored 110 Congressional Fellows. This is a most impressive legacy, which by providing selected psychologists with a "hands on" public policy experience, forever shapes their views of the political/public policy process. Such interaction between mental health professionals and the policy landscape is essential for advancing the agenda of mental health care across the nation, and advocates for rural mental health are sorely needed. Former APA Congressional Science Fellow Neil Kirschner commented on his experiences as follows:

> More often than not, research findings in the legislative arena are only valued if consistent with conclusions based upon the more salient political decision factors. Thus, within the legislative setting, the research data is not used to drive decision-making decisions, but is more frequently used to support decisions based upon other factors. As psychologists, we need to be aware of this basic difference between the role of research in science settings and the legislative world. It makes the role of the researcher who wants to put 'into play' available research results into a public policy deliberation more complex. Data needs to be introduced, explained or framed in a manner cognizant of the political exigencies. Furthermore, it emphasizes the importance of efforts to educate our legislators on the importance and long-term effectiveness of basing decisions on quality research data . . . . If I've learned anything on the Hill, it is the importance of political advocacy if you desire a change in public policy. (N. Kirschner, personal communication, August 2003)

Another APA Congressional Science Fellow Gregory Hinrichsen et al. (2010) enumerated a number of specific suggestions for effective advocacy on behalf of the elderly, which are highly relevant for those concerned with the needs of rural America. "Aging of the U.S. population raises numerous public policy issues about which gerontological researchers, policy experts, and practitioners have much to contribute. However, the means by which aging-related public policy is influenced are not always apparent" (Hinrichsen et al., 2010, p. 735). They go on to note that: "(P)olitical agendas are typically established when problems are recognized, and there is growing consensus that some action should be taken" (p. 737). Their suggestions for advancing the aging policy agenda (which is highly relevant to the rural agenda) include:

- Bring aging friendly legislators out of the closet.
- Listen and you are more likely to be heard.
- Emphasize local issues and access local avenues for policy advocacy.
- Build relationships to influence public policy, including establishing connections with local, state, and federal offices. Learn about the legislator and one's priorities (especially your own elected officials). Make yourself useful and memorable. And, utilize other avenues for influencing policy, such as professional organizations and advocacy groups.
- Follow up with staff.
- Be attuned to the importance of timing in policy making.
- Find new channels for policy advocacy.
- Work with local groups.
- Expand the policy research of national member organizations representing aging (rural) researchers and practitioners.
- Use current and past policy Fellows as a resource.

For those interested in advocacy for rural health care, the National Association of Community Health Centers (NACHCs) can also be an influential partner.

RECRUITING AND RETAINING RURAL MENTAL HEALTH WORKERS

A persistent problem affecting the delivery of mental health and behavioral health services in rural areas is the lack of trained mental health providers. The HRSA has identified primary care, dental, and mental health provider shortage areas (HPSAs), that is, areas where the number of providers are insufficient to meet the needs of the residents. More than one-third of rural residents live in a federally designated HPSA (Rabinowitz, Diamond, Markham, & Wortman, 2008) and more rural than urban counties are designated as mental health HPSAs and dental HPSAs (National Advisory Council on Rural Health and Human Services, 2008). These health professional shortages contribute to rural Americans not having access to care or entering care late with more advanced symptoms, and thereby requiring more intensive and expensive forms of treatment.

Several federal and state programs have been developed to increase the recruitment and retention of mental health providers. One of the earliest federal programs was the National Health Service Corps (NHSC), created in 1970 to improve health care for the underserved in areas of critical need (National Advisory Council on the National Health Service Corps, 2000). This program was created to deal with the shortage of physicians in rural communities due to retirements and moves to urban areas in the 1950s and 1960s. Physicians were drawn to urban areas because of the higher compensation, availability of facilities with advanced medical technologies, greater interaction with colleagues, the proximity of educational and cultural venues, and job opportunities for their spouses. Also during this time in medicine, more physicians were moving away from primary care practice into specialty care.

To address these shortages, the NHSC developed two major programs. The NHSC Scholarship program is a competitive program that pays tuition and a stipend to students enrolled in accredited medical (MD or DO), dental, nurse practitioner, certified nurse midwife, and physician assistant training (but not mental health training). In return, upon graduation, scholarship recipients work between 2 and 4 years in a community-based NHSC-approved site in an HPSA.

The NHSC Loan Repayment Program, begun in 1987, is available to behavioral and mental health professionals, including health service psychologists, licensed clinical social workers, marriage and family therapists, and licensed professional counselors. It offers fully trained primary care physicians (MD or DO), primary care nurse practitioners, certified nurse midwives, primary care physician assistants, dentists, and dental hygienists as well as primary care behavioral and mental health clinicians up to $60,000 tax-free to repay student loans in exchange for 2 years serving in an NHSC-approved community-based site in an HPSA. A recent change to the program allows some recipients to receive $170,000 for 5 years of service.

More than 37,000 primary care providers have served in the National Health Service Corps since its inception. In 2000, the NHSC had 2,439 clinicians in service across the country, but the National Advisory Council on the NHSC stated that the nation needed "20,000 more clinicians, properly distributed in currently underserved areas, to completely redress these access issues" (National Advisory Council, 2000, p. 17). A big push in the right direction came when nearly $200 million from the American Recovery and Reinvestment Act of 2009 was used to significantly augment the number of NHSC awards. Recovery Act funding enabled the NHSC to make over 4,000 new loan repayment awards and 250 new scholarship awards between 2009 and 2011. Unfortunately, these funds represented a temporary boost to the program that will require continued advocacy to sustain.

According to the HRSA Data Warehouse, as of July 6, 2011, there were 3,729 Mental Health HPSAs in the nation, with 61% in nonmetropolitan areas (U.S. Department of Human Services, 2011a). To meet the mental health needs, 4,771 mental health practitioners would be required. The NHSC mental health field strength in 2011 was 2,580 practitioners, meaning that the NHSC has fulfilled 54% of mental health manpower needs in these shortage areas. This shows impressive improvement from the year 2000 when the NHSC was filling only 6% of the mental health manpower shortage. Additionally, in comparison, the NHSC has filled only 21% of the primary care need and 9% of the dental need.

Today over 8,446 NHSC primary health care clinicians are working in underserved communities and more than 7 million people, many without health insurance, rely on NHSC clinicians for their health, dental, and mental health care. The NHSC providers currently are about equally split between rural and urban underserved areas. As of February 2011, 29% of the NHSC workforce were behavioral and mental health workers (including psychiatrists), closely followed by physicians (25%), nurse practitioners (16%), physician assistants (14%), dentists (12%), dental hygienists (2%), and nurse midwives (2%) (Dey, 2011). In 2007, among the NHSC behavioral health providers, 37.8% were clinical psychologists, 25% social workers, 17.1% licensed professional counselors, 10.9% psychiatrists, and less than 5% each of marriage/family counselors and psychiatric nurses/nurse practitioners.

In addition to the NHSC programs, the HRSA State Loan Repayment Program (SLRP) provides grants to 31 states to operate their own loan repayment programs. These state programs offer loan repayments to primary care providers working in HPSAs. Requirements vary by state, but mental health professionals are eligible in some states. Currently more than 500 providers are serving in 31 states. Further, the Indian Health Service (HIS) provides a loan repayment program to recruit health professionals who are committed to working in American Indian and Alaska Native communities, with preference given to American Indian and Alaska Native applicants. For many, this means that the financial support offered allows them to return to their home communities and provide needed services there.

Even beyond its major goal of improving the health care of those in underserved areas through the recruitment and retention of trained health professionals, programs such as the NHSC have made another major contribution to health care in America, especially in its relationship to mental health care. The NHSC has advocated for "the development of new systems of health care delivery in communities of greatest need," stating "planning and development shall be based on the interdisciplinary model of health care delivery; communities shall be encouraged to avail themselves of the broadest array of health care clinicians to meet their needs in the most creative and cost-effective manner" (National Advisory Council on NHSC, 2000, p. 18). Through its advocacy of interdisciplinary models of health care and funding of mental health providers, behavioral and mental health treatment is being integrated into primary care settings and regarded as an essential component of quality health care. This approach has provided many more points of access for mental health care for rural residents and significantly reduced the stigma and other barriers associated with seeking mental health services. Additional discussion on integrated care and its impact on rural mental health can be found in Chapter 9.

THE PATIENT PROTECTION AND AFFORDABLE CARE ACT

The enactment of President Obama's landmark health care reform legislation, the Patient Protection and Affordable Care Act ([PPACA) (P.L. 111-148 and the P.L. 111-152 amendments), could potentially have an extraordinarily positive impact upon rural America. The law's emphasis upon improving access to primary care services, as well as preventive and public health care, directly addresses many of the needs of rural Americans. By 2014, this legislation will ensure that all Americans have access to high-quality, affordable, and comprehensive health insurance plans that cannot include lifetime or annual dollar limits on benefits. The law also includes a number of rural provisions, such as expanding rural demonstration initiatives, modifying programmatic Medicare reimbursement levels, and calls for a MedPAC (Medicare Payment Advisory Commission) comprehensive study of the adequacy of Medicare payments for health care providers serving in rural areas. It further reauthorized the NHSC until 2015 and authorized $1.5 billion in funding during that time period.

The significant additional resources ($11 billion over 5 years) provided for the systematic expansion of federally qualified community health centers (FQCHCs) represents a major strategic component, with approximately half of the current centers already serving rural populations. Of particular interest, the legislation created a new Title VII (health professions) grant program for training mental and behavioral health providers. President Bush's (2001) New Freedom Commission on Mental Health (Executive Order # 13217) had found that there was a shortage of behavioral health care providers and that this shortage was notably severe in rural areas, as we noted above. In 2008, for example, HRSA reported that there were 3,059 HPSAs (Health Professional Shortage Areas) for behavioral health, with a total of 77 million people living in these areas. Sixty-six percent of the behavioral health HPSAs were in rural areas. PPACA authorizes the Secretary to award grants to institutions of higher education to support the recruitment and education of students in social work programs, interdisciplinary psychology training programs, and internships or other field placement programs related to child and adolescent mental health, as well as state-licensed mental health organizations to train paraprofessional child and adolescent mental health workers. The chronic health care needs of the residents of rural America should be well served by the Administration's emphasis on integrated, holistic, and coordinated care provided by teams of interdisciplinary health care providers; for example, in Accountable Care Organizations (ACOs) which are functionally, rather than disciplinarily, conceptualized.

ACOs are expected to address all facets of a patient's condition and foster shared accountability for overall quality and costs encompassing a larger range of providers. It is important for organized psychology to affirmatively enter into the ongoing policy debates, at both the local and federal level, especially in determining whether these initiatives will be physician-dominated "medical homes" or more broadly conceptualized as interdisciplinary "health homes." Health homes offer a full array of coordinated primary and specialty services, including behavioral health and long-term community-based services, in a person-centered system of care. ACOs are an alternative to medical homes, which tend to be defined on the basis of the patient's last episode of care. These new entities are provider-led organizations that share, with the government, insurers, and other entities, accountability for achieving quality improvement and spending growth reductions. Unlike the notion of the medical home, ACOs are not necessarily physician focused and "address all facets of a patient's condition and foster shared accountability for overall quality and costs encompassing a larger range of providers" (McClellan, McKethan, Lewis, Roski, & Fisher, 2010, p. 985). Similarly, the new Nurse-Managed Health Clinics provision of the law would provide comprehensive primary health care and wellness services to vulnerable or underserved populations, providing care to all patients regardless of income or insurance status. Another authorized initiative seeks to encourage educational institutions in the delivery of primary care. Specifically, the Teaching Health Centers section urges the establishment of newly accredited or expanded primary care residency programs.

Reflecting ongoing changes occurring at the national health policy level, there has been a gradual realization within the profession of psychology that many exciting opportunities exist within rural America (DeLeon, 2000b) and within the nation's primary health care system (i.e., ACOs and other integrated care models). DeLeon et al. (2011) note that many concerning statistics essentially mandate that psychologists play an active role in health reform, including the fact that mental health and substance-use problems are the leading cause of combined disability and death in women, second highest in men, and by 2020 will be in the top five leading causes of morbidity, mortality, and disability among children in the United States. Reflecting the view that the locus of services must be flexible, PPACA authorized a new grant program for colocating primary and specialty care in community-based mental health settings, under which individuals with mental illness and co-occurring primary care conditions and chronic diseases would be served.

The ability for psychologists to prescribe psychoactive medication is also a much-discussed current policy issue. McGrath and Sammons (2011) capture the close relationship between systematically learning more about clinical psychopharmacology in depth and, ultimately, obtaining prescriptive authority which is a highly relevant legislative agenda for psychology. "Prescribing psychology and primary care psychology represent complementary paths to re-engineering the future of professional health care practice in psychology.

The greatest advantage of primary care psychology over prescribing psychology as a goal is its reliance on the traditional tools of the psychologist as a psychosocial care provider, making it more palatable to key audiences within psychology and medicine. Furthermore, it requires no legislative action. On the other hand, prescriptive authority involves service to the same patient population that is most familiar to psychologists. Although the legislative barriers can be daunting, once overcome, the shift in psychologists' roles is inevitable. There is an existing funding stream for medication management that becomes available to psychologists through third-party payers so that the authorized prescribers can quickly create practice opportunities" (p.117).

Again reflecting gradual societal changes and the critical nature of viewing mental health and substance-use care as important elements of our nation's overall health care system, the President of the Institute of Medicine (IOM) stated: "(I)mproving our nation's general health and the quality problems of our general health care system depends upon equally attending to the quality problems in health care for mental and substance-use conditions. The committee calls on primary care providers, other specialty health care providers, and all components of our general health care system to attend to the mental and substance-use health care needs of those they serve. Dealing equally with health care for mental, substance-use, and general health conditions requires a fundamental change in how we as a society and health care system think about and respond to these problems and illnesses. Mental and substance-use problems and illnesses should not be viewed as separate from and unrelated to overall health and general health care. Building on this integrated concept ... the Institute of Medicine will itself seek to incorporate attention to issues in health care for mental and substance-use problems and illnesses into its program of general health studies" (IOM, 2006, p. x). Such programs, as discussed in Chapters 9 and 12, are critical in addressing the mental health care needs of rural residents.

TECHNOLOGY EFFECTIVELY ADDRESSING THE IMPACT OF HISTORICAL ISOLATION

Perhaps the two most significant obstacles to providing high-quality mental and behavioral health care in rural America are the persistent shortage of trained specialists and professional/personal isolation. Over time, with carefully crafted rural-oriented health professions training initiatives, there will be a substantial increase in the number of rural providers of all disciplines, especially as our nation's training institutions begin to accept their societal responsibility for addressing this pressing need. The time has long passed for challenging the historically isolated, silo-oriented separation between town and gown. More immediately, however, the unprecedented advances occurring within the communications and technology fields have the potential for revolutionizing the delivery of care throughout America, including in isolated rural areas.

A fundamental issue in the delivery of mental health and behavioral health services in rural areas is how to provide treatment to individuals disbursed throughout large geographical areas who would have to travel long distances to a central town or city. Several outreach strategies have been used to address this challenge, including "circuit riders," mental health professionals who would travel from town to town, or the later concept of "mobile vans" in which a health care team would travel together to remove rural areas, or the use of paraprofessional outreach workers. HRSA's Office of Rural Health Policy (ORHP) earlier on had an outreach grant program for extending rural health care. In doing so, they were one of the forerunners in the efforts to use technology to provide access to health and mental health care for rural residents. Initiatives in telehealth, which is use of technology to deliver health care, health information, or health education at a distance, are still a part of the ORHP through the Office for the Advancement of Telehealth (OAT). They provide support and grants to rural communities to create and evaluate telehealth programs, as well as promote information about "best telehealth practices." One very useful guide developed by the ORHP is the "Rural Health IT Toolbox" (http://www.hrsa.gov/healthit/toolbox/RuralHealthITtoolbox/About/index. html) that provides a number of resources for planning, implementing, and evaluating the various forms of information technology, including telehealth applications, for rural settings. Below are some of the particular policy-relevant aspects of telehealth and telepsychology; additional details on telehealth and its evidence base can be found in Chapter 10.

In 2004, President George W. Bush signed Executive Order # 13335 highlighting his Administration's commitment to the promotion of health information technology (HIT) in order to lower costs, reduce medical errors, improve the quality of care, and provide better information for patients and providers. The newly established Office of the National Coordinator for Health Information Technology was charged with developing a blueprint for a nationwide interactive health information infrastructure and coordinating health information technology policies and programs across the federal government. The foundation was being laid for a new era in health care, one of unprecedented accountability and data-driven decision making.

With a similar orientation, President Obama's PPACA legislation incorporated the Health Information Technology for Economic and Clinical Health (HITECH) Act with the vision of promoting the widespread adoption of health information technology for the electronic sharing of clinical data among hospitals, health care providers, and other healthcare stakeholders. At that time, only approximately 5% of physicians had fully functional electronic health records (EHR) systems, with no available comparable information on the percentage of psychologists using EHRs. The Obama Administration's goal is to bring utilization up to 70% for hospitals and 90% for physicians by

2019. The President's Economic Stimulus legislation (P.L. 111-5) increased the HIT National Coordinator's budget from approximately $66 million in Fiscal Year 2009 to $2 billion, with numerous health policy experts suggesting that the federal government's overall investment for HIT under the legislation exceeded $19 billion. The Stimulus bill also provided $1.1 billion for Comparative Clinical Effectiveness Research (CCER). The underlying objective of this particular initiative is to scientifically evaluate the relative effectiveness of various health care services and treatment options, as well as to encourage the development and use of clinical registries, clinical data networks, and other forms of electronic data to generate outcomes data. PPACA included a section which authorized the establishment of a private, nonprofit, tax-exempt corporation called the Patient-Centered Outcomes Research Institute. The goal is to assist patients, clinicians, purchasers, and policy makers in making informed health decisions by advancing the quality and relevance of clinical evidence through research and evidence synthesis.

The potential impact of the unprecedented advances occurring in technology upon the health care arena is once again not a new realization. More than a decade ago, the Pew Health Foundations Commission futuristically noted: "The successful practitioner of the next century will need to master information technologies in order to effectively manage the care of their patients. As the microscope allowed practitioners in an earlier era to see the microbial agents of infection, the computer allows today's generation to aggregate data about populations and understand broader patterns of health and illness. But the computer will also change the patient. As patients arrive with better and more information, health care professionals may find themselves increasingly in the role of counselor and consultant" (O'Neil & Pew, 1998, p. 18).

THE ADVENT OF TELEPSYCHOLOGY AND LICENSURE MOBILITY

There can be little question that the advances occurring within the telehealth field have the potential for truly revolutionizing psychology's presence in rural America. Its efficacy has already been demonstrated by the various federal agencies, including the Department of Defense, Department of Veterans Affairs, and the Indian Health Service (Folen, Jones, Stetz, Edmonds, & Carlson, 2010). Substantive articles are increasingly being published in the professional literature, including psychology's training journals. Intensely aware of the clinical, research, and educational implications, in February 2011 the APA Council of Representatives approved the creation of a Telepsychology Task Force, co-chaired by Linda Campbell and Fred Millan, to be composed of four APA representatives, four Association of State and Provincial Psychology Boards (ASPPB) representatives, and two American Psychological Association Insurance Trust (APAIT) representatives. One of the critical issues that the task force will undoubtedly face is interjurisdictional practice/licensure mobility.

In the spring of 2011, HRSA released its Health Licensing Board Report To Congress (U.S. Department of Health and Human Services, 2011b). Requested by the FY' 2010 Senate Appropriations bill, the report updated efforts being made on licensure portability and the level of cooperation between health licensing boards, the best models for such cooperation, and the barriers to cross-state licensing arrangements. HRSA focused on physicians and nurses since in its view these are "the two professional groups for which there is the most information on alternative approaches to overcoming licensing barriers to cross-state practice" (USDHHS, p. 6). Utilizing funding from FY' 2006, HRSA created its licensure portability grant program, which has subsequently funded projects submitted by the Federation of State Medical Boards (FSMB) and the National Council of State Boards of Nursing (NCSBN), as well as the State of Wisconsin Department of Regulation and Licensing.

"Licensure portability is seen as one element in the panoply of strategies needed to improve access to quality health care services through the deployment of telehealth and other electronic practice services (e-care or e-health services) in this country. But licensure portability goes beyond improving the efficiency and effectiveness of electronic practice services. Overcoming unnecessary licensure barriers to cross-state practice is seen as part of a general strategy to expedite the mobility of health professionals in order to address workforce needs and improve access to health care services, particularly in light of increasing shortages of health care professionals. It is also seen as a way of improving the efficiency of the licensing system in this country so that scarce resources can be better used in the disciplinary and enforcement activities of state boards, rather than in duplicative licensing processes" (HRSA, 2011b, p. 5).

The primary purpose of licensing health care professionals is to protect the public from incompetent or impaired practitioners. A licensure system must be able to administer and enforce its standards. The basic standards for medical and nursing licensure have become largely uniform across all states. Physicians and nurses must graduate from nationally approved educational programs and pass a national licensure examination. However, there are significant differences in administrative and filing requirements among the states. The American Bar Association Health Law Section in its 2008 report proposed a model for allowing the cross-state licensure of physicians, which was approved by the ABA House of Delegates. The Federal Communications Commission (FCC) released its National Broadband Plan in 2010 urging states to revise licensure requirements to enable "e-care." Noting that current licensure requirements limited practitioners' ability to treat patients across state lines, which hindered access to care, the FCC urged increased collaboration. If the states failed to develop reasonable licensing policies to facilitate electronic practice over the next 18 months, the FCC recommended that Congress ensure that Medicare and Medicaid beneficiaries are not denied the benefits of "e-care." Clinical pharmacy reports that: "(R)eciprocity of pharmacy licensure is possible across all the states, Puerto Rico, and the District of Columbia and is facilitated by a national licensure transfer process and a national jurisprudence exam. There is no multi-state compact; however, as in nursing. The National Association of Boards of Pharmacy (NABP) provides these national mobility resources as a service to member state boards of pharmacy and to licensees. NABR also provides the Model Pharmacy Practice Act and updates it regularly. The Model Act addresses key issues, including the regulatory framework for collaborative drug therapy management agreements between pharmacists and physicians, nurse practitioners, and other prescribers. This facilitates pharmacists' patient management activities which include the initiation, modification, and cessation of medications" (Lucinda Maine, personal communication, June 10, 2011). Over the years, psychology's elected leadership has increasingly called for focused attention upon the importance of facilitating licensure mobility (DeLeon, 2000a). Stan Moldawsky obtained the endorsement of the APA Council of Representatives during its February 2000 meeting and mobility was a significant topic at James Bray's 2009 Presidential Summit on the Future of Psychology. Although licensure has historically been a state responsibility regardless of professional discipline, some health policy experts have been calling for the federal government to enact national licensure.

CONCLUSION

Although the rural population in the United States continues to gradually decrease, the health of rural communities and their people remains a vital concern to our country. Rural communities play a critical role in America's economy, growth, preservation, and identity. President Obama's creation of the White House Rural Council underscores the importance of rural counties for America's future and the significant involvement of the federal government in addressing rural issues.

Rural areas vary significantly in demographics, economics, industry, and degree of isolation, but the major barriers to providing physical, mental, and behavioral health care in rural America are similar: low population density, long distances from metropolitan areas, large geographical areas with poor transportation, and limited manpower and financial resources. While the challenges in rural health care have not changed dramatically, the national conversations about health care have. In the health care reform discussions, a fundamental issue was: How can this nation provide access to, and pay for, quality health care for all citizens? How can the United States provide health care in a cost-effective manner? These issues have long consumed rural America, but now a broad spectrum of health care stakeholders was involved in the conversations.

While the discussions did not result in as major or as comprehensive an overhaul in the health care system as some had hoped, participants identified current policies and programs effective in increasing access and controlling costs, and they resolved to expand them. Programs that were the mainstay of rural health care, such as the federally qualified community health centers and the National Health Service Corps that have produced significant results, were targeted for increased funding in the health care reform legislation. Rural communities will immediately reap the benefits of these expansions.

Additionally, health care reform discussions concluded that the U.S. health care system needed new cost-effective strategies. One of the strategies was the better use of technology to deliver health information and services, as well as track and share health information and outcomes. Interestingly, tele-health applications, originally developed to address rural access obstacles, were offered as an effective strategy to deal with health care issues for all Americans. Integrated health care systems also were proposed as effective strategies because of the established positive connection between physical and mental health and the importance of behavioral aspects of health, especially in chronic diseases and in prevention. Furthermore, since integrated health care centers use an interdisciplinary model, each profession can be used to its fullest capacity, maximizing the use of the health provider workforce. Greater implementation of this model will provide rural residents with a culturally appropriate and more easily accessible way for receiving behavioral and mental health services, thereby improving both physical and mental health.

As national groups continue to recognize these new health care strategies, we are confident that the momentum will build to resolve the policy, professional, training, and funding issues that have historically hindered the implementation of alternative health care models. These issues include cross-state licensing, initial capital investment costs, poor interprofessional collaboration in health care settings, and providers unprepared for minority populations/settings (including rural) and many more. As the strategies and obstacles are articulated, other stakeholders in America's health system are beginning to weigh in. Federal and state grants and supports are being established to deal with these issues, health professions associations are examining actions they might take (i.e., regarding licensure mobility), and health profession educators are considering how to prepare their graduates for new health care initiatives and opportunities.

In summary, the national conversations about health care reform brought to light both promising practices in rural areas and continuing problems and challenges plaguing many underserved populations, most centrally, access to affordable care. The discussions and resulting legislation set in motion a number of promising initiatives. As a result, positive movement is afoot to enhance the health and mental health of rural Americans.

The goal of accessible, quality mental and behavioral health care for rural Americans is achievable. Progress has been made. However, many different stakeholders in the health care system—health providers and organizations, educators, professional associations, state and federal governments—must continue to work together to outline the steps to reach that goal. They must advocate for the necessary changes, and then act to accomplish them. Collaboration and a steady focus on the goal are needed. Such partnerships and persistence will produce better health outcomes for rural Americans.

REFERENCES

Agency for Healthcare Research and Quality (AHRQ). (1996). *Improving health care for rural populations. Research in Action Fact Sheet (AHCPR Publication No. 96-P040).* Rockville, MD: Agency for Health Care Policy and Research. Retrieved from http://www/ahrq.gov/research/rural.htm

Anderson, N. B., & Anderson, P. E. (2003). *Emotional longevity: What really determines how long you live.* New York: Viking, The Penguin Group.

Bush, G. W. (2001, June 18). Executive Order # 13217. Community-based alternatives for individuals with disabilities. *Federal Register, 66*(120), 33155–33156.

Bush, G. W. (2004, April 30). Executive Order # 13335. Incentives for the use of health information technology and establishing the position of the National Health Information Technology Coordinator. *Federal Register, 69*(84), 24058–24061.

DeLeon, P. H. (2000a). The critical need for licensure mobility. *Monitor on Psychology, 31*(4), 9.

DeLeon, P. H. (2000b). Rural America: Our diamond in the rough. *Monitor on Psychology, 31*(7), 5.

DeLeon, P. H., Giesting, B., & Kenkel, M. B. (2003). Community health centers: Exciting opportunities for the 21st century. *Professional Psychology: Research and Practice, 34*(6), 579–585.

DeLeon, P. H., Kenkel, M. B., Oliveira Gray, J. M., & Sammons, M. T. (2011). Emerging policy issues for psychology: A key to the future of the profession. In D. H. Barlow (Ed.), *Handbook of clinical psychology* (pp. 34–51). New York: Oxford University Press.

DeLeon, P. H., Wakefield, M., & Hagglund, K. (2003). The behavioral health care needs of rural communities in the 21st century. In B. H. Stamm (Ed.), *Rural behavioral health care: An interdisciplinary guide* (pp. 23–31). Washington, DC: American Psychological Association.

Dey, D. R. (2011, April). *National Health Service Corps. Presentation at the National Oral Health Conference.* Retrieved from http://www.aacdp.com/docs/2011Dey.pdf

Folen, R., Jones, S., Stetz, M., Edmonds, B., & Carlson, J. (2010). Behavioral telehealth: Lessons learned from the Pacific. *Register Report, 36*, 8–15.

Hinrichsen, G. A., Kietzman, K. G., Alkema, G. E., Bragg, E. J., Hensel, B. K., Miles, T. P., Segev, D. L., & Zerzan, J. (2010). Influencing public policy to improve the lives of older Americans. *The Gerontologist, 50*(6), 735–743.

Institute of Medicine (IOM). (2006). *Improving the quality of health care for mental and substance-use conditions: Quality chasm series.* Washington, DC: National Academies Press.

McClellan, M., McKethan, A. N., Lewis, J. L., Roski, J., & Fisher, E. S. (2010). A national strategy to put accountable care into practice. *Health Affairs, 29*, 982–990.

McGrath, R. E., & Sammons, M. T. (2011). Prescribing and primary care psychology: Complementary paths for professional psychology. *Professional Psychology: Research and Practice, 42*(2), 113–120.

National Advisory Council on the National Health Service Corps. (2000). *A National Health Service Corps for the 21st century.* Retrieved from http://nhsc.hrsa.gov/about/NAC.pdf

National Advisory Council on Rural Health and Human Services. (2008). *Report to the Department of Health and Human Services Secretary.* Rockville, MD: U.S. Department of Health and Human Services, Office of Rural Health Policy. Retrieved from http://www.hrsa.gov/advisorycommittees/rural/2008secreport.pdf

Obama, B. (2011, June 14). Executive Order #13575. Establishment of the White House Rural Council. *Federal Register, 76*(114), 34840–34843.

O'Neil, E. H., Pew Health Professions Commission. (1998). *Recreating health professional practice for a new century: The fourth report of the Pew health professions commission.* San Francisco: Pew Health Professions Commission.

Puente, A. E. (2011). Psychology as a health care profession. *American Psychologist, 66*(8), 781–792.

Rabinowitz, H. K., Diamond, J. J., Markham, F. W., & Wortman, J. R. (2008). Medical school programs to increase the rural physician supply: A systematic review and projected impact of widespread replication. *Academic Medicine, 83,* 235–243.

Ricketts, T. C., III (Ed.). (1999). *Rural health in the United States.* New York: Oxford University Press.

The American Recovery and Reinvestment Act of 2009 [ARRA]. [P. L. 111-5]. (H.R. 1). 123 STAT. 115-521, 26 USC 1 (February 17, 2009).

The Balanced Budget Act of 1997. [P. L. 105-33]. 111 Stat. 251 (August 5, 1997). H. Conf. Rpt. # 105-217.

The Omnibus Budget Reconciliation Act of 1987. [P.L. 100-203]. (OBRA'87). (H.R. 3545). 101 Stat. 1330-472, 42 USC 1395 (December 22, 1987).

The Patient Protection and Affordable Care Act [PPACA]. [P.L. 111-148]. (H.R. 3590). March 23, 2010).

The Paul Wellstone Mental Health and Addiction Equity Act of 2008. [P.L. 110-343]. (H.R. 1424). (October 3, 2008).

Office of Technology Assessment (OTA), U.S. Congress (1990). *Health care in rural America. (OTA-H-434).* Washington, DC: U.S. Government Printing Office.

U.S. Department of Health and Human Services (HHS). (1991). *Healthy people 2000: National health promotion and disease prevention objectives.* DHHS Pub. No. (PHS) 91-50212(3). Washington, DC: U.S. Government Printing Office.

U.S. Department of Health and Human Services (HHS). (2011a). *Health professional shortage areas; Metropolitan/non-metropolitan classification as of June 30, 2011.* Retrieved from http://datawarehouse.hrsa.gov/quickaccessreports.aspx

U.S. Department of Health and Human Services (HHS). (2011b). *HRSA Health Licensing Board Report to Congress.* Retrieved from http://www.hrsa.gov/ruralhealth/about/telehealth/licenserpt10.pdf

3

Rurality as a Diversity Issue

K. BRYANT SMALLEY AND JACOB C. WARREN

INTRODUCTION: THE IMPORTANCE OF CULTURE IN MENTAL HEALTH

"*C*ulture" is defined as "a unique meaning and information system, shared by a group and transmitted across generations, that allows the group to meet basic needs of survival, pursue happiness and well-being, and derive meaning from life" (Matsumoto & Juang, 2007, p. 12). At the individual level, a person's "culture" fundamentally represents characteristics in personality, personal preferences, and worldview shaped by that person's upbringing within a group of similar people. Frequently, when we think of cultural or multicultural issues, images of race, ethnicity, religion, and sexual orientation typically come to mind. Each of these groups has strong associated cultures that make their life experiences and worldviews different from individuals with a different background. These cultures help to make our world diverse, and represent the spectrum of human experience.

The field of psychology has long recognized the importance of considering cultural/diversity issues in the training of future clinicians. Accreditation criteria from the American Psychological Association require that programs "engage in actions that indicate respect for and understanding of cultural and individual diversity" (APA, 2011, p. 6). As a result, most programs in clinical psychology incorporate training in multicultural issues into every trainee's curriculum to expand their horizons and knowledge base of the various cultures that may be encountered in their professional practice. This helps therapists better understand their clients' culturally influenced decision-making and overall approach to mental health services.

The concept of "cultural competency" has received much recent attention, defined as acknowledging and incorporating "the importance of culture, assessment of cross-cultural relations, vigilance toward the dynamics that result from cultural differences, expansion of cultural knowledge, and adaptation of services to meet culturally unique needs" (Betancourt, Green, Carrillo, & Ananeh-Firempong, 2003, p. 294). Cultural competency has been recognized as being so important in the field of mental health that the ethical codes of the American Psychological Association (Section 2.01b), the National Association of Social Workers (Section 1.05), and the American Counseling Association (Section A.2.c) incorporate an ethical mandate to be culturally sensitive and competent when working with clients (American Counseling Association, 2005; American Psychological Association, 2010; National Association of Social Workers, 2008).

Failure to fully understand the cultural realities of clients can lead to mistrust, can damage the rapport that is so important to effective therapy, and can lead to fundamental misunderstandings of the factors that may underlie an individual's mental health needs (Sue, 1998). For instance, failure to recognize the continued discrimination and stereotyping that African Americans face may leave therapists ill-equipped to address some of the larger social issues that may be influencing the emotional well-being of their African American clients. The ability to be culturally sensitive and aware is so valued within clinical training programs and clinical practice that individuals who demonstrate an inability to gain cultural competence and sensitivity can be held back or even dismissed from training programs (Chronicle of Higher Education, 2010; Inside Higher Ed, 2010).

The focus on cultural competence has a strong evidence base. The ability of a therapist to be aware of and sensitive to the cultural influences acting on their clients impacts not only the client s perceptions of the therapist s ability to help, but also the actual outcomes of therapy (Sue, 1998, 2003). Therefore, awareness of important cultural influences is more than educative; it is vital to effective clinical practice. Cultural-tailoring of treatment plans and other interventions has also resoundingly been proven more effective than a "one-size-fits-all" approach to numerous outcomes, including depression and chronic disease management (Cooper et al., 2003; Givens, Houston, Van Voorhees, Ford, & Cooper, 2007; Kalichman, Kelly, Hunter, Murphy, & Tyler, 1993; Kreuter, Lukwago, Bucholtz, Clark, & Sanders-Thompson, 2003; Primm, Cabot, Pettis, Vu, & Cooper, 2002; Utz et al., 2008).

WHAT ABOUT RURAL?

Despite the abundant evidence pointing to the importance of considering and incorporating cultural themes into mental health treatment, the recognition of rurality as a *bona fide* multicultural issue has not been embraced by the mental health field. More than one in five Americans live within a rural area (U.S. Census Bureau, 2010), where economic, religious, historical, and geographic factors combine to create a unique culture that has been shown to influence mental health outcomes, physical health conditions, and health behaviors (Georgia

Health Equity Initiative, 2008; Pathman, Konrad & Schwartz, 2001; Pearson & Lewis, 1998; Tai-Seale & Chandler, 2003). It is surprising, then, that rurality has traditionally not been viewed as a diversity issue worthy of inclusion with other recognized multicultural groups (Harowski, Turnder, LeVine, Schank, & Leichter, 2006). There are actually more rural residents than any racial, ethnic, or sexual orientation minority group, representing a large group of individuals being strongly influenced by culture, but without professional recognition of the importance of that culture in influencing their mental health.

We posit that rurality should be recognized as its own unique culture that merits inclusion into the traditional notions of multiculturalism—in essence, that rurality is a diversity issue. While a concise definition of rural is elusive (see Chapter 1), and has been debated in the literature since at least the 1930s (Jordan & Hargrove, 1987), this lack of a consistent definition does not mean that rurality has any less of an influence on an individual's cultural heritage.

THE CULTURE OF RURAL LIVING

While there are no clear definitions of rurality, the fact remains that the rural environment creates a unique culture that influences all aspects of an individual's life (as does any other culture). For rural residents, this culture is shaped by several key factors: population density and geography, agricultural heritage, economic conditions, religion, behavioral norms, mental health stigma, and distance to care. These factors combine to impact not only on their potential need for mental health care but also on the ways in which clients will be receptive or resistant to mental health treatment. By considering the cultural factors associated with rural living that follow, mental health professionals may be able to improve both rapport and outcomes in therapy.

Remoteness and Isolation

The most intuitive concepts of rurality stem from ideas of "open land" that are typically associated with rural living—farmlands, fields, prairies, and mountain valleys (Smith & Parvin, 1973). Many definitions of rurality are based upon similar notions of population size or density—for instance, the Census has long defined rural areas as anything that is nonurban, which it has variously defined as populations of 2500 or less (ca. 1970; Smith & Parvin, 1973) or census blocks that have a population density of less than 500 people per square mile (ca. 2000; U.S. Census Bureau, 2002). Another frequent measure is that used by the Federal Office of Management and Budget, which specifies urban areas as cities with more than 50,000 residents (U.S. Department of Agriculture [USDA], 2008). Regardless of the measure used, while the mental image is of wide-open spaces, the underlying implication is a dispersed population separated from other residents (sometimes by miles) and other population centers (sometimes by dozens if not by hundreds of miles).

In addition to the separation this creates from other community members, geographic isolation also contributes to the potentially life-threatening distance to medical and mental health care that is available. Many definitions of rural incorporate some measure of distance from medical care providers or emergency care (Connor, Kralewski, & Hillson, 1994; Weinert & Boik, 1995); while these are typically looked at in terms of physical health care providers, the shortages for mental health care in rural areas are just as severe and likely foster notions of having to be self-reliant for physical and mental health issues. Also, because of the increased travel distance associated with mental health treatment in rural areas (HRSA, 2005), rural residents likely perceive receiving mental health treatment as even more of an inconvenience and burden to friends and families. For clinicians, it will be even more important to emphasize to rural clients the importance of continuing treatment to help ensure that they remain motivated throughout the difficult process of commuting to and from a mental health professional who is frequently many miles away.

This geographic separation from other individuals and from care providers has a distinct influence upon the culture of rural areas. Rural residents are often portrayed as independent and self-sufficient (Long & Weinert, 1989; Weinert & Long, 1987)—characteristics that stem from necessity when geographically isolated from other groups of people and from service providers. These norms of self-reliance can directly impact on an individual's willingness to seek psychological help and progression through therapy. Resistance to therapeutic techniques and to revealing to friends and families the presence of a mental illness will be amplified in rural settings, and clinicians must understand that the reasons behind such resistance may well be based in cultural, rather than cognitive, decision-making processes.

Agriculture

Associated with notions of "wide-open spaces" is the frequent agricultural nature of rural areas. Farming has long been seen as a rural pursuit because of the requisite land for successful farm operation. In fact, one of the earliest discussions on rurality argued that all the cultural and economic conditions present in rural areas stem from their direct tie to agriculture (Sorokin & Zimmerman, 1929 as cited in Jordan & Hargrove, 1987). Early sociological reviews on the measurement of rurality continued to put forth the percentage of residents whose employment is agriculturally based as a crude measure of rurality (Stewart, 1958). While not all rural areas are agricultural, there is an undeniable influence of farm-living on many rural residents. As with geographic isolation, farm-living fosters a sense of independence, strong work ethic, and personal responsibility that will likely spill over into general personality

3 Rurality as a Diversity Issue 41

characteristics. It may also influence the view rural residents have on the role of children in supporting a household, as farm families typically rely on children within the family to help operate the farm.

Poverty

Rural areas have long been recognized as having high rates of poverty and unemployment that directly impact on the mental health of their populations; in fact, the connection between poverty and mental health has been described as "one of the most well established in all of psychiatric epidemiology" (Belle, 1990, p. 385). Because rural economies often center on agriculture, a highly volatile market (Giot, 2003; Koekebakker & Lien, 2004), economic uncertainty is almost a staple in rural communities. Poverty is also strongly associated with a lack of health insurance, further making affordable mental health services harder to reach for rural residents (DeNavas-Walt, Proctor, & Lee, 2006). As such, individuals from rural backgrounds may be unwilling to spend money on psychological treatment, especially when such treatment remains highly stigmatized (Health Resources and Service Administration [HRSA], 2005; Letvak, 2002; see Chapter 4).

The impact of poverty on both mental and physical health status has been well recognized, and poverty has long been one of the largest focuses of social justice movements seeking equality in health for all (Murali & Oyebode, 2004; Patrick, Stein, Porta, Porter, & Ricketts, 1988). While publically supported services are sometimes available (but still limited in rural areas), individuals living in poverty have been shown to have a mistrust of public services and a general fear regarding the stigma associated with having to seek public assistance (Canvin, Jones, Marttila, Burstöm, & Whitehead, 2007).

Religion

As discussed in more detail in Chapter 6, religion plays an extremely prominent role in rural areas, particularly in the rural South. Rural residents are more likely to regularly attend church (Farley & Ruesink, 1997), and many aspects of religious beliefs can impact on an individual's approach to and perception of mental health treatment. For instance, rural religious individuals are more likely to believe that the church can answer life's problems and that psychological problems should be handled within the family or church (Fox, Merwin, & Blank, 1995; Glenna, 2003). In addition, nearly 3/4 of all Americans use their faith as a way to cope with stressful life experiences (Weaver, Flannelly, Garbarino, Figley, & Flannelly, 2003). Increasingly, the role of religion has been recognized as an important factor in the psychological treatment of rural clients (Hook et al., 2010; Post & Wade, 2009), but traditionally mental health professional training has steered away from incorporating religion into therapy. It may be particularly important when working with rural clients to check in with them about their religious views and how those views may be integrated into the therapy process. This does not require a Christian counseling approach; rather, exploration of religious themes and influences can be used to inform the therapeutic process.

Behavioral Norms

There are many health-related behavioral norms that will also impact on mental health treatment. Rural residents (and rural youth in particular) are more likely to engage in alcohol and substance use partially due to permissive cultural norms regarding such use in rural settings (see Chapter 12). Addressing these cultural norms can be very difficult, but should be considered if working with rural clients with substance abuse concerns. Similar health risk-taking behaviors such as smoking and sedentary lifestyle are also more prevalent in rural settings (Doescher, Jackson, Jerant, & Hart, 2006; Tai-Seale and Chandler, 2003), and may make it even more difficult when working with clients wanting to address these issues.

Stigma

As discussed in Chapter 4, there is generally a negative perception toward those receiving mental health services in rural areas. This stigma has a direct impact on not only rural residents' likelihood to seek care in the first place, but also their likelihood of continuing in care for the recommended course of treatment (Parr & Philo, 2003). Unfortunately, it also impacts on rural clients' willingness to share their mental health struggles with individuals outside of the therapeutic relationship. Similarly, if social support is needed as a part of the treatment planning process, clients may not be as open to discussing their needs with friends and family members. Rural practitioners must consider the impact of the culture of stigma surrounding rural regions and be prepared to pursue unique ways of counteracting its effects.

IMPLICATIONS FOR TRAINING PROGRAMS

As presented in this chapter, rurality is most definitely a diversity issue that warrants equal focus in the diversity literature as race, ethnicity, gender, religion, sexual orientation, and other well-established diversity groups. Given that the rural population represents a larger subgroup in the United States than any racial or ethnic group, it is exceedingly important for psychology trainees to gain at least a basic understanding of the cultural aspects of rural living that can impact on the therapeutic process. Specific focus should be given to each of the above-mentioned factors that are important in helping psychologists-in-training become culturally competent with respect to rural culture.

Initial reactions may hold that if a therapist is likely to practice in an urban setting there is no need to gain competence in working with rural populations; however, individuals from rural backgrounds will be encountered in practice regardless of the therapist's location, similar to encountering individuals from multiple countries of origin even if practicing solely in the United States. By expanding current cultural training to encompass rural culture, practitioners can be more prepared for what they may face in therapy with rural clients, and may also be more willing to seek opportunities to work in rural communities.

IMPLICATIONS FOR PRACTICING THERAPISTS

By viewing rurality as a diversity issue, practicing therapists can frame their approach to learning more about rural clients in a similar way they would for an individual from an unknown world culture. Clinicians who find themselves working with an individual from a rural background may wish to explore the client's upbringing and childhood experiences to see how they might be influencing the client's current mental state and perceptions of the therapeutic process itself. For individuals from an even more specialized rural culture, such as Appalachian or frontier, learning more about the culture itself can benefit the therapeutic relationship. As with any cultural group, it is important not to fall into the trap of assuming all individuals from that background share the same experiences and mindset; however, exploring the potential impact of their rural heritage upon their current mental state could prove very valuable.

Recommendations for therapists who work with clients from a rural background include:

1. Remember that not all rural cultures are the same—an African American client from the rural Deep South likely had a very different childhood experience from a Caucasian client from a frontier Midwest area. Ask the client about her or his upbringing to learn about their own region and the influence it may have on their presenting symptoms.
2. Given its widespread importance in rural areas, explore religion as appropriate with rural clients. Do not assume that clients are or are not religious, but be mindful of the fact that religious beliefs may enter the therapeutic discussion and be prepared to handle these discussions in a respectful, nondismissive way. Also keep in mind that the client may have originally sought help from a religious leader.

3. Be aware of the potential effects of rural living upon personality characteristics, including self-reliance and avoidance of help-seeking behaviors.
   These can impact on the course of therapy.
4. Because of the high rates of poverty in rural areas, do not assume a rural individual's current socioeconomic status reflects the SES of their original home-
   life, but simultaneously do not assume that because the individual is rural
   that they grew up in poverty. Explore their current and previous SES as
   appropriate given their presenting problems.
5. Keep in mind that rural clients are less likely to have insurance, are traveling
   longer distances to receive mental health care than their urban counterparts, and that in general rural areas have more stigma toward receipt of
   mental health services. This may make it even more crucial to establish
   good rapport, demonstrate early in therapy the potential benefits of
   ongoing therapy, and continually highlight progress being made.

CONCLUSION

There are many factors that prove that rurality is a cultural diversity issue that
merits full recognition within not only the field of mental health, but across
medical and social fields. By recognizing its importance in personal decision
making, worldview, and interaction patterns with other people, the helping professions can begin to culturally tailor their messages, approaches, and interventions in a way that will be maximally impactful for rural populations. Training
programs should begin to incorporate basic knowledge of rural culture into
their curriculum—not only within rural-focused programs, but more importantly
outside of such programs where rural competency might not otherwise be
acquired. With 20% of the U.S. population being rural, and even more than that
coming from a rural background, every clinician will face the influence of rural
culture. Equipping clinicians-in-training with an understanding of rural culture
can help them ensure that they deliver the best possible care to their clients.

REFERENCES

American Counseling Association. (2005). *American Counseling Association code of
ethics.* Retrieved from http://www.counseling.org/Files/FD.ashx?guid=ab7c1272-
71c4-46cf-848c-f98489937dda
American Psychological Association. (2010). *Ethical principles of psychologists and
code of conduct.* Retrieved from http://www.apa.org/ethics/code/index.aspx
American Psychological Association. (2011). *Guidelines and principles for accreditation of programs in professional psychology.* Retrieved from http://www.apa.
org/ed/accreditation/about/policies/guiding-principles.pdf
Belle, D. (1990). Poverty and women's mental health. *American Psychologist, 45*(3),
385–389.

Betancourt, J. R., Green, A. R., Carrillo, J. E., & Ananeh-Firempong, O. (2003). Defining cultural competence: A practical framework for addressing racial/ethnic disparities in health and health care. *Public Health Reports, 118*, 293–302.

Canvin, K., Jones, C., Marttila, A., Burstöm, B., & Whitehead, M. (2007). Can I risk using public services? Perceived consequences of seeking help and health care among households living in poverty: A qualitative study. *Journal of Epidemiology & Community Health, 61*, 984–989.

Chronicle of Higher Education. (2010). *Augusta State U. is accused of requiring a counseling student to accept homosexuality.* Retrieved from http://chronicle.com/article/Augusta-State-U-Is-Accused-of/123650/

Connor, R. A., Kralewski, J. E., & Hillson, S. D. (1994). Measuring geographic access to health care in rural areas. *Medical Care Review, 51*(3), 337–377.

Cooper, L. A., Gonzales, J. J., Gallo, J. J., Rost, K. M., Meredith, L. S., Rubenstein, L. V., ... Ford, D. E. (2003). The acceptability of treatment for depression among African American, Hispanic, and White primary care patients. *Medical Care, 41*(4), 479–489.

DeNavas-Walt, C., Proctor, B. D., & Lee, C. H. (2006). *Income, poverty, and health insurance coverage in the United States: 2005.* Washington, DC: U.S. Census Bureau.

Doescher, M. P., Jackson, E., Jerant, A., & Hart, G. L. (2006). Prevalence and trends in smoking: A national rural study. *The Journal of Rural Health, 22*, 112–118.

Farley, G. E., & Ruesink, D. C. (1997). Churches. In G. A. Goreham (Ed.), *Encyclopedia of rural America: The land and people* (Vol. 1, pp. 102–105). Santa Barbara, CA: ABC-CLIO.

Fox, J., Merwin, E., & Blank, M. (1995). De facto mental health services in the rural south. *Journal of HealthCare for the Poor and Underserved, 6*, 434–468.

Georgia Health Equity Initiative. (2008). *Georgia health disparities report.* Atlanta, GA: Author.

Giot, P. (2003). The information content of implied volatility in agricultural commodity markets. *The Journal of Futures Markets, 23*(5), 441–454.

Givens, J. L., Houston, T. K., Van Voorhees, B. W., Ford, D. E., & Cooper, L. (2007). Ethnicity and preferences for depression treatment. *General Hospital Psychiatry, 29*(3), 182–191.

Glenna, L. (2003). Religion. In D. L. Brown, & L. E. Swanson (Eds.), *Challenges for rural America in the twenty-first century* (pp. 262–272). University Park, Pennsylvania: The Pennsylvania State University Press.

Harowski, K., Turnder, A. L., LeVine, E., Schank, J., & Leichter, J. (2006). From our community to yours: Rural best perspectives on psychology practice, training, and advocacy. *Professional Psychology: Research and Practice, 37*(3), 158–164.

Health Resources and Services Administration. (2005). *Mental health and rural America: 1994–2005.* Rockville, MD: Author.

Hook, J. N., Worthington, E. L., Jr. Davis, D. E., Jennings, D. J., II, Gartner, A. L., & Hook, J. P. (2010). Empirically supported religious and spiritual therapies. *Journal of Clinical Psychology, 66*(1), 46–72.

Inside Higher Ed. (2010). *Legal loss for anti-gay student.* Retrieved October 2, 2011 from http://www.insidehighered.com/news/2010/08/23/psych

Jordan, S. A., & Hargrove, D. S. (1987). Implications of an empirical application of categorical definitions of rural. *Journal of Rural Community Psychology, 8*, 14–29.

Kalichman, S. C., Kelly, J. A., Hunter, T. L., Murphy, D. A., & Tyler, R. (1993). Culturally tailored HIV-AIDS risk-reduction messages targeted to African American urban women: Impact on risk sensitization and risk reduction. *Journal of Consulting and Clinical Psychology, 61*(2), 291–295.

Koekebakker, S., & Lien, G. (2004). Volatility and price jumps in agricultural futures prices: Evidence from wheat options. *American Journal of Agricultural Economics, 86*(4), 1018–1031.

Kreuter, M. W., Lukwago, S. N., Bucholtz, D. C., Clark, E. M., & Sanders-Thompson, V. (2003). Achieving cultural appropriateness in health promotion programs: Targeted and tailored approaches. *Health Education and Behavior, 30*(2), 133–146.

Letvak, S. (2002). The importance of social support for rural mental health. *Issues in Mental Health Nursing, 23,* 249–261.

Long, K. A., & Weinert, C. (1989). Rural nursing: Developing the theory base. *Research and Theory for Nursing Practice, 3*(2), 113–127.

Matsumoto, D., & Juang, L. (2007). *Culture and psychology* (4th ed.). Belmont, CA: Thomson Wadsworth.

Murali, V., & Oyebode, F. (2004). Poverty, social inequality and mental health. *Advances in Psychiatric Treatment, 10,* 216–224.

National Association of Social Workers. (2008). *Code of ethics of the National Association of Social Workers.* Retrieved October 2, 2011 from http://www.socialworkers.org/pubs/code/code.asp

Parr, H., & Philo, C. (2003). Rural mental health and social geographies of caring. *Social & Cultural Geography, 4*(4), 471–488.

Pathman, D. E., Konrad, T. R., & Schwartz, R. (2001). Findings brief: The proximity of rural African American and Hispanic/Latino communities to physicians and hospital services. Retrieved September 19, 2008 from http://www.shepscenter.unc.edu/research_programs/rural_program/fb65.pdf

Patrick, D. L., Stein, J., Porta, M., Porter, C. Q., & Ricketts, T. C. (1988). Poverty, health services, and health status in rural America. *The Milbank Quarterly, 66*(1), 105–136.

Pearson, T. A., & Lewis, C. (1998). Rural epidemiology: Insights from a rural population laboratory. *American Journal of Epidemiology, 148*(10), 949–957.

Primm, A. B., Cabot, D., Pettis, J., Vu, H. T., & Cooper, L. A. (2002). The acceptability of a culturally-tailored depression education videotape to African Americans. *Journal of the National Medical Association, 94*(11), 1007–1016.

Post, B. C., & Wade, N. G. (2009). Religion and spirituality in psychotherapy: A practice-friendly review of research. *Journal of Clinical Psychology, 65,* 131–146.

Smith, B. J., & Parvin, D. W. (1973). Defining and measuring rurality. *Southern Journal of Agricultural Economics, 5*(1), 109–113.

Stewart, C. T. (1958). The urban–rural dichotomy. *American Journal of Sociology, 64,* 52–58.

Sue, S. (1998). In search of cultural competence in psychotherapy and counseling. *American Psychologist, 53*(4), 440–448.

Sue, S. (2003). In defense of cultural competency in psychotherapy and treatment. *American Psychologist, 58*(11), 964–970.

Tai-Seale, T., & Chandler, C. (2003). Nutrition and overweight concerns in rural areas. In L. D. Gamm, L. Hutchison, B. Dabney, & A. Dorsey (Eds.), *Rural Healthy*

People 2010: A companion document to Healthy People 2010 (Vol. 1). College Station, TX: The Texas A&M University System Health Science Center, School of Rural Public Health, Southwest Rural Health Research Center.

U.S. Census Bureau. (2002). Census 2000 urban and rural classification. Retrieved October 1, 2011 from http://www.census.gov/geo/www/ua/ua_2k.html

U.S. Census Bureau. (2010). American FactFinder. Retrieved 7-22-2010 from http://factfinder.census.gov/servlet/DCGeoSelectServlet?ds_name=DEC_2000_SF1_U

U.S. Department of Agriculture. (2008). *What is Rural?* Retrieved October 2, 2011 from http://www.nal.usda.gov/ric/ricpubs/what_is_rural.shtml

Utz, S. W., Williams, I. C., Jones, R., Hinton, I., Alexander, G., Yan, G. et al. (2008). Culturally tailored intervention for rural African Americans with type 2 diabetes. *The Diabetes Educator, 34*(5), 854–865.

Weaver, A. J., Flannelly, L. T., Garbarino, J., Figley, C. R., & Flannelly, K. J. (2003). A systematic review of research on religion and spirituality in the Journal of Traumatic Stress: 1990–1999. *Mental Health, Religion, & Culture, 6*(3), 215–228.

Weinert, C., & Boik, R. J. (1995). MSU rurality index: Development and evaluation. *Research in Nursing and Health, 18*, 453–464.

Weinert, C., & Long, K. A. (1987). Understanding the health care needs of rural families. *Family Relations, 36*(4), 450–455.

4

The Impact of Mental Health Stigma on Clients From Rural Settings

JONATHON E. LARSON, PATRICK W. CORRIGAN, AND
THOMAS P. COTHRAN

INTRODUCTION

*T*he stigma of mental illness presents a complex phenomenon that negatively impacts on rural residents like a double-edged sword. On one side,
public stigma leads to discrimination, which takes away opportunities to
reach and maintain life goals. On the other, mental illness self-stigma consists
of internalized public stigma that leads to reductions in self-esteem and self-
efficacy. Interventions hoping to reduce the burden of mental health stigma
upon rural residents require addressing both sides of the equation. In this
chapter, definitions of public stigma and self-stigma are reviewed, with focus
placed on how both types of stigma impact residents of rural areas. We then
conclude with a case illustration of how the effects of stigma can be explored
in therapy.

PUBLIC STIGMA

Public stigma consists of three components: stereotypes, prejudice, and discrimination. Stereotypes are social and efficient knowledge structures
learned by members of a social group (Hilton & von Hippel, 1996; Judd &
Park, 1996; Krueger, 1996). Stereotypes include a social component because
they represent collectively agreed upon notions of types of people. They
also provide an efficient manner to organize our complex world; individuals
quickly generate impressions and expectations of individuals belonging to a
stereotyped group (Hamilton & Sherman, 1994). Prejudice describes endorsement of negative stereotypes generating negative emotional reactions (Devine,

1989; Hilton & von Hippel, 1996; Krueger, 1996). In essence, stereotyping includes awareness of negative labels while prejudice contains both awareness *and* agreement leading to negative emotional responses, that is, disgust, anger, fear, and blame (Allport, 1954/1979; Eagley & Chaiken, 1993).

Everyone develops cognitive sets of stereotypes; however, this does not imply they agree with them (Jussim, Nelson, Manis, & Soffin, 1995). For example, persons may identify stereotypes about different racial groups but do not agree that the stereotypes are valid. On the other hand, people with prejudicial attitudes endorse these negative stereotypes and generate negative emotional reactions (Devine, 1989; Hilton & von Hippel, 1996; Krueger, 1996). In contrast to stereotypes, which are acknowledgements, prejudicial attitudes involve an evaluative component generally leading to negative viewpoints (Allport, 1954/1979; Eagley & Chaiken, 1993).

Discrimination describes behavioral reactions connected to the negative emotional responses produced by prejudice (Crocker, Major, & Steele, 1998). While prejudice involves awareness and agreement of negative stereotypes, discrimination contains both prejudice and an *action* connected to negative emotional reactions produced by prejudice. Prejudice (yielding disgust, anger, fear, and blame) leads to hostile reactions, avoidance, and/or behaviors of withholding resources and opportunities for individuals with severe mental illness, thus resulting in discrimination against those individuals (Corrigan, 2000; Corrigan & Penn, 1999; Weiner, 1995).

Consider an insurance company owner in a small town who reads a local newspaper and mentions to her business partner, "This article says individuals with mental illness can be unpredictable and dangerous" (stereotype). She continues, "From my experience, I agree and I'm fearful of people with mental illness" (prejudice). She finishes, "I'm not going to hire anyone with mental illness because I'm afraid of what they might do while they are working with our clients" (discrimination).

SELF-STIGMA

Individuals with mental illness adapt and cope with symptoms, functional limitations, and "disability stigma" associated with their "spoiled identity" (Goffman, 1963). Disability stigma leads to reduced well-being, social rejection, and discrimination within housing, employment, and health care settings (Bordieri & Drehmer, 1986; Link, 1982, 1987). Link (1987) described a modified labeling theory stating that stigmatized individuals constrict their social opportunities in anticipation of rejection due to stigma; this process leads to increased social isolation, decreased employment opportunities, and reduced incomes. The resulting self-isolation and limited social contact results in self-esteem and self-efficacy decrements (Link, Cullen, Frank, & Wozniak, 1987; Markowitz, 1998) that directly impact on mental health. The stigma appears to connect with internal processes leading to accepting and applying negative labels and its accompanying stereotypes as self-relevant. This process has been referred to as "self-stigma."

Traditional theories of stigma maintain that individuals will experience lower self-esteem due to self-stigma when they belong to a group that is stigmatized (Allport, 1954/1979; Erikson, 1956; Jones et al., 1984). However, more recent evidence suggests that this is not a uniform response across people with stigmatized conditions or within individuals across time (Deegan, 1997; Gilmartin, 1997). Many members of stigmatized groups do not suffer a loss of self-esteem due to stigma. Some people react to stigma by becoming energized and empowered while others remain relatively indifferent and unaffected (Chamberlin, 1978; Corrigan & Watson, 2002; Deegan, 1990; Lee, Kochman, & Sikkema, 2002).

In general, self-stigma consists of individuals internalizing public stigma by accepting and applying negative stereotypes to themselves. Individuals experiencing self-stigma face reduced self-esteem, lower social interactions, diminished relationships, and increased unemployment (Allport, 1954/1979; Corrigan & Penn, 1999; Link, Cullen, Struening, Shrout, & Dohrenwend, 1989). Individuals may endorse and demonstrate self-stigma through harmful self-thoughts and negative behaviors turned inward. Furthermore, they may avoid seeking mental health services in order to avoid a negative label of mental illness. Self-stigma negatively impacts on individuals in many aspects of life, including employment, housing, politics, education, relationships, and health care goals. When bombarded with public stigmatizing images and behaviors, individuals may endorse these notions, turn them inward, and experience minimal self-esteem, self-efficacy, and confidence, which may lead to the lack of drive to pursue life goals. By internalizing stigma, individuals may believe that they are less valued in society.

Self and public stigma contain the same components (stereotypes, prejudice, and discrimination), but the constructs interact differently. Initially, the self-stigma process includes an awareness of negative stereotypes. An individual may mention, "I'm aware that parts of society think that individuals with my mental condition are dangerous and incapable of doing things" (stereotype awareness). The next self-stigma step includes self-prejudice or agreeing and applying the stereotype to the self. An individual might say, "People at the coffee shop say I'm incompetent because of my illness; I believe it and I feel worthless" (self-prejudice). Self-prejudice leads to self-disgust, low self-esteem, and limited self-efficacy. The final stage of self-stigma consists of self-discrimination leading to avoidance behaviors. An individual states, "I'm useless and dangerous so I'm not going to apply for the grain elevator job. They won't hire me anyway, so why try" (self-discrimination). Low self-efficacy and demoralization have been associated with self-discrimination behaviors of avoiding employment opportunities and evading the pursuit of independent living at which individuals might otherwise succeed (Link, 1982, 1987).

Research offers the equation:

self-stereotype + self-prejudice + self-discrimination = self-stigma

Research indicates that self-stigma predicts anguish (Ritsher & Phelan, 2004); conversely, decreased self-stigma alienation is associated with increased sense of hope (Lysaker, Buck, Hammoud, Taylor, & Roe, 2006). Positive identification with others suffering from mental illness and viewing stigma as illegitimate provides a buffer against self-stigma (Watson, Corrigan, Larson, & Sells, 2007); however, in rural settings identifying others who are facing the same mental health concerns is very difficult (Pullman, VanHooser, Hoffman, & Heflinger, 2010).

STIGMA IN RURAL SETTINGS

There are a variety of barriers that make it difficult for persons living in rural settings to access mental health services. Human and Wasem (1991) categorized these barriers in terms of accessibility, availability, and acceptability. Accessibility concerns barriers such as the distance a person from a rural setting has to travel to receive treatment. Rural settings are heterogeneous and vary in terms of physical remoteness and isolation which impacts on accessibility of mental health services. Availability concerns barriers such as the prominent lack of specialized mental health practitioners in rural settings (Heflinger & Christens, 2006). Jameson and Blank (2007) noted a report from the United States Department of Health and Human Services that indicated that about half of rural counties did not have a master's-level or doctoral-level social worker or psychologist in residence.

Acceptability concerns barriers such as stoic attitudes toward the necessity of mental health treatment and fears related to stigma of mental illness. Brems, Johnson, Warner, and Roberts (2006) noted that according to a sample of health care providers, the stigma of mental illness may affect rural communities differently according to the size of the population. They found that perceived stigma as a barrier was greatest in communities with populations ranging from 3,500 to 14,999. Perceived stigma was downplayed among healthcare providers in rural settings populated by less than 3,500. These authors suggested that the social cost of ostracizing even a single community member becomes too great within intensely interdependent communities in increasingly remote locales.

On the other hand, Hoyt, Conger, Valde, and Weihs (1997) found that level of rurality was directly related to stigmatized attitudes about mental illness. They defined size of community in terms of six categories ranging from farm-based households to rural population centers with more than 50,000 residents. Persons from the smaller, rural settings were more likely to hold stigmatizing attitudes toward the label of mental illness and mental health treatment. In yet another study, Komiti, Judd, and Jackson (2006) found that attitudes and perceived stigma were prevalent within rural contexts but did *not* differ by population size. In contrast to their expectations, they did not find that perceived stigma negatively influenced help-seeking for psychological symptoms, either. More research is needed to determine whether the difference in these findings is due to the difference in perspectives between providers of mental health services and residents of rural communities on the impact of stigma on help-seeking. Additionally, Komiti et al. (2006) suggest that there may be other unidentified moderating variables that affect the relationship between perceived stigma and help-seeking for psychological symptoms in rural settings.

Nevertheless, negative attitudes concerning the efficacy of mental health treatment and concerns related to mental illness stigma may render mental health treatment unacceptable for persons struggling with psychiatric symptoms in rural settings. Parr and Philo (2003) present a manner of conceptualizing rural and urban communities along the continuums of population density and social involvement. Rural settings are characterized by a population that is physically distant but socially proximate, whereas urban settings involve a population that is physically proximate but socially distant. Due to the social proximity of rural community members, persons struggling with psychiatric symptoms may believe they are unable to access mental health services anonymously. They may fear being recognized entering a mental health clinic and having that information spread rapidly through local gossip networks. Additionally, negative attitudes concerning mental health treatment among persons in closed emotionally proximate social circles may make it less likely that a person will be able to see the benefit of mental health treatment.

The threat of perceived stigma may not only affect the individual in need of services, but may also influence the individual's family members. Heflinger and Christen (2006) discuss the familial level of response to mental illness. They describe the family as the gateway to the initiation of mental health treatment, serving as a support and as a liaison to mental health providers. Families may discourage a person from seeking treatment if they do not recognize the need, or they may place the needs of the family above the needs of the individual. As an example, consider a farming family who may postpone seeking help for a member until after the fall harvest. Franz et al. (2010) found evidence to suggest that perceived threat of stigma was related to a raised threshold for treatment initiation among families in rural settings. These families appeared to adopt coping strategies such as denial and minimization in order to avoid labeling their loved one with a mental illness. These strategies ultimately prolong the time between the affected family member's onset of symptoms and the initiation of treatment, which can have negative implications for prognosis (Gaynor, Dooley, Lawlor, Lawoyin & O'Callaghan, 2009; Keshavan et al., 2003).

Among practitioners, a major concern in rural settings is the likelihood of frequent interactions outside the therapy context (Brems et al., 2006), discussed in detail in Chapter 7. In rural communities, persons receiving mental health services run the risk of unplanned interactions with their providers in the community. In rural life, these providers are more than anonymous specialists who are never seen beyond the parameters of an office. They may be embedded in the social foundation of a socially proximate community. The provider's profession may be common knowledge among the community. Consider Joaquin, a 24-year-old Hispanic male living in a village in northern Maine. While grocery shopping with a new girlfriend, he encounters his therapist in aisle 7. Joaquin struggles with the thought that being recognized in the community by a mental health professional is a "dead giveaway" of his mental health status by observers of the interaction. Situations such as these place both parties in a precarious predicament. Not only might the encounter be uncomfortable for Joaquin, but it is argued that these potential encounters are considered a disincentive for providers to establish a practice in rural settings (Brems et al., 2006; Jameson & Blank, 2007; Nelson, Pomerantz, & Schwartz, 2007). Clients may travel to services outside their local community to avoid shame, guilt, and other problems associated with stigma and unplanned self-disclosure. Of course, urban patients face self-stigma; however, they maintain a higher level of privacy and less likelihood of unplanned disclosure than do their rural counterparts.

Many members of stigmatized groups are aware of the stereotypes that exist about their group, such as, individuals with mental illness are incompetent and dangerous (Hayward & Bright, 1997). However, it should be noted that awareness of stigma and associated stereotypes does not necessarily lead to internalizing the negative stereotype (Crocker & Major, 1989). Individuals with mental illness do report being aware of negative stereotypes (Bowden, Schoenfeld, & Adams, 1980; Kahn, Obstfeld, & Heiman, 1979; Shurka, 1983; Wright, Gronfein, & Owens, 2000) but do not necessarily agree with these stereotypes (Hayward & Bright, 1997). This provides an opportunity for rural mental health professionals to address issues surrounding mental health stigma during the course of therapy in a way that will hopefully prevent the internalization of public stigma.

TREATMENT OF SELF-STIGMA IN RURAL SETTINGS

Psychological interventions for people with serious mental illness typically focus on psychosocial factors, emphasize symptom reduction, and utilize cognitive-behavioral methods (Hayward & Bright, 1997). Improving psychosocial factors (e.g., unemployment, low economic status, minimal education) increases life satisfaction that, in turn, combats self-stigma. Treatments target symptoms of self-worth and self-efficacy that directly address self-stigma rather than targeting diagnostic categories. Cognitive approaches can challenge and change negative self-stigma thoughts. Interventions reduce self-stigma by enhancing empowerment through identifying life goals, cultivating strengths, and building personal skills.

Opportunities to discuss the pros and cons of disclosure of the client's mental health condition to others also prove effective. This may include components of motivational interviewing (MI) to explore costs and benefits of disclosure and identify strategies either to disclose or to remain silent.

Research on treatments for reducing self-stigma has demonstrated positive results for cognitive therapies; as an example, a six-week course combining cognitive and psycho-educational methods significantly reduced self-stigma (Macinnes & Lewis, 2008). A group-based cognitive-behavior therapy program focusing on self-stigma produced significantly improved self-esteem (Knight, Wykes, & Hayward, 2006). Acceptance and Commitment Therapy (ACT), which focuses on accepting problems and developing a commitment for change, has also been shown to reduce self-stigma in substance abuse (Luoma, Kohlenberg, Hayes, Bunting, & Rye, 2008). Initial results of a Resisting Internalized Stigma (RIS) intervention, which challenges internal negative thoughts, appear promising (Calmes, 2009; Lucksted et al., 2009).

Case Illustration

Following is a hypothetical case illustration demonstrating how addressing issues of public and self-stigma during the course of treating a depressed rural client can be used to increase self-awareness and improve outcomes.

Presenting Problem and Client Description

H.M. is a 50-year-old, divorced Caucasian man who has lived in the same northern Midwestern rural community for his entire life, except for attending an urban university where he earned a BA in business. He was married for 20 years before divorcing over ongoing relationship and financial conflicts. His ex-wife has remarried and lives 50 miles away. H.M. has an 18-year-old daughter and 20-year-old son from his marriage. Both children are attending out-of-state universities and visit H.M. on the weekends once a month. His girlfriend lives and works in a nearby city during the week and commutes to live with H.M. on the weekends.

H.M. owns a farm house two miles from a rural community of 3,000 people. He owns and operates a stock portfolio trading company that specializes in grain and food commodities. He and his four employees have mostly operated a profitable business since 1986. However, his company has seen a drastic downturn in profits over the past 2 years.

He has been an active community member, serving on a local city planning committee and the school board. He facilitates a local book club, plays poker with his friends, and attends a monthly "cuisine from around the world" party. His personal goals include re-engaging with his friends and business contacts, pursuing an MBA degree, developing his relationship with his girlfriend, improving financial stability, and losing weight.

H.M. entered the psychotherapist's office with complaints of moderate anxiety, severe depression, and feelings of shame related to his depression. He expressed self-disgust about his inability to control his depression and a strong feeling of being shunned by distant family members aware of his depression. He reported low self-esteem and feelings of worthlessness. He experienced bouts of anxiety related to the fear of people discovering his mental illness. He reported poor sleep patterns, periodic irritability, and low energy. Over his lifetime, he reported being admitted to psychiatric hospitals six times, once for a suicide attempt and five times for major depression. He revealed he went to a mental health facility in urban suburbs to avoid people in his community finding out about his illness. He reported utilizing various psychotropic medications for depression and anxiety over the years, all of which he found helpful. Throughout his adulthood, he periodically received outpatient psychotherapy. H.M. asked for help with two main problems. First, he was avoiding efforts to obtain new business clients and attend his usual social activities. Second, he had experienced an increase in self-disgust and a decrease of self-esteem, related to experiencing self-stigma.

During the initial session H.M. reported that he was experiencing trouble dealing with the "secret" about his depression which he had kept "since college." He revealed that only his ex-wife and girlfriend knew about his mental illness. He reported that he had "mentioned it" to his children, but that they knew "not to tell other people and to keep it in the family." He never spoke with his friends about his hospitalizations, his symptoms, or the fact that he takes medications. He reported that currently his symptoms are "in check" but that he feels as though his secret is "wearing [him] out."

H.M. told the therapist that he is afraid of the consequences that may occur if he is "found out." He is fearful that because he lives in a rural community any news of his mental illness would spread quickly. He is concerned that he would then lose friends and business clients. At a recent "Cuisine Around the World" meal there was a discussion about college shootings like those at Virginia Tech or Northern Illinois University. H.M. heard his friends make comments like, "people with mental illness are crazy and dangerous and incompetent" and "they don't take care of themselves." He heard them argue that people with mental illness are a burden to taxpayers and that "these people just need to pull themselves up by the bootstraps and move on." During this conversation H.M. was silent, but he felt a range of negative emotions including fear, shame, anger, disgust, and guilt. He felt even more convinced that if people found out about his secret he would lose business relationships and friendships.

After this social occasion, H.M. felt a strong sense of worthlessness. He felt confused by this feeling because he had been fairly successful. However, despite his accomplishments in life he was beginning to agree with the notion that people with mental illness were incompetent and weak. He also found that he was avoiding people. He reported not readily understanding this avoidance. With H.M.'s permission, the therapist offered the suggestion that his secret and feelings of worthlessness were connected to avoiding people. The therapist worked with H.M. to identify problem areas, many of which were directly related to self-stigma. During this initial session, the therapist did not mention self-stigma, instead using H.M.'s language to frame his problems rather than using technical language.

Case Formulation

H.M's secret is leading to fatigue, anxiety, and fear. He is experiencing an increase in thoughts of worthlessness, leading to self-disgust, and he has been avoiding people. The vignette below illustrates the case formulation shared in the second session. The therapist began by summarizing the first session and seeking clarification around the main points. Next, the therapist presented three target areas to work on: secret, worthlessness, and avoidance. H.M. chose to first work on avoiding people. In the vignette, we provide therapist skills in *italics* and self-stigma components in ***bold italics***.

Therapist: OK. I'd like to start with a few questions to lead us into working on avoidance.

H.M.: That's fine.

Therapist: What are some of the things that people say about people with mental illness? (***Exploring Stereotype Awareness***)

H.M.: Well, over the years, I've read and heard things like—those crazy people are dangerous and unpredictable and can't take of themselves and they always need help to get by. (***Stereotype Awareness***)

Therapist: What are your immediate or automatic thoughts about that? (*Exploring Automatic Thoughts*)

H.M.: Hmmm . . . I've never said this to anyone, but there are times that I think they may be right. I mean, there have been times that I couldn't take care of myself and I needed help. (***Agreeing and Applying Stereotypes***)

Therapist: Tell me more. (***Exploring Stereotype Agreement, Application, and Self-Prejudice***)

H.M.: Nobody knows that there are times when I've needed help with my depression. I'm afraid that if people find out then they'll think I'm worthless and incompetent and they'll treat me differently. Now that we are talking about it, I think I'm starting to agree with them. I'm disgusted with myself because I just can't get over this on my own and I must be weak and worthless. (***Self-Prejudice***)

Therapist: Let me know if I'm on the right track. You are sensing yourself agreeing with the stereotypes of worthlessness and incompetent and you are feeling self-disgust. (*Check Back and Reflection*) (**Highlighting Self-Prejudice Process**)

H.M.: Yeah.

Therapist: How does avoiding people fit into this? (*Socratic Questioning*) (**Eliciting Self-Discrimination**)

H.M.: At first, I thought I started avoiding people because I was scared they might find out my secret and that may be part of the problem. But now I think it may be something else. It may be that I feel weak in the mind and worthless or unequal to other people and I don't deserve to be around them so I avoid them. I'm worthless and weaker and more incompetent than they are, and I just don't want to be reminded of that so I don't spend time with them. I don't know . . . it seems confusing. (**Self-Discrimination**)

Therapist: Could I offer some observations? (*Asking Permission*)

H.M.: Sure.

Therapist: Over the years, you've heard bad things about people with mental illness like worthlessness and incompetence and now you think they apply to you. And you feel self-disgust because there are times that you seem to fit the stereotypes, like when you need help and you can't fix it on your own. And now you think you are worthless and incompetent and avoid being around people because being around them reminds you of being weak. (**Observations to Explain Self-Stigma Process**)

H.M.: Sounds like one way to explain my current problems. What do we do about it?

Therapist: In our next session, we will practice some skills and talk about ways to deal with the worthlessness thoughts and avoiding people.

In this vignette, H.M. and the therapist agreed upon problem areas and identified avoiding people as the first target. Once identifying a target problem, the therapist started the self-stigma framework by asking, "What are some of the things that people say about people with mental illness?" This question raised H.M.'s awareness of his perspectives on mental illness stereotypes. The therapist noticed that H.M. is internalizing stereotypes and making self-prejudice statements, "I think I'm starting to agree with them. I'm disgusted with myself because I just can't get over this on my own and I must be weak and worthless." The therapist moved to identifying self-discrimination by exploring the connection between worthlessness and avoiding people, "How does avoiding people fit into this?" H.M. identified connections between his self-prejudice and self-discrimination. The therapist clarified the self-stigma process for H.M. When working with H.M, the therapist framed the client's problems in stereotype awareness, stereotype agreement, stereotype application, self-prejudice, and self-discrimination; however, the therapist utilizes H.M.'s words to explain the process.

Course of Treatment

During session 3, the therapist employs techniques to address H.M's self-stigma and related problems. The therapist began with a cognitive probe to identify thoughts related to avoidance behavior. H.M. reported that he is worthless because he has depression. The therapist then elicited discussion about situations that trigger thoughts related to avoidance behavior. H.M. identified feeling worthlessness first thing in the morning, when he is home alone, and when he is getting ready to talk to people. H.M. said that he does not feel as worthless when his girlfriend is home and when he is busy at the office. Next, the therapist probed any personal beliefs that may influence H.M.'s thought of worthlessness. H.M. believed that he should be "strong enough to kick this funk." H.M. believes other people are strong enough to avoid depression. He also thought that people were right that he was "weak and worthless" and unable to take care of himself. The therapist utilized reflection to encourage H.M. to fully explore these topics.

H.M. discussed feeling disgusted with himself and fear that he will "stay this way." He reported sadness because he is unable to get over these "bothersome and busy thoughts." He identified physical sensations associated with these thoughts such as cold hands, tension in his neck and back, and the feeling that his stomach is "all tied up." H.M. indicated that these thoughts were not related to his depression. He stated, "My self-esteem has never been this low before but my depression seems to be under control right now." In the following vignette the therapist summarizes H.M.'s negative thoughts and shifts the session toward the topic of self-stigma.

Therapist: Busy and bothersome thoughts of worthlessness and depression lead to feelings of disgust, fear, and sadness. You feel there is more going on with you than depression. And you avoid people and experience body stress. Could we call your different experience as self-stigma? (*Summary and Asking Permission*)

H.M.: Yeah. What is self-stigma?

Therapist: It differs from depression in that you have internalized mental illness stereotypes that you have heard from people over the years. And this leads to you avoiding people. So we are going after your self-stigma to see if we can improve your life.

H.M.: Hmmm, so it is more than depression. I'm beating myself up because of self-stigma.

Therapist: Correct. So, let's look at your thought—I'm worthless because of self-stigma. Give me some evidence that this is true. (*Cognitive Challenge*)

H.M.: Well . . . (pause) I've been experiencing self-stigma and beating myself up and avoiding people. I see myself as worthless and I can't get out of this funk. I can't think of anything else supporting my thought.

Therapist: Give me evidence that you are worthy. (*Cognitive Challenge*)

H.M.: My kids are doing well in college, I own my own home, my business has been successful for the most part, good friends, my employees rely on me for a job. At times, I can really focus on my business. I helped a lot of clients earn money, and things are going well with my girlfriend.

Therapist: So you see evidence on both sides of your thought of worthlessness because of self-stigma. With your thought, what is the worst case scenario? (*Cognitive Reframing*)

H.M.: Well, things will continue and get worse. I can get into a bigger funk and then feel even more desperate and worthless.

Therapist: What is the best case scenario? (*Cognitive Reframing*)

H.M.: I get out of this funk and my thoughts of worthlessness and self-stigma go away and I get back to myself.

Therapist: What's the probable scenario? (*Cognitive Reframing*)

H.M.: I think that I may continue with this thought and eventually it will get weaker and go away. I see a little hope now that I'm talking about all this stuff.

Therapist: You are hopeful and see worst, best, and probable case scenarios. Let's practice some mindfulness with your current thought of worthlessness. (*Reframing Summary and Offering Practice*)

H.M.: OK. How do we do it?

Therapist: First, I'd like to explain the steps and then we'll practice mindfulness to deal with your bothersome thoughts. Being mindful includes focusing on only one thought at a time. We don't say the thought is good or bad; we just accept that we are having the thought. We want to effectively deal with the thought and efficiently work through it. Instead of having the thought, we take a step back and notice that we are having a bothersome thought. Any questions so far? (*Explanation of Mindfulness*)

H.M.: Yeah, so I don't want to tell myself to stop having the thought. I thought that I would want to tell my thought to go away and I can't have that thought.

Therapist: How well has that worked in the past? (*Cognitive Challenge*)

H.M.: Not real well. Avoiding the thought or telling it to go away seems to make it stronger.

Therapist: Yes, with some bothersome thoughts, the more we fight it and try to stop it the more we have it. So in mindfulness, in a non-judging way, we accept that we are having a bothersome thought. We work the thought through three steps. First, we become aware that we are having the worthless thought and we may say something like—"hmmm, there's that thought, what's that about?" Second, we describe the thought; "it is painful and being alone brings it on; I feel anxious, scared, sad; I avoid people; and my body gets tense." Last, we participate with the worthless thought. We notice having the thought and picture coming into our head, observing it, and seeing it leave. It may come back, and we continue to notice it, describe it, and participate with it. (*Skill Explanation*)

H.M.: That's a lot to take in. How do we start practicing this mindfulness?

Therapist: Our first step is to practice some breathing exercises to get your body and mind to a calm and alert state so you are at a good place to be mindful with bothersome thoughts. Then we will learn mindfulness skills to notice your thoughts rather than having your thoughts. In following sessions, we will practice additional skills to deal with your secret, your worthlessness thoughts, and avoiding people.

Throughout H.M.s remaining sessions, continued use of cognitive therapy, motivational interviewing, and mindfulness techniques challenged and reframed his self-stigma automatic thoughts. He continued to learn finer points of cognitive therapy and mindfulness. He learned basic biofeedback techniques using skin temperature, skin moisture, and heart rate to maintain a relaxed physical state. Role-plays were conducted during sessions to practice mental illness disclosure to close friends. At home with his girlfriend, he practiced disclosure discussions, and he eventually talked to a close friend about his mental illness. He began using a positive statement log, each day listing three good things that happened. He also listed reasons of why those things went well for the day. He used breathing skills in the mornings and used cognitive skills throughout the day to address self-stigma thoughts. He set and followed a specific bed time and a specific wake up time. He used a 1–10 scale (1 = low, 10 = high) to rate his level of worthlessness and self-disgust. It took 25 one hour sessions and numerous situational experiments to incorporate these cognitive and behavioral skills into his daily routine.

CONCLUSION

The stigmatization of mental illness impacts on mental health service delivery across the spectrum in rural areas by impacting on willingness to seek therapy, ability to disclose ongoing mental illness, and the level of support an individual is able to receive from their family and peers. The case of H.M. demonstrates numerous clinical methods to address self-stigma among rural clients. From the empirical research and our experience, individuals facing self-stigma typically benefit from cognitive treatments that specifically target bothersome thoughts, emotions, behaviors, and body tension related to experiences of self-stigma. Self-stigma becomes apparent and addressed when making connections among automatic thoughts, public stigma awareness, stereotype agreement, emotional reactions, and behavioral reactions.

REFERENCES

Allport, G. W. (1979). *The nature of prejudice*. New York: Doubleday Anchor Books. (Original work published in 1954).

Bordieri, J., & Drehmer, D. (1986). Hiring decisions for disabled workers: Looking at the cause. *Journal of Applied Social Psychology, 16*, 197–208.

Bowden, C. L., Schoenfeld, L. S., & Adams, R. L. (1980). Mental health attitudes and treatment expectations as treatment variables. *Journal of Clinical Psychology, 36*, 653–657.

Brems, C., Johnson, M. E., Warner, T. D., & Roberts, L. W. (2006). Barriers to healthcare as reported by rural and urban interprofessional providers. *Journal of Interprofessional Care, 20*(2), 105–118.

Calmes, C. (2009). Resisting internalized stigma intervention. *MIRECC Matters, 10*(2), 1–2.

Chamberlin, J. (1978). *On our own: Patient-controlled alternatives to the mental health system*. New York: McGraw-Hill.

Corrigan, P. W. (2000). Mental health stigma as social attribution: Implications for research methods and attitude change. *Clinical Psychology: Science & Practice, 7*, 48–67.

Corrigan, P. W., & Penn, D. L. (1999) Lessons from social psychology on discrediting-psychiatric stigma. *American Psychologist, 54*(9), 765–776.

Corrigan, P. W., & Watson, A. C. (2002). The paradox of self-stigma and mental illness. *Clinical Psychology: Science & Practice, 9*, 35–53.

Crocker, J., & Major, B. (1989). Social stigma and self-esteem: The self-protective properties of stigma. *Psychological Review, 96*, 608–630.

Crocker, J., Major, B., & Steele, C. (1998). Social Stigma. In D. Gilbert, S. T. Fiske, & G. Lindzey (Eds.), *The handbook of social psychology* (4th ed., Vol. 2, pp. 504–553). New York: McGraw-Hill.

Deegan, P. E. (1990). Spirit breaking: When the helping professions hurt. *Humanistic Psychologist, 18*, 301–313.

Deegan, P. E. (1997). Recovery and empowerment for people with psychiatric disabilities. *Social Work in Mental Health Care, 25*(3), 11–24.

Devine, P. G. (1989). Stereotypes and prejudice: Their automatic and controlled components. *Journal of Personality and Social Psychology, 56*, 5–18.

Eagley, A. H., & Chaiken, S. (1993). *The social psychology of attitudes*. Fort Worth, TX: Harcourt Brace Javanovich, Inc.

Erikson, E. (1956). The problem of ego identity. *Journal of the American Psychoanalytic Association, 4*, 56–121.

Franz, L., Carter, T., Leiner, A. S., Bergner, E., Thompson, N. J., & Comptom, M. T. (2010). Stigma and treatment delay in first-episode psychosis: A grounded theory study. *Early Intervention in Psychiatry, 4*, 47–56.

Gaynor, K., Dooley, B., Lawlor, E., Lawoyin, L. R., & O'Callaghan, E. (2009). Cognitive deterioration and duration of untreated psychosis. *Early Intervention in Psychiatry, 3,* 157–160.

Gilmartin, R. M. (1997). Personal narrative and the social reconstruction of the lives of former psychiatric patients. *Journal of Sociology & Social Welfare, 25*(2), 77–103.

Goffman, E. (1963). *Stigma: Notes on the management of spoiled identity.* Englewood Cliff, NJ: Prentice-Hall.

Hamilton, D. L., & Sherman, J. W. (1994). Stereotypes. In R. S. Wyer Jr. & T. K. Srull (Eds.), *Handbook of social cognition* (2nd ed., Vols. *1–2,* pp. 1–68). Hillsdale, NJ: Lawrence Erlbaum Associates, Inc.

Hayward, P., & Bright, J. A. (1997). Stigma and mental illness: A review and critique. *Journal of Mental Health, 6,* 345–354.

Heflinger, C. A., & Christens, B. (2006). Rural behavioral health services for children and adolescents: An ecological and community psychology analysis. *Journal of Community Psychology, 34*(4), 379–400.

Hilton, J., & von Hippel, W. (1996). Stereotypes. *Annual Review of Psychology, 47,* 237–271.

Hoyt, D. R., Conger, R. D., Valde, J. G., & Weihs, K. (1997). Psychological distress and help-seeking in rural America. *American Journal of Community Psychology, 25*(4), 449–470.

Human, J., & Wasem, C. (1991). Rural health in America. *American Psychologist, 46*(3), 232–239.

Jameson, J. P., & Blank, M. B. (2007). The role of clinical psychology in rural mental health services: Defining problems and developing solutions. *Clinical Psychology: Science and Practice, 14*(3), 283–298.

Jones, E. E., Farina, A., Hastorf, A. H., Markus, H., Miller, D. T., & Scott, R. A. (1984). *Social stigma: The psychology of marked relationships.* New York: Freeman.

Judd, C., & Park, B. (1996). Definition and assessment of accuracy in stereotypes. *Psychological Review, 100,* 109–128.

Jussim, L., Nelson, T. E., Manis, M., & Soffin, S. (1995). Prejudice, stereotypes, and labeling effects: Sources of bias in person perception. *Journal of Personality & Social Psychology, 68*(2), 228–246.

Kahn, M. W., Obstfeld, L., & Heiman, E. (1979). Staff conceptions of patients' attitudes toward mental disorder and hospitalization as compared to patients' and staff's actual attitudes. *Journal of Clinical Psychology, 35,* 415–420.

Keshavan, M. S., Haas, G., Miewald, J., Montrose, D. M., Reddy, R., Schooler, N. R., & Sweeney, J. A. (2003). Prolonged untreated illness duration from prodromal onset predicts outcome in first episode psychoses. *Schizophrenia Bulletin, 29,* 757–769.

Knight, M. T., Wykes, T., & Hayward, P. (2006). Group treatment of perceived stigma and self-esteem in schizophrenia: A waiting list trial of efficacy. *Behavioural and Cognitive Psychotherapy, 34*(3), 305–318.

Komiti, A., Judd, F., & Jackson, H. (2006). The influence of stigma and attitudes on seeking help from a GP for mental health problems: A rural context. *Social Psychiatry and Psychiatric Epidemiology, 41*(9), 738–745.

Krueger, J. (1996). Personal beliefs and cultural stereotypes about racial characteristics. *Journal of Personality & Social Psychology, 71,* 536–548.

Lee, R. S., Kochman, A., & Sikkema, K. J. (2002). Internalized stigma among people living with HIV-AIDS. *AIDS and Behavior, 4*(6), 309–319.

Link, B. G. (1982). Mental patient status, work and income: An examination of the effects of a psychiatric label. *American Sociological Review, 47*, 202–215.

Link, B. G. (1987). Understanding labeling effects in the area of mental disorders: An assessment of the effects of expectations of rejection. *American Sociological Review, 52*(1), 96–112.

Link, B. G., Cullen, F. T., Frank, J., & Wozniak, J. F. (1987). The social rejection of former mental patients: Understanding why labels matter. *American Journal of Sociology, 92*, 1461–1500.

Link, B. G., Cullen, F. T., Struening, E. L., Shrout, P. E., & Dohrenwend, B. P. (1989). A modified labeling theory approach to mental disorders: An empirical assessment. *American Sociological Review, 54*(3), 400–423.

Lucksted, A., Drapalski, A., Boyd, J., DeForge, B., Calmes, C., & Forbes, C. (2009). *Resisting internalized stigma: A nine session class for individuals receiving mental health services*. Baltimore, MD: VA VISN-5 MIRECC.

Luoma, J. B., Kohlenberg, B. S., Hayes, S. C., Bunting, K., & Rye, A. K. (2008). Reducing self-stigma in substance abuse through acceptance and commitment therapy: Model, manual development and pilot outcomes. *Addiction Research & Theory, 16*(2), 149–165.

Lysaker, P. H., Buck, K. D., Hammoud, K., Taylor, A. C., & Roe, D. (2006). Associations of symptoms, psychosocial function and hope with qualities of self-experience in schizophrenia: Comparisons of objective and subjective indicators of health. *Schizophrenia Research, 82*(2-3), 241–249.

Macinnes, D. L., & Lewis, M. (2008). Evaluation of a short group programme to reduce self stigma in people with serious and enduring mental health problems. *Journal of Psychiatric and Mental Health Nursing, 15*, 59–65.

Markowitz, F. E. (1998). The effects of stigma on the psychological well-being and life satisfaction of persons with mental illness. *Journal of Health & Social Behavior, 39*, 335–347.

Nelson, W. A., Pomerantz, A., & Schwartz, J. (2007). Putting "Rural" into psychiatry residency training programs. *Academic Psychiatry, 31*, 423–429.

Parr, H., & Philo, C. (2003). Rural mental health and social geographies of caring. *Social & Cultural Geography, 4*(4), 471–488.

Pullman, M. D., VanHooser, S., Hoffman, C., & Heflinger, C. A. (2010). Barriers to and supports of family participation in a rural system of care for children with serious emotional problems. *Community Mental Health Journal, 46*, 211–220.

Ritsher, J. B., & Phelan, J. C. (2004). Internalized stigma predicts erosion of morale among psychiatric outpatients. *Psychiatry Research, 129*(3), 257–265.

Shurka, E. (1983). The evaluation of ex-mental patients by other ex-mental patients. *International Journal of Social Psychology, 29*, 286–291.

Watson, A. C., Corrigan, P. W., Larson, J. E., & Sells, M. (2007). Self stigma in people with mental illness. *Schizophrenia Bulletin, 33*(6), 1312–1318.

Weiner, B. (1995). *Judgments of responsibility: A foundation for a theory of social conduct*. New York: Guilford Press.

Wright, E. R., Gronfein, W. P., & Owens, T. J. (2000). Deinstitutionalization, social rejection, and the self-esteem of former mental patients. *Journal of Health Social Behavior, 41*, 68–90.

5

Loneliness and Isolation in Rural Areas

JACKSON P. RAINER AND JOHNATHAN C. MARTIN

INTRODUCTION

*I*n any discussion on rural mental health, loneliness and the experience of emotional and social isolation must be figurally considered. By definition and connotation, rurality speaks about the contemporary problem of separateness. In the rural landscape, there are fewer people, spread out over wider spaces, with sparse social and cultural resources. The Population Reference Bureau (2010) reports that 79% of United States citizens reside in urban areas, with a yearly rate of change for urban settings of 1.3%. With the vast and fast-paced amounts of urbanization today, it is easy to forget about the modern social conveniences, for example, access to health care, entertainment, and commodities that are not afforded to the remaining 21% (or ~65 million) of residents who constitute the demographics of rural areas. Pertinent to this chapter is the provision of mental health and psychotherapy services, which remain a persistent problem affecting rural areas; there is a notable lack of trained mental health professionals offering counseling and therapy. As stated in other places in this book, the Health Resources and Services Administration (HRSA) has identified primary care, dental, and mental health provider shortage areas (HPSAs), that is, areas where the number of providers is insufficient to meet the needs of the residents. More than one-third of rural residents live in federally designated HPSAs (Rabinowitz, Diamond, Markham, & Wortman, 2008) and more rural than urban counties are designated as mental health HPSAs (National Advisory Council on Rural Health and Human Services, 2008). These health professional shortages contribute to rural Americans' lack of access to care and later entrance into care when symptoms are more advanced and pronounced, requiring more intensive and expensive forms of treatment. This chapter addresses one specific complaint common to rural residents needing mental health care—that of loneliness and isolation—and the process of psychotherapy for such individuals who present with this concern as a primary treatment issue.

LONELINESS AS A PSYCHOTHERAPY ISSUE

People have a basic predisposition to search for human connection and roots. When an individual feels alienated, anxious, or cut off from society, the pain of loneliness ensues. Loneliness is a terrible experience and contributes to a range of psychological difficulties. "Isolation" is a negative correlate of loneliness and is defined as the lack of affiliative behavior (Suedfeld, 1974). In the absence of meaningful societal connection, it is not uncommon for an individual to experience varied emotions, such as depression or anxiety. Rollo May (2009) suggested that this results as a manifestation of, or as an antecedent to, feelings of alienation or being "on the outside."

The feeling of belonging is a multidimensional social construct of relatedness to persons, places, or things, and is fundamental to personality and social well-being (Hill, 2006). The antithesis of the feeling of belonging is the sense of loneliness characterized by social isolation. Social isolation is defined by loss of place within one's group. This isolation may be voluntary or involuntary, and is characterized by the distancing of an individual, psychologically or environmentally, from the preferred network of needed relationships with others. It is typically accompanied by feelings related to loss or marginality. As an example of the impact of isolation upon mental well-being in rural areas, a rural client of the authors described her symptoms as she presented for treatment, saying, "I am now living on the edge of the world. I moved here to be closer to my adult children, but didn't account for how much I always relied on the resources of my home community to feel vital and alive. If it is possible to grieve the loss of a place, then that's where I am. I miss the resources of the city. I'm no longer in the mainstream, not even in this little town. While it's very pretty and seems nice enough, I just can't find my place."

In its broadest sense, loneliness involves a sense of deprivation in social relationships (Murphy & Kupshik, 1992). Peplau and Perlman (1986) suggest that loneliness occurs when an individual perceives social relationships as not containing the desired quality or quantity of social contacts. In this context, relational feedback is considered a foundation that provides the feeling of normalcy. Feedback gives the individual an opportunity to learn and adapt. Individuals cycle through feedback loops as learning occurs, contrasting their personal experience with those they observe in others. This process includes adopting standards and norms used to judge typical experiences in relation to those of others. So, loneliness may be considered as a feedback gap. For lonely individuals, there is insufficient interaction with the environment to confirm or disconfirm how the world works and is working for that person; this becomes even more pronounced in rural areas where such inter-actions are even more sparse and difficult to come by even for those not experi-encing psychological distress.

Loneliness has been referred to as an alienation of the self and is some-times seen as global, generalized, disagreeable, uncomfortable, and more terri-ble than anxiety (Austin, 1989). Loneliness differs from depression. The lonely individual attempts to integrate back into new relationships; the depressed individual surrenders to distress.

As an affective state, loneliness exists on a continuum rather than a dichotomy. The consideration of loneliness is better thought of in terms of qualitative differences. Circumstances and environment generally contribute great influence on defining various individual needs, and given the purpose of this chapter, it is appropriate to frame loneliness in a therapeutic fashion. To do so, it may be pragmatic to consider the continuum of loneliness in what Gestalt theorists would call a figure-ground model, noting the degree of the lonely individual's "unmet needs" for social contact. In this model, needs for social connection become more figural for and more readily perceived by the individual, due in large part to the individual's awareness of relational needs. Not uncommonly, such awareness emerges from an experience of pain or discomfort rather than via cognition.

WHEN LONELINESS BECOMES A PROBLEM

Apartness, or aloneness, is often described as a desirable state known as soli-tude. Solitude is accompanied by positive feelings and is most often voluntarily initiated by an individual. If privacy or being alone is actively chosen, enhancing the individual psyche is likely to ensue. Loneliness, on the other hand, is isolat-ing, and is negatively viewed because of the pain occurring in the lack of social connection. Pain is an experience that is generally avoided by the majority of people in our society. However, there is a great degree of utility found in this experience. Though it is avoided, pain serves as a warning signal that waves a red flag in the forefront of the individual's thoughts as a means of signifying need for change. Like nutritional requisites, people become more aware of the need to ingest some form of sustenance as hunger pangs gradually become more pronounced. In order to lessen the discomfort, food is ingested, and the ache of hunger gives way. As people become aware of the need to eat, the amount of pain symbolizes the extent of the hunger sensation.

The same is true with loneliness. As a way of understanding the severity of loneliness, cognitive theorists provide a lens that conceptualizes its scope. Beck and Young (1978) distinguish between three types of loneliness: chronic loneliness, which evolves from social deficits continuing over a period of years; situational loneliness, which usually results at the termination of a relationship; and transient loneliness, which refers to the short bouts of loneliness that most people experience periodically as a result of brief periods of social deficiency. Transient loneliness is so commonplace that it is simply accepted as a part of everyday life.

Social deficiency, as a concept, is as elusive a term as the word "normal." Complex social norms are pervasive, situationally and ecologically bound, and culturally driven. "Normal" connotes conformity. However, behavior that may conform in one situation may be deviant in another. Therefore, simple departure from what is socially appropriate is a poor defining characteristic of loneliness. A stigma exists for the individual lacking in an adequate number and type of social relationships. Not all solitary individuals, however, define themselves as lonely. Simply stated, being alone is not a precursor of feeling lonely. There are psychological encounters, presenting themselves as developmental transitions and detours away from, or outside of, the desired destination of personal fulfillment. The more accurate concept of loneliness comes from self-defining characteristics that the individual interprets as difference from the norm, consequently resulting in pain and isolation. This type of attribution error carries a sense of inadequacy, dependence, and impotence.

The client who described living "on the edge of the world" continued to speak. "I'm getting older, and that's OK. But I felt like I needed to be closer to those who could care for me when I needed more hands-on aid and assistance. My family welcomed me, and I am far from being handicapped or infirm yet. I've joined groups here in this new rural community—it is about a thousand miles from nowhere—but find that the people of my age and state of life already have established routines and groups. They are nice enough, but seem to be much more self-sufficient than I am. I wonder how it is that I could get along on my own all of my adult life when I lived in the suburb of a medium sized city, but feel completely inept here in this lovely little mountain town."

Attribution theory hinges on the belief that an individual has personal mastery over the environment. The sense of being-in-charge is essential to effective daily functioning. Known as self-efficacy, this belief encourages people to be more willing to attempt new solutions and to do so with greater persistence to continuing problems. Self-efficacy is adaptive, and attribution theory suggests that people's search for a sense of mastery is a lifelong quest.

The implication for loneliness in attribution theory is found in the feeling that an individual lacks sufficient mastery to provide for personal and social needs. This elicits cognitive dissonance and is alarming, since most people have a strong desire to feel in charge of their day-to-day experience. However, individuals tend to live the way they believe others want them to; feeling lonely is not consistent with this cognition of self-control. To reconcile this state of being, individuals must look either to the environment for a solution ("There are no people here for me to be related") or to admit to themselves the lack of personal efficacy ("I don't know how to be related"), which can damage self-esteem and cause distress and disability.

As noted, the pain of loneliness often arises from this fundamental attribution error. In social situations, individuals tend to create skewed perceptions about others' behavior, based on an overestimation of the other's disposition and an underestimation of situational causes. For individuals who describe loneliness in terms of isolation, it seems that cognitive distortions of personal behavior may aggravate psychic pain and lead to polarization on the attribution continuum. This type of response is basic to social learning theory (Bandura, 1977), which describes the importance of opportunities to observe others. Such observation provides a demonstrative model for appropriate behaviors, emotional reactions, and attitudes. The theory brings new meaning to the old adage "When in Rome, do as the Romans do." With limited social contact, the lonely individual has a heightened tendency to lose sight of self, abilities, and worth.

Early in therapy, the aforementioned client told this story. "I expected that since I play bridge, I would be able to find company and friends quickly. That just hasn't been the case, much to my dismay. The senior center here has an organized group that plays blackjack with eight decks of cards. The people who play it, love it. I hate it. I tried to learn it, but find the rules frustrating and the game much too aggressive for my taste. But it seems to be this or not playing cards anymore. Generally speaking, people in this town seem to think that I'm a snob because I want to play bridge, rather than this funny game. I've started to feel crazy because of a hobby that I enjoy."

Because of this definition, it is unwise to dichotomize loneliness. There are multiple contributors and events in the environment, with gradients and hues of connectivity that influence individual experience. Rather than categorizing an experience as lonely/not lonely, there is greater wisdom in examining the degree of loneliness along a continuum; the basis of the individual's position on the continuum is based on the degree of social deficit experienced. Additionally, the individual is influenced by fears of having broken social norms, and that in the experience of loneliness, will be experienced as odd or unusual. Such influence amplifies the affective experience and cognitive dissonance. If the individual cannot attribute the feeling of loneliness to factors other than the self, an energetic push into deeper feelings of loneliness escalates, and the feedback loop becomes regrettably self-sustaining.

The client continued. "I decided if I couldn't do social activities, like bridge, then I'd just get a job. So now, I'm teaching English as a second language. It is rewarding, but I've started hesitating telling people what I do. There is such a political backlash about immigrants. More than once, I've felt liked I've been 'lumped in' to a political stand that really isn't accurate at all. I take the class on public field trips to practice the language and find as many people rude as welcoming. I don't find that this community has much room for difference, and this makes me feel bad about myself and my work."

How is it that social deficiency manifests into an amplified state of loneliness? Further appreciation of the fundamental attribution error can be seen from the perspective of the locus of control of the individual. The rudiments of this theory coincide insomuch that one's perception of the degree of mastery over the environment colors the sense of efficacy. As in any crisis situation, a picture of one's descent into loneliness—whether chronic, situational, or transient—can be captured by understanding the individual's sense of control over the environment. The greater the individual's self-efficacy, the greater that individual's proficiency and capacity becomes for coping with stressors. As the individual begins to feel overwhelmed by external factors, self-efficacy is diminished, generating more feelings of emotional stress. Emotional stress triggers the warning signal of pain. Psychic stress, like physical pain, can be utilized as a tool for motivation, prodding the individual to dismiss maladaptive behavior and seek healthier, more meaningful behavior. This occurs, though, only with the proper amount of stress.

The Yerkes–Dodson Law indicates that as stress increases, so does performance (Yerkes & Dodson, 1908). However, this is the case only to a certain point. With a surplus of stress, a parabolic feature of behavior occurs, where performance or the motivation to perform (i.e., cope with stressors) begins to wane. Stressors held in isolation become physically and emotionally exhausting over time, creating a psychic emptiness within the individual. In isolation, although facing challenges of daily living was once manageable, the adaptation of healthy cognition and behavior needed to deal with stress effectively becomes increasingly unreliable because of the lack of an intrinsic sense of efficacy. Tried-and-true coping strategies become ineffective and futile, and this intrinsic state of exhaustion has the potential to lead to what can be thought of as *psychological drift*.

The Yerkes–Dodson Law lends itself to this notion of drift. For the lonely individual, resources of connection and meaning are perceived on a psychological continuum ranging from sparse to nonexistent. This may be amplified in a rural environment. As the faulty belief begins to settle within the individual, it takes root as an unmet need and the motivation to seek resources for satisfaction dwindles. Fewer resources and connections are sought and what may have begun as a transient or situational type of loneliness can manifest in chronic distress. From this perspective, it becomes clearer how the individual's psyche (i.e., the individual's worldview and degree of motivation) causes a drift into social deficiency, escalated loneliness, and isolation. Without proper treatment, hazards and adverse implications for loneliness become defined by this maladaptive behavior and these distorted cognitions.

It should be noted that over the past few decades, *social drift* theorists have proposed various explanations for behavioral, physical, mental, and economic health. Since their inception, notions of social drift have focused primarily on criminal behavior (Matza, 1964) and the influence of social class on severe forms of mental illness, such as schizophrenic disorders (Fox, 1990; Goldberg & Morrison, 1963). With respect to mental illness, Goldberg and Morrison (1963) debated that a downward shift in social class (e.g., one's vocation) was considered as a causal factor in the onset of severe mental illness. Opposing this view, Fox (1990) purported that a downward shift in social class was a latent effect of mental illness, with a decline in vocational and economic status following onset. The notion of psychological drift in the presence of loneliness pays homage to these theories of social drift, but is distinctly different. It is of utmost importance to recognize this theory of psychological drift as contending that social class is not a necessary element with respect to mental health issues. However, it is noteworthy to consider that the lack of social resources, commonly found in rural areas, may contribute to this notion of drift.

In the rural community, the environment itself can be a stressor and the initiating aggravator of loneliness, despite one's social class. Like a widower or last surviving member of a family, there is a nomothetic undercurrent that carries many residents of rural areas into existential and behavioral challenges. At another point in the loneliness continuum, for example, the same can be said for community leaders who disclose, "It's lonely at the top," after reaching a high-status position. Therefore, it can be seen that social class is not a necessary element of loneliness and isolation, as individuals ranging from lower to upper social class status can find themselves without social connection. For rural residents, this lack of connection is significantly enhanced, in part, due to geography. Because of the lack of physical proximity, social isolation is more prevalent, and the energy and motivation to seek social connection begin to define psychological drift. The fundamental work of Festinger, Schachter, and Back (1950) supports this notion. The Effect of Propinquity is concerned with the effects of proximity on social encounters and on the establishment of relationships. It has been demonstrated that the closer individuals reside or work with each other (in terms of geographic proximity), the greater the likelihood for the formation of relationships. The effect works inversely, as well. It can easily be recognized in persons who live great distances from neighbors and community resources. With more physical space in between, the greater the tendency for less social interaction. Less social interaction holds the potential for increasing social deficit, intrinsic emptiness, and subsequently, deeper psychological drift.

How is social deficit measured? Again, a viable clinical answer is found in foundational literature. The JoHari Window (see Table 5.1), developed in the mid-20th century by cognitive psychologists Luft and Ingham (1955), is a

TABLE 5.1

JoHari Window

	Known By Individual	Unknown By Individual
Known By Others	*"Public"*	*"Blindspot"*
Unknown By Others	*"Private"*	*"Unknown"*

model that provides a framework conceptualizing an individual's personal and social awareness, which serves as a guide to encourage increased communication. The model (shown p. 73) consists of four quadrants representing the Self: (1) information known by the individual and others, (2) information unknown to the individual, but known to others, (3) information known by the individual but not known to others, and (4) information unknown by both the individual and others. The quadrants shift in size as new information is gathered and shared. The dynamic structure of the model creates a self-sustaining feedback loop. For an individual feeling lonely and experiencing the pain of isolation, the need for interaction and feedback from others becomes figural. With a growing social deficit, the "unknown" quadrant (representing the individual's untapped characteristics, i.e., secrets and possibilities) increases, thereby increasing the risk of isolation.

ISOLATION AND THE PAIN OF YEARNING

What does it mean to be lonely in a social world? How does loneliness muster in a rural environment to the point that it becomes symptomatic of distress for an individual? Loneliness becomes an issue of serious concern when it settles long enough to create a persistent, self-reinforcing loop of negative thoughts, sensations, and behaviors. It is the antithesis of being satisfied and secure in personal bonds with others and in social connection. Roots of the human impulse for social connection run at great depth, and the pain of loneliness is a deeply disruptive, aching hurt. Both psychological and physiological, the disruption can turn an unmet need for connection into a chronic condition. As a general rule, people care about how others think of them, and feeling isolated can undermine the ability to think clearly. Feedback gives the individual an opportunity to learn and adapt, which is at the core of intelligence and critical thinking.

According to researchers Cacioppo and Patrick (2008), the powerful effects of loneliness stem from the interplay of three complex factors. The first is identified as the level of vulnerability to social disconnection. The researchers postulate that each individual has a genetic inheritance for a certain level of need for social inclusion, expressed as sensitivity to the pain of social exclusion. Each individual's propensity operates like a thermostat, turning on or off distress signals whether or not the individual need for connection is being met. The second effect is defined by the ability to self-regulate the emotions associated with feeling isolated. Successful self-regulation means being able to cope with challenges while remaining on an even keel. As loneliness increases and persists, a disruption of ability occurs that leaves the individual more vulnerable to stressors and less efficient in carrying out soothing and healing functions, such as sleep. Finally, the long-term effects of loneliness disturb mental representations, expectations, and reasoning about others.

When loneliness takes hold, social cognitions, including the ways self and others are seen, are heavily influenced by feelings of unhappiness, threat, and the impaired ability to self-regulate.

The energy of longing, also known as yearning, drives an individual from one place to another, from one desire to a different one and then another one, in search of fulfillment to satisfy and finally silence the inner voice that never seems satisfied with anything. Lonely individuals who feel isolated report, as one client said, ". . . however hard I try, I still have this sense that something is missing."

The Greek word for longing is *thumos*, meaning the presence of life itself. It is the raw presence in the psyche that senses and feels, and in its original translation, is defined as the massed power of individual emotional being. Not only is it the energy of longing, but also the energy of passion and appetite. The energy is viewed without cognition. Therefore, when left to itself, the energy moves without reason. Feeling dislocated by geography or circumstance heightens the tendency for this energy of longing to be experienced as pain rather than power. In pain, the individual is unable to see the self clearly, nor to attribute favorable meaning to experience. The experience of being outside, that is, lonely, becomes embittering and rejecting. Because of its self-regulating tendency, the pain of isolation is found in the self as distancing from the experience of loneliness. As another client reported, "The strange thing is that the negativity isn't the depression itself but in running from the depression. What I imagine that I'm afraid of isn't what I'm really afraid of at all. I get afraid of the feeling of longing for something because I make no allowances for what I think or what I care for. The longing wants all of me and consumes me. I lose my sense of safety and start to look outside of myself. But then, there is nothing there because I am in such a remote place with myself."

THE TREATMENT OF LONELINESS AND ISOLATION

Contemporary life expects that happiness and joy are found primarily in relationship to others. Certainly love and friendship are important components of what makes life worthwhile. However, they are not the only source of happiness and satisfaction. Humans come into this world alone and will leave it in a similar way. Between the entrance and the exit, most people spend a great deal of time searching for companionship. Such essential loneliness can be reframed, allowing the individual to embrace, rather than escape, the experience. Rather than recognizing loneliness as an isolating incompleteness, that something is lacking, it can be integrated with the sense of aloneness as an affirmation of unique individuality.

A middle-aged male client came requesting psychotherapy using the exquisite metaphor, "I'm surrounded by water and dying of thirst." He described working in an environment that 'feels mechanical.' My work encroaches

on my whole sense of who I am. I work with others, but feel like I am completely by myself. I don't ever get feedback. Meaningful communication has
become an impossible task. I've worked hard for this arrangement, and am
really disappointed that I feel like my environment is cruel. I am productive
and should take pride in my achievements. Instead, I am craving to be attached
to something real. I've degenerated into a profound depression, and it is affecting everything in my life."

The man realized that his loneliness was isolating, even in the presence of
others. This jumbled heap of affect and attribution left him feeling dissatisfied
with his productivity and flattened by his inability to connect to what he considered authentic. Because of his brilliant verbal skills, his ability to introspect,
and his precipitating complaints, a course of interpersonal humanistic psychotherapy was initiated. The client reported a good deal of inner turmoil,
which was exacerbated by multiple technological interruptions, for example,
telephone, email, text messages. Focus was initially on helping the client find
a sense of peace in his aloneness so that his experience might be reframed
as solitude. He was guided to structure the tethers of his day so that he became
more in charge of intrusions. As he felt more of a sense of mastery over his time,
he was able to attend to the self-talk contributing to his unhappiness.

Such introspection led the client into a general sense of anxiety characterized by feelings of fragmentation. He said, "The disorganization I felt on the
outside is a mirror of what I have been feeling on the inside. It is really hard
for me to be quiet and with myself, since I feel like I could disintegrate if I get
still. I feel like I've been drifting toward nothingness for a long time." The
client was able to form a strong and malleable relationship with his therapist.
Through reframing, the client came in contact with his aloneness as imaginative,
rather than fragmenting. He progressively came to see his solitary time as a
means of maintaining contact with his inner world of imagination. Even with
his sense that his ability to engage in intimate relationships was damaged, the
development of a creative imagination exercised a healing function. As he felt
a sense of order in his intrapersonal life, he was able to seek interpersonal
relationships, reflecting a self-described sense of maturity and harmony.

As in all effective psychotherapy interventions, choice and autonomy
reside within the client. While there may be best practices related to
symptom resolution and readiness for change, much of the work related to
the psychotherapy of loneliness and isolation lives in the subjective realm of
individual experience. Therefore, treatment goals and trajectories will vary.
Certain useful techniques and strategies can be generalized.

Psychotherapy for loneliness should assess for the distinction between
solitude and isolation. The clinician can observe for three distinct features:
(1) negativity, (2) involuntary, or self-imposed disconnections from contact,
and (3) declining quality and numbers within the individual's social network
(Larson & Lubkin, 2009). Isolated loneliness should be distinguished from
depression, though both are often accompanied by anxiety, desperation,

self-pity, and boredom. It is not unusual that an isolated individual will attempt to mollify the pain of loneliness through self-destructive behavioral means, such as substance use and abuse. The individual should be evaluated in context of culture, heritage, and personal history. Readiness for change should also be assessed in terms of treatment goals initially revolving around relief.

Treatment proceeds in an integrative framework that combines primary cognitive and existential approaches. The client can be instructed on the nature of loneliness and its correlates. The client examines existing social ties and networks and determines how effectively and ineffectively they work in service to the individual. Teaching the concepts of solitude versus isolation—both as components of loneliness—aids in reframing the experience of the individual. Cognitive interventions target symptoms to change awareness, perceptions, and behaviors. Additionally, reward structures, secondary gain, and a heightened understanding of social networks and resources may help define the problem and potential solutions.

Psychologist Jeffrey Young (1986) describes a paradigm for treating chronically lonely adults using a cognitive-behavioral approach. In working with clients, the primary focus revolves around the lonely person's desires to build better social relationships. He describes moving through six stages of personal growth, moving from less complicated to more complicated tasks. The goals of the stages are as follows:

1. To overcome anxiety and sadness about spending time alone
2. To engage in activities with a few casual friends
3. To engage in mutual self-disclosure with a trustworthy individual
4. To meet a potentially intimate, appropriate partner
5. To begin to develop intimacy with an appropriate partner, usually through disclosure and sexual contact
6. To make an emotional commitment to an appropriate partner for a relatively long period of time

Psychologist Rae Andre (1992) translated Young's behavioral hierarchy into a rubric that reframes isolation into positive solitude. Andre suggested six similar stages:

1. To feel physically safe when alone, both at home and outside the home
2. To overcome anxiety and sadness about spending time alone
3. To learn to feel comforted and not anxious when one is both tired (and sick) of being alone
4. To understand the principle of the feedback gap and to find interesting, personally enriching things to do every day when alone
5. To build solace, tradition, and other long-term enrichments into day-to-day living
6. To demonstrate to the self that life, lived alone, has meaning

Existentially, psychotherapy helps the individual to find intrapersonal meaning in a life alone. Questions are raised such as, "By whose standards are we to decide what a fulfilling life is?" and "What is enough contact for satisfaction and satiation?" Only the person responsible for running his or her life can judge the nature of fulfillment. Ultimately, each individual must develop beliefs and goals that make sense of "who I am" in aloneness. No one else can allay personal doubts about meaningfulness or meaninglessness of life. Answers are found in the development of a personal philosophy for being alone. Exploring basic beliefs and goals is essential to the successful experience of aloneness, and holding a personal rubric for being alone is the ultimate antidote to loneliness. Formulating and addressing such beliefs and goals is important to well-being since the belief system is the basis from which all other approaches to loneliness are derived. Without a coherent philosophy, the individual is vulnerable to pain, which leads to isolation. As a counterbalance, the lonely individual can learn to articulate the "whys" of being alone, what is positive about the experience, and what is negative about it. New understandings strengthen change.

During exploration, three themes will emerge. The first theme is related to the search for meaning. Clients will ask themselves questions such as, "What is really meaningful to me?" and "What is important to my life?" A second theme emerges in terms of relationship with others. Questions are formed, such as, "Now that I understand and can live with solitude, what is to be my relationship with other people? What does love mean to my life? What is the role of responsibility? What do others contribute to me, and what do I give to them?" Finally, the third theme revolves around the potential for self-fulfillment. Questions emerge such as, "In a life lived alone, how can I become more creative and self-actualized? What new avenues are open to me?" (Andre, 1992)

In existential psychotherapy, the client may be taught solace. In cognitive-behavioral terms, this practice is facilitated as self-soothing strategies. Experientially, solace is the emotional experience of a soothing presence. It is what gives an individual composure in the presence of adversity or turbulence, and is a reminder to be contented when alone. It may be speculated that one of the reasons that people say they are lonely is because of the absence of solace. Without a capacity to self-soothe when in distress, an individual can move quickly into states of desperation and despair. Ego psychology refers to the experience of solace as transitional relatedness. Internal contentment is seen as an unconscious process that is evoked by internal, symbolic objects derived from early secure attachments. Memories of these soothing relationships are then symbolized by things in the environment.

Using cognitive and existential approaches facilitates the overarching goal of helping the client to stay interested in life. Since all people face periods of aloneness and connectedness, both conditions must be acknowledged and energized. Isolated loneliness is disruptive, while the aloneness of solitude is creative. The two may become confused. A client reported, "The only isolation I have known in my lifetime I felt in the presence of others." A therapeutic task, therefore, is to help the client to sort affective experiences into what one client called "pockets." As she became able to distinguish differences between isolation and solitude, she said, "I live by myself a good deal of the time. I work by myself and live in the country without close contact of others. I've learned lessons of solitude, though. When I am lonely, I think my way through it. Loneliness does not have to destroy me. It's my attitude toward it, what I bring to it, that matters. That attitude can't be fear. I choose much of my aloneness. So, when I begin to feel disconnected and isolated, I consider questions of morality and responsibility. I meditate, ask big questions, and get busy with myself. This helps me move from that ache into a sense of peace. I have found that what grows in solitude then goes back into community, and I can reconnect with others as I need."

CONCLUSION

The need to purposefully connect and reconnect is an experience far too familiar for residents of rural areas. Urban development continues to gain the bulk of attention in terms of policy and focus on health; the rapid movement for advancements and services in urban areas can quickly and literally leave rural populations "in the dust." Rural residents drift further and further away from needed services as this societal gap grows between urban and rural settings. Distance between services bears considerable weight on the issue of personal loneliness and isolation. Addressing loneliness holds the implication of diversity for rural populations in general, equal to the implications it carries as a mental health treatment issue. Recognition of these implications is warranted as is the need to monitor and increase integrated societal feedback loops for rural individuals and groups. This recognition will resonate and provide significant steps toward conceptualization and treatment of residents in need of reassurance as well as a resource that supports a lifestyle of solitude.

REFERENCES

Andre, R. (1992). *Positive solitude*. New York: Harper Perennial.

Austin, D. (1989). Becoming immune to loneliness: Helping the elderly fill the void. *Journal of Gerontological Nursing, 15*(9), 25–28.

Bandura, A. (1977). *Social learning theory*. New York: General Learning Press.

Beck, A. T., & Young, J. E. (1978, September). College blues. *Psychology Today,* 83–92.

Cacioppo, J. T., & Patrick, W. (2008). *Loneliness: Human nature and the need for social connection*. New York, NY: W. W. Norton & Company.

Festinger, L., Schachter, S., & Back, K. (1950). The spatial ecology of group formation. In L. Festinger, S. Schachter, & K. Back (Eds.), *Social pressure in informal groups* (pp. 141–161). Palo Alto, CA: Stanford University Press.

Fox, J. W. (1990). Social class, mental illness, and social mobility: The social-selection drift hypothesis for serious mental illness. *Journal of Health and Social Behavior, 31*(4), 344-353.

Goldberg, E. M., & Morrison, S. L. (1963). Schizophrenia and social class. *The British Journal of Psychiatry, 109,* 785-802.

Hill, D. L. (2006). Sense of belonging as connectedness, American Indian worldview and mental health. *Archives of Psychiatric Nursing, 20*(5), 210-216.

Larson, P. D., & Lubkin, I. M. (2009). *Chronic illness: Impact and intervention* (7th ed.). Boston, MA: Jones and Bartlett.

Luft, J., & Ingham, H. (1955). *The JoHari Window: A graphic model for interpersonal relations.* Los Angeles, CA: University of California Western Training Lab.

Matza, D. (1964). *Delinquency and drift.* New York: John Wiley and Sons, Inc.

May, R. (2009). *Man's search for himself.* New York: W. W. Norton & Company, Inc.

Murphy, P. M., & Kupshik, S. (1992). *Loneliness, stress, and well-being.* New York: Routledge.

National Advisory Council on Rural Health and Human Services (2008). *Report to the Department of Health and Human Services Secretary.* Retrieved from Health Resources and Services Administration website: http://www.hrsa.gov/advisory committees/rural/2008secreport.pdf

Peplau, L. A., & Perlman, D. (Eds.). (1986). *Loneliness: A sourcebook of current theory, research, and therapy.* New York: John Wiley and Sons.

Population Reference Bureau. (2010). *Demographic Highlights.* Retrieved from http://www.prb.org/Datafinder/Geography/Summary.aspx?region=72&region_type=2

Rabinowitz, H. K., Diamond, J. J., Markham, F. W., & Wortman, J. R. (2008). Medical school programs to increase the rural physician supply: A systematic review and projected impact of widespread replication. *Academic Medicine, 83,* 235-243.

Suedfeld, P. (1974). Social isolation: A case for interdisciplinary research. *Canadian Psychologist, 15*(1), 1-15.

Yerkes, R. M., & Dodson, J. D. (1908). The relation of strength of stimulus to rapidity of habit-formation. *Journal of Comparative Neurology and Psychology, 18,* 459-482.

Young, J. (1986). Loneliness, depression, and cognitive therapy: Theory and application. In L. A. Peplau, & D. Perlman (Eds.), *Loneliness: A sourcebook of current theory, research, and therapy* (pp. 379-405). New York: John Wiley and Sons.

6

Religion and Rural Mental Health

JAMIE ATEN, PATRICK HALL, ISAAC WEAVER, MICHAEL MANGIS,
AND CLARK CAMPBELL

INTRODUCTION

*T*he purpose of this chapter is to introduce readers to the role of religion in rural areas and the influence of religion on mental health in rural communities. This chapter draws from the rural mental health literature, as well as from our psychotherapy, consultation, teaching, and research experience in rural areas. Moreover, most of us grew up in rural communities, so this chapter reflects our own personal experiences—including Western Frontier, Appalachian mountain, Midwest farming, and Deep South rural communities. First, we begin the chapter by defining religion and spirituality, as well as contextualizing religion in the psychological sciences. Second, we provide an overview of the role and influence of religion in rural communities. Third, we provide a series of applied recommendations for working with rural religious clients.

RELIGION

Currently in the psychological literature, over 200 different terms on the definition of religion have been offered (Zinnbauer & Pargament, 2005). The proliferation of definitions is likely a testament to the complexity and nuances of religion. Over 1,200 different religions currently are being practiced worldwide (Aten & Leach, 2009). Moreover, a great deal of diversity can be found in how people think about and practice each of these religions. Historically, within the field of professional psychology, religion was the primary term for describing devotion to and practice of a particular worldview. However, in recent years, the term spirituality appears to be more commonly embraced by mental health professionals. In most cases, the terms religion and spirituality are often used interchangeably. Yet, more researchers have begun to note that there is an overlap between religion and spirituality, as well as distinctions that warrant attention.

Spirituality is often conceptualized as a broad concept, encompassing one's thoughts, feelings, and behaviors in relation to the transcendent (Hill et al., 2000). Further, spirituality has been described as feeling connected to the sacred, or as the personal expression of faith. On the other hand, religion is more commonly defined as the corporate expression of faith, such as worshiping in a community of believers. Religion is also commonly associated with an adherence to a specific core set of beliefs, doctrines, or orthodoxy, as prescribed by a particular worldview.

Despite some who have argued that religion and spirituality are distinct constructs, several researchers have cautioned against superficial separation between religion and spirituality. For example, several studies have shown that people often define themselves as both religious and spiritual or as spiritual and religious (Aten & Leach, 2009). Worthington and Aten (2009) have offered a conceptualization that may help add greater clarity to understanding the complex relationship between religion and spirituality. According to Worthington and Aten (2009), spirituality can be categorized into four types, with each type being defined by the object the individual views as sacred: (a) religious spirituality, (b) humanistic spirituality, (c) nature spirituality, and (d) cosmos spirituality. Spirituality, then, can include both religious and nonreligious aspirations. The concept of religion, however, has a narrower semantic range than spirituality, as it refers to a specific system of beliefs and behaviors that are sanctioned by a community and/or tradition (Hill et al., 2000). The distinction between religion and spirituality is important because in rural communities, people are more likely to describe themselves as religious rather than spiritual.

IMPACT OF RELIGION ON WELL-BEING

A recent Gallup poll of over 500,000 Americans found that, even after controlling for demographic factors, "very religious" individuals reported higher levels of well-being than moderately religious or nonreligious individuals (Gallup Organization, 2010). Moreover, Moreira-Almeida, Neto, and Koenig (2006) conducted a literature review of over 850 studies on the religion–mental health relationship and reported that the majority of well-conducted studies found a positive correlation between high levels of religious involvement and indicators of psychological well-being. Those who were more involved in religious practices and behaviors enjoyed higher levels of happiness, morale, positive affect, and general life satisfaction. Their review also concluded that high religiosity generally had an inverse relationship with depression, substance abuse, and suicidal ideation and behavior. In terms of overall health, it has been demonstrated that religiosity is positively correlated with better eating habits, exercise, and on average 7 years greater life expectancy than those who are nonspiritual. Religious involvement is also negatively correlated with tobacco use, alcohol consumption, and unprotected sexual activity (Gallup Organization, 2010; Plante, 2008).

In addition to the emotional and physical benefits of religiosity, the literature also suggests that religion serves as an effective coping behavior. Moreira-Almedia et al. (2006) found that the positive outcomes of religiosity were even more pronounced for people who were experiencing stressful circumstances. Other studies have reported that over 70% of Americans identify with some faith community and use their faith as a means to cope with life experiences, especially following disasters (Weaver, Flannelly, Garbarino, Figley, & Flannelly, 2003). Religion and spirituality are also thought to help establish meaning and provide purpose in life, fulfill human needs for relationships, and offer support during times of illness or suffering (Darling, Hill, & McWey, 2004; Guthrie & Stickley, 2008).

The data from the above studies of well-being are drawn from both rural and urban populations. Several studies of exclusively rural populations confirm similar trends. For example, a multistate investigation of rural low-income mothers found that both religious beliefs and faith involvement were inversely related to lower depressive symptoms (Garrison, Marks, Lawrence, & Braun, 2005). Another study of elderly individuals in rural areas of West Virginia and North Carolina also revealed a negative relationship between religiosity and depression (Dong Pil, 2006).

ROLE AND INFLUENCE OF RELIGION IN RURAL COMMUNITIES

Rural churches were usually the first foothold established by Europeans settling North America (Burkart, 1997). The influence of the church was so significant that they were often the primary catalyst for building and establishing communities among immigrant groups (Swierenga, 1997). Until the late 19th and early 20th centuries most Americans either lived in or held family roots in rural communities. Religion, therefore, is still deeply embedded in the cultural landscape of most rural communities. Throughout the rural South, for example, roads are commonly named according to churches (e.g., Ephesus Church Road, Mount Zion Church Road, Mount Olive Church Road; Hatch & Lovelace, 1980). Rural people have traditionally been more likely than urban people to be connected to and regularly attend a church (Farley & Ruesink, 1997). They are more likely than urban dwellers to believe that religion can answer life's problems, are more likely to attend church, to read the Bible, and to hold socially and politically conservative beliefs and values (Glenna, 2003). For rural residents, religious institutions are more than a mere place of weekly worship;

for many communities, these churches are an integral aspect of the rural culture, providing important spiritual, educational, social, political, and economic resources (Aten, Mangis, & Cambell, 2010). Rural residents tend to integrate their religious lives into their already well-established civic lives. In urban communities, on the other hand, religion plays a different role. Urban dwellers tend to join religious organizations "in an attempt to create a sense of community in an environment largely void of real community" (Burkart, 1997, p. 608).

Popular beliefs that are more mythical than factual cloud cultural understandings of how religion operates in a rural setting. Two pervasive myths regarding rural life that are pertinent to the discussion on religion are: (1) the Myth of utopia, and (2) the Myth of primitivism. The myth of a utopian countryside is often portrayed in media depictions of the rural life as a pristine respite from the busy-ness of city-life. This myth plays upon our need for nostalgia. The second myth is the myth of primitivism, the idea that healthy life is unsustainable in rural areas due to the character flaws and ignorance of its inhabitants. In many cases, rural faith communities are also often depicted in an oversimplified manner, sometimes even in a negative light, such as assuming they are overly conservative or fundamentalist. Neitz (2005) claims that the image of the simple country church on the decline is so prevalent in the media that it actually precludes an accurate portrayal of the current strengths and weaknesses of the rural church.

Nearly 95% of the U.S. population reports to believe in God (Gallup, 2002). At least 80% of individuals claim that religion plays a "fairly" or "very" important role in their lives (Gallup Organization, 2009). Among religious believers, the vast majority participate in a Judeo-Christian tradition. Although the number of individuals in non-Judeo-Christian faiths has increased three- to fourfold since 1970, these religions still comprise less than 3% of the American population (Smith, 2002). Moreover, in rural populations there tends to be an even higher prevalence of religiosity than in their urban counterparts (Aten et al., 2010; Chalfant & Heller, 1991). Overall, religion plays a major role in most rural areas across the United States and has a significant influence on everyday life.

More specifically, an investigation by Chalfant and Heller (1991) found significant differences between the religious behavior of urban and rural residents and between rural residents located in different regions of the country. Their study defined religiosity in terms of three dimensions:

1. Ritualistic—frequency of church attendance and prayer;
2. Experiential—perceived closeness to God; and
3. Ideological—tendency to view the Bible literally.

Using nationwide data gathered from the General Social Survey of the National Opinion Research Center, three of their four measures found that rural residents attend church more often, feel closer to God, and are more likely to view the Bible as the literal word of God. They did not find a significant differ-ence in frequency of prayer for rural–urban residence. Notably, their investi-gation found still stronger regional effects over rural–urban effects for each of these measures, including prayer frequency. In general, rural residents in the South and Midwest displayed higher levels of religiosity than their counter-parts residing in the East and West. This pattern was particularly strong for church attendance, a little less so for prayer, and even less for feeling of close-ness to God.

A recent Gallup poll (Gallup Organization, 2009) interviewing over 350,000 participants reported similar regional patterns in religiosity. By a significant margin, rural Southerners were the most likely to view the Bible as the literal word of God, followed closely by Midwesterners, and, to a lesser degree, residents in the East and West Regions. Another study found similar results among African American populations. After surveying 400 African American individuals in the southeastern United States, results indi-cated that African Americans in rural areas tended to feel and express their faith more than their urban counterparts (Holt, Schulz, & Wynn, 2009). These regional findings may, in part, account for the historically stronger Pro-testant presence in the South and Midwest in comparison with the Northeast where Catholicism has been more dominant and in the West where a dominant traditional group has not been established (Chalfant & Heller, 1991). Taken together, these results underscore the importance of understanding the reli-gious cultural variability that exists in both rural–urban and regional contexts. When conceptualizing the religious life of clients in rural communities, it may be helpful to recognize that there are significant differences from urban popu-lations, and that often there is even greater variability among rural individuals who reside in different areas of the country.

THE ROLE OF THE CHURCH IN THE RURAL COMMUNITY

Participation in church life provides a sense of personal identity and security for many rural residents. Congregational involvement has been found to help individuals achieve greater social status and a sense of belonging within the community. These religious communities are typically "tight-knit" and those who are outside these social circles may be viewed with reticence or suspicion (Aten et al., 2010). Leaders in these faith communities are considered people of considerable respect and influence. Pastors and other church leaders are selected carefully and recruited in limited numbers (Woodberry & Smith, 1998). These authority figures are usually the first place people turn to for advice and guidance. For example, in times of crisis or extreme duress, churches are often the first place residents turn to for support (Aten, Topping, Denney, & Bayne, 2010). In addition to their influence within the church, clergy, church leaders, and elders are often embedded within the power structures of the greater community. As a result, religion often has strong influence on the overall social and political ethos of rural communities.

RURAL RELIGIOUS WORLDVIEWS

Although adherents to a wide ideological range of world religions can be found in rural areas of this country, the majority of rural residents are Christians who adhere to a traditional and conservative belief system. For example, Dillon and Savage (2006) found that rural Americans were more religious than those in metropolitan areas in relation to church attendance and being "born-again," a term more likely to be used by those in rural and small town areas. Likewise, much of rural community and church life is permeated with a traditional gender structure (Glenna, 2003). While the strength of their conservatism varies, what fundamentally ties these rural religious individuals together is that they place a high value on religious authority, evangelism, living by defined moral codes of behavior, and the authority of scripture (Aten et al., 2010).

An important practice of this belief system is to pray for and convert others who do not share one's faith (Woodberry & Smith 1998). While rural believers tend to be relatively private, most still feel strongly about sharing their faith with others. This form of proselytizing is primarily motivated by a concern for others' spiritual well-being and not as an aggressive or hostile act.

Among rural religious populations there is also a common expectation that people conform to the established behavioral and social practices of their respective communities. Most members in these communities understand that there are certain "do's and don'ts" to how one dresses, behaves, and interacts with others. Those who ascribe to different beliefs or whose lifestyle is incongruent with these norms may find social integration difficult.

Perhaps the strongest unifying characteristic of religious rural populations, especially predominately Christian rural populations, is their insistence for all of life to be understood in the light of scripture (Hood, Hill, & Williamson, 2005). Reading, interpreting, and applying the Bible is done from a more literal perspective. Researchers have found that rural believers most often look through the framework of scripture to find emotional comfort, discover proper ways of living and thinking, understand relationships, and seek guidance on life decisions. For example, children are often read scripture by family members from a very young age and later encouraged to learn and even memorize portions of scripture. For these rural religious populations, this belief structure serves to provide an identity, meaning, and a sense of purpose in life. Psychologically, it offers stability, certainty, and coherence, in an otherwise turbulent and unpredictable environment (Hood et al., 2005).

Despite the prevalence of this conservative *belief* system, there is a wide diversity of religious *expression* in rural areas. Within the rural context, in addition to mainline Christian denominations, Amish, Mennonite, Shaker, Pentecostal, serpent-handling sects, rural African American Christians, Native American communities, and Catholic Latinos are common representative religious groups (Campbell, Gordon, & Chandler, 2002). There has also been a recent upsurge in religious minority groups living in rural areas, such as an increase in rural Muslim residents. This upsurge mimics national immigration patterns.

To bring attention to examples of the rich and often misunderstood worldviews that clinicians may encounter in rural areas, we now briefly highlight three of these religiously diverse groups.

Amish Religious Worldview

An often caricatured rural fundamentalist group is the Amish, for whom biblical principles, tradition, and folklore—not the scientific method—comprise a guiding metanarrative (Cates & Graham, 2002). The Amish may be reticent to participate in mental health care for reasons including: (a) belief that bishops or ministers should serve as counselors; (b) aversion toward working with agnostic and atheistic counselors; and (c) emphasis upon the "untrained mind" or "humility" as a religious value. Each of these factors may lead the Amish to avoid exploring the complexity of psychological issues (Cates, 2005). When participating in therapy, the Amish may expect more self-disclosure on the part of the clinician than would a typical client. A therapist working with this population needs to be open to working with clients who have a highly fundamentalist religious worldview, recognizing that fundamentalist beliefs are often connected to a complex worldview and larger belief system. Only through a careful consideration of these religious vantage points may one avoid the temptation to categorize them as premodern, and in fact see the relevance they have for people living in rural areas (Glenna, 2003).

Appalachian and Serpent-Handling Religious Worldviews

Appalachian religion has been criticized for its seemingly fatalistic bent, yet critics have failed to understand how Appalachian religion was a reflection of the grueling conditions in which many of this particular population lived (Jones, 1994). The religion of this region is not only a reflection of this reality, but also is a way of coping with it. Churches like the Pentecostal church allow its members to access a source of power unavailable to them in secular society, and for this reason is very popular (Keefe, 2002).

Another maligned religious group is the serpent-handling sect currently found sparsely throughout the Appalachian region. This practice is based upon a controversial passage at the end of the Gospel of Mark, and during the practice this group takes up venomous snakes during worship, believing that God, who is all powerful, holds their fate in his hands (Handwerk, 2007). Although many theologians might regard this practice as radically unorthodox at best, and primitively repulsive at worst, there are contextual reasons for its significance within Appalachian culture. Daughtery (1978) claimed that snake-handling has served as a process for the Appalachian poor to both memorialize and confront the harsh reality of living in the poor and remote regions of Appalachia. Even so, although this practice was developed in a context of poverty, its practice is no longer limited to rural areas (Handwerk, 2007).

MENTAL HEALTH CARE IN THE RURAL CONTEXT

Because of the unique blend of the rural and religious characteristics found in rural populations, providing psychological services to these individuals can be challenging. The worldview that has been established in many rural areas may clash with the notion of seeking outside mental health treatment. Rural religious individuals considering enlisting the help of an outside therapist often face a number of cultural obstacles that may hinder them from actually seeking help from a mental health professional.

Life in these communities is typically conducted within a "closed system," where those outside the system may be viewed with reticence and suspicion. Psychological concerns are typically viewed as personal problems, which should remain within the traditional confines of family and church (Fox, Merwin, & Blank, 1995). In addition, it is often believed that scripture is capable of providing for all one's spiritual, emotional, and relational needs. Some within the community may perceive those who seek additional sources of help as spiritually weak. For example, each of the authors has heard reports of rural clergy preaching sermons reflecting the belief that all mental health problems are caused by lack of faith or unresolved sin. Such experiences could cause rural clients struggling with emotional issues to experience a higher degree of personal shame and they might also fear diminished social status among their peers if others knew of their struggles.

MENTAL HEALTH CARE WITH RURAL RELIGIOUS CLIENTS

To help rural practitioners overcome the aforementioned obstacles, we offer a series of treatment recommendations which may promote more effective and culturally appropriate care of rural religious clients.

1. *Therapists need to be aware of their own perceptions and potential biases about rural clients.* Psychology tends to be a metropolitan and urban

profession. Overall, there is a shortage of practicing mental health professionals in rural areas. The majority of training programs in professional psychology are also primarily located in metropolitan or urban areas. On the whole, therapists may have fewer experiences with rural clients or populations. Therefore, we encourage therapists to engage in reflexivity practices to garner a deeper understanding into how they view rural life.

First, do not be biased by either utopian or dystopian myths about rural life. Rural residents are no less likely than urban residents to be troubled by mental health difficulties because of their "simple and stress-free" lifestyle. In fact, some stressors are greater for rural communities, especially in light of economic and political inequities in American society (Brown & Swanson, 2003). Rural Americans, for example, are significantly overrepresented in the United States military, and therefore suffer disproportionately from combat-related difficulties.

Second, as a profession, mental health professionals tend to be less religious than other professions, and by far less religious in comparison with their potential rural clientele. Recent research shows a positive trend among psychologists with regard to greater appreciation and acceptance toward client religiosity. However, research has shown that some psychologists continue to hold a skewed view of religious clients, and may over-pathologize religious clients or view religious clients less optimistically. Thus, therapists may benefit from self-awareness tools like the spiritual genogram or spiritual journaling (Wiggins, 2009).

2. *Clinicians should assess rural clients' religiosity and conservatism from the onset of treatment.* According to Belaire and Young (2002), highly conservative Christians expect significantly more in-session religious behavior from clinicians (scripture usage, prayer, and religious language) than moderately conservative groups. Furthermore, members of more conservative groups are more likely to expect mental health professionals to involve their ministers in the counseling process. These findings would suggest that for clinicians working with religious clients, it would be important to assess the strength of their conservatism and to discuss any religious behaviors the client may expect in session, and to agree upon ways in which both parties feel comfortable addressing these expectations (Belaire & Young, 2002). Post and Wade (2009) contend that it is important to address these issues early in treatment and that one of the most effective ways to do this is to include a religious/spiritual assessment, which can be formal (using standardized interview protocols and normed scales) or informal (using open-ended questions).

Similarly, mental health professionals can use their assessment skills for helping identify mental health needs in local congregations. For example, consider the summary offered by Benes, Walsh, McMinn, Dominguez, and Aikens (2000) on how clergy and mental health professionals collaborated in an underserved part of rural Nebraska through the Catholic

Social Services located in Lincoln, Nebraska. Before collaborating with clergy, the researchers conducted a needs assessment with congregation members. Based on this needs assessment, they decided to establish a parish-based indirect services model as opposed to a direct remedial services model. Establishing bidirectional referrals contributed to a lessening of stigma regarding mental health and supported the prevention process. The authors suggested that a needs assessment is useful not only for psychologists, but also in reassuring clergy of their roles as professionals and establishing the initial relationship between psychologists and clergy.

3. *Therapists should consider utilizing evidence-based spiritually oriented interventions and practices with rural religious clients.* The majority of guiding ethics codes among the mental health professions encourage clinicians to consider and accommodate clients' culture and diversity, including religiosity (e.g., American Counseling Association, 2005; American Psychological Association, 2010). Current guidelines on evidence-based practice in professional psychology also recommend that treatments and interventions be selected in light of clients' values as well. In general, it appears that many clients are interested in bringing spirituality into therapy sessions (Aten, McMinn, & Worthington, 2011). Rose, Westefeld, and Ansley (2001) examined the preferences of religiously diverse clients (40% claiming no religious affiliation) at nine different agencies and reported that the majority (63%) believe it is appropriate to discuss religious issues in therapy, over half (55%) claimed that they wanted to discuss these concerns, and only 18% indicated that they preferred not to do so. They noted that personal spiritual experience was the strongest factor for explaining preferences.

In a recent review of the literature, Post and Wade (2009) also found that for religious clients, especially highly religious clients, evidence-based interventions and practices that incorporate clients' faith tend to be as effective, if not more effective, than nonreligious accommodative approaches. Overall, researchers have identified over 30 evidence-based spiritually oriented interventions and practices that have received strong empirical support (Hook et al., 2010).

Gill, Barrio Minton, and Myers (2010) examined how spirituality and religiosity affected the wellness of low-income rural women from a rural southeastern state. Three specific factors related to spirituality and religiosity were found to affect wellness in a positive manner:

1. Purpose and meaning in life;
2. Unifying interconnectedness; and
3. Private religious practices.

The authors suggest that effective interventions for this group of rural women can be shaped around these three factors. For instance, they note that in order to improve wellness, rural clients could participate in "prayer, meditation, and reading of sacred texts in an informal manner outside the public domain" (Gill et al., 2010, p. 300).

4. *Therapists need to consider collaborative efforts with rural churches and church leadership.* Religious institutions are an integral part of mental health care delivery in rural settings. Within these communities, clergy are uniquely positioned to have a significant impact on mental health outcomes. In fact, Wang, Berglund, and Kessler (2003) analyzed data from a nationally representative population survey of over 8,000 respondents that indicated that those with a serious mental disorder contacted clergy (23.5%) in higher proportions than psychiatrists (16.7%) and physicians (16.7%). The ratios were similar in both rural and urban settings. Chalfant et al. (1990) found that approximately 40% of those seeking treatment for psychological problems sought out clergy. Many times, clergy are the only human services resource available in rural areas (Kirchner, Farmer, Shue, Blevins, & Sullivan, 2011). Yet, research examining the role of clergy in mental health service delivery is limited, and the literature investigating this relationship in rural contexts is virtually nonexistent. Taylor, Ellison, Chatters, Levin, and Lincoln (2000) identified four important reasons why ministers play a vital role in mental health service delivery:

1. The senior pastor holds a critical leadership role within the congregation, a position which is intricately involved in both congregational programming and collaborative efforts with service organizations outside the church;
2. Ministers play a number of roles in church-based programs and interventions, particularly when it involves initiatives that target behavioral and/or social change;
3. Clergy often function as gatekeepers to formal mental health services; and
4. The pastor is often the first and only professional that many individuals will engage.

For these reasons, along with the personal nature of their pastoral relationships, clergy can have a significant impact on the psychological, physical, and spiritual trajectory of members in their congregation.

McMinn, Campbell, Chaddock, Edwards, and Limb's (1998) research gives insight into enhancing therapist–clergy collaboration, including the following findings:

1. Skills that psychologists can bring to improve the life of the church include program evaluation, suicide prevention, education, and consultation;
2. Psychologists in the survey reported a higher rate of referral, revealing that psychologists and clergy often have different understandings of what it means to refer;

3. Factors leading to collaboration include the reputation of the professional, having an established relationship, a recommendation of the professional, and shared beliefs and values; and
4. Clergy emphasized the importance of theological awareness.

Although the aforementioned survey was conducted primarily with metropolitan and urban churches, several suggestions for collaborating with clergy evolved from their findings that appear relevant to rural communities:

1. Consider exemplars of psychologist–clergy collaborations;
2. Consider how unidirectional referral may preclude truly mutual collaboration; and
3. Consider ways to enhance trust (proximity and familiarity) in the clergy–psychologist relationship.

Establishing and maintaining successful clergy–mental health collaborations in rural contexts can be a challenging endeavor. Yet, for the emotional well-being of the millions of rural religious people across the United States, it behooves mental health professionals and clergy to work diligently to achieve a productive relationship. Studies have found that many ministers are prepared to collaborate with mental health professionals, especially when practitioners make efforts to establish relationships (McMinn, Runner, Fairchild, Lefler, & Suntay, 2005). Campbell et al. (2002) also suggest that psychologists provide a "theological rationale" (p. 330) for their services in order to overcome possible stigma and connect with pastors. Specifically, Campbell and colleagues call on more clinical graduate programs to unify efforts to train students in spiritual and religious competence and send more students with this competence to work in rural areas.

The Clergy Outreach and Professional Engagement (C.O.P.E.) model is another helpful model that developed in an urban setting but would appear promising for aiding therapists working with clergy in rural areas. Milstein, Manierre, Susman, and Bruce (2008) developed C.O.P.E., a multidisciplinary, multifaith, and research-focused program, to "improve the care of individuals by reducing the care giving burdens of clergy and clinicians through consultation and collaboration." This promising model has expanded to a number of different settings and has facilitated collaboration between clinicians and clergy from a variety of religious backgrounds (e.g., Hindu, Muslim, Reform Jewish), as well as Evangelical and mainline Protestants, which are common in most rural communities.

5. *Therapists should consider using faith-based community psychology approaches for addressing mental health needs.* Blank, Mahmood, Fox, and Guterbock (2002) maintain that stigma may lead rural residents, especially minority residents, to somaticize symptoms, seek hospital care, and minimize symptoms while accessing informal support systems. As a

result, researchers have suggested that community psychology approaches should be considered in addition to more traditional individual approaches. Thus, in addition to collaborating with rural churches and church leaders, it may also be advantageous for mental health professionals working in rural areas to consider how they might leverage resources and networks to implement community psychology interventions.

Within the psychological and health care literature, examples of behavioral health care interventions have been successfully implemented utilizing a community psychology approach in collaboration with rural churches to address a wide range of emotional and behavioral health care problems. For example, Davis-Smith (2007) examined a diabetes prevention program that was successfully implemented within the context of a rural African American Church. Another example is found in Schoenburg et al. (2009), who developed a faith-based cervical cancer intervention. Likewise, Aten et al. (2010) have reported developing faith-based emotional interventions to address the long-terms needs of Hurricane Katrina in rural communities through community psychology approaches such as: (a) community outreach and education, (b) town hall meetings, (c) psychoeducational conferences, (d) learning collaborative, and (e) training-the-trainer.

6. *Mental health professionals should consider the possibility of offering psychological services in primary care settings for rural religious clients.* As noted earlier, many rural religious clients may be hesitant to seek out mental health services for a wide range of reasons, such as religious stigma or belief that emotional problems should only be addressed by the church. Another likely reason that some rural religious clients may be hesitant about seeking services may stem from the historical tenuous relationship between psychology and religion. Historically, the resistant stance of clinicians on incorporating religion and spirituality into therapy can be seen as emanating from an adversarial relationship between psychology and religion. With notable exceptions (e.g., William James), the majority of early influential figures in psychology largely viewed religion in a negative light. Freud, Skinner, Watson, and Ellis, for example, each voiced their share of antagonistic remarks toward religion (though Ellis would later retract many of his remarks; Plante, 2008).

However, while the relationship between psychology and religion has been less than ideal at times, there appears to have been a renewed interest and acceptance of the role of faith in the treatment process (Aten & Leach, 2009). Still, in many rural churches, remnants of the storied past between psychology and religion can and do continue to influence choices and may even prevent some rural religious clients from seeking mental health services.

However, practices of faith do not always preclude those from rural areas from seeking *medical* interventions. Through a focus group study conducted in southern West Virginia, Coyne, Demian-Popescu, and Friend

(2006) discerned that even though West Virginians relied on their faith in God when facing medical problems, this did not stop them from seeking medical attention. They concluded that a lack of health-seeking behaviors was most related to an insufficient amount of knowledge regarding health care, and not the substitute of religion as a coping mechanism. Therefore, therapists practicing in integrated care settings (see Chapter 9) may have the opportunity to reach rural religious clients who might otherwise not set foot in a mental health center.

McAuley, Pecchioni, and Grant (2000) suggested recommendations for addressing religion in a culturally sensitive health care environment. Such an approach would allow for the discussion on religion in terms of:

1. Their attitudes about locus of responsibility and locus of control over illness;
2. Their understanding of the god/patient/physician relationships (and the role that religious leaders play in these perceived relationships;
3. Their expectations about the outcomes of medications and therapies; and
4. Their compliance with recommendations (pp. 32–33).

Practitioners already offering services in primary care settings may be able to garner lessons from the following study to help inform their work with religious clients. Arcury, Quandt, McDonald, and Bell (2000) explored how rural older adults made use of faith to maintain health. Data were collected by the Rural Health and Nutrition (RUN) project in two rural counties in North Carolina over the course of 3 years. Members of this study came from Southern Baptist, Primitive Baptist, Disciples of Christ, African Methodist, Episcopal, and Presbyterian PCA denominations. In examining the stories of these older adults, researchers came to understand that there were both *emic* and *etic* ways to understand how these older adults integrated religion and health. In the *emic* sense, religion was understood by the participants not as a tool to manage health, but as a way of life. Using an *etic* perspective, however, the researchers noted three themes related to health self-management emanating from the participants' Christian faith: prayer, reading the Bible, and church services.

CONCLUSION

The purpose of this chapter was to introduce mental health professionals to the role and influence of religion on rural communities and everyday rural life, and to explore intersections where faith and mental health connect. It is our hope that mental health professionals will feel more informed about the important role religion plays in rural communities. Likewise, we hope that professionals will benefit from the treatment recommendations for working with rural clients and communities. Religion plays a major role in most rural communities and in the everyday life of most rural residents. Within rural communities, mental health professionals will encounter a richly diverse religious experience. By being more aware of the impact of religion in rural areas, mental health professionals will be able to provide more holistic and culturally sensitive services to rural clients and communities.

REFERENCES

American Counseling Association. (2005). *ACA code of ethics*. Alexandria, VA: Author.

American Psychological Association. (2010). *The APA code of ethics*. Washington, DC: Author.

Arcury, T. A., Quandt, S. A., McDonald, J., & Bell, R. A. (2000). Faith and health self-management of rural older adults. *Journal of Cross-Cultural Gerontology, 15,* 55–74.

Aten, J., & Leach, M. (2009). Spirituality and mental health research: A primer. In J. Aten, & M. Leach (Eds.), *Spirituality and the therapeutic process: A comprehensive resource from intake through termination* (pp. 9–24). Washington, DC: American Psychological Association.

Aten, J. D., Mangis, M. W., & Campbell, C. (2010). Psychotherapy with rural religious fundamentalist clients. *Journal of Clinical Psychology, 66*(5), 513–523.

Aten, J., McMinn, M., & Worthington, E., Jr., (2011). Spiritually oriented interventions: Introducing the issues. In J. Aten, M. McMinn, & E. Worthington Jr. (Eds.), *Spiritually oriented inventions for counseling and psychotherapy* (pp. 3–12). Washington, DC: American Psychological Association.

Aten, J., Topping, S., Denney, R., & Bayne, T. (2010). Collaborating with African American churches to overcome disaster mental health disparities: What mental health professionals can learn from Hurricane Katrina. *Professional Psychology: Research and Practice, 41,* 167–173.

Belaire, C., & Young, J. (2002). Conservative Christians' expectations of non-Christian counselors. *Counseling & Values, 46*(3), 175.

Benes, K. M., Walsh, J. M., McMinn, M. R., Dominguez, A. W., & Aikens, D. C. (2000). Psychology and the church: An exemplar of psychologist–clergy collaboration. *Professional Psychology: Research and Practice, 31,* 515–520.

Blank, M., Mahmood, M., Fox, J. C., & Guterbock, T. (2002). Alternative mental health-services: The role of the Black church in the South. *American Journal of Public Health, 92,* 1668–1672.

Brown, D. L., & Swanson, L. E. (2003). *Challenges for rural America in the twenty-first century.* University Park, PA: The Pennsylvania State University Press.

Burkart, G. (1997). Religion. In G. A. Goreham (Ed.), *Encyclopedia of rural America: The land and people* (pp. 605–609). Santa Barbara, CA: ABC-Clio Inc.

Campbell, C. D., Gordon, M. G., & Chandler, A. (2002). Wide open spaces: Meeting mental health needs in underserved rural areas. *Journal of Psychology and Christianity, 21,* 325–332.

Cates, J. A. (2005). Facing away: Mental health treatment with the Old Order Amish. *American Journal of Psychotherapy, 59,* 371–383.

Cates, J. A., & Graham, L. L. (2002). Psychological assessment of the Old Order Amish: Unraveling the enigma. *Professional Psychology: Research and Practice*, *33*, 151–161.

Chalfant, H., & Heller, P. L. (1991). Rural/urban regional differences in religiosity. *Review of Religious Research*, *33*(1), 76.

Chalfant, H., Heller, P. L., Roberts, A., Briones, D., Aguirre-Hochbaum, S., & Fan, W. (1990). The clergy as a resource for those encountering psychological distress. *Review of Religious Research*, *31*(3), 305.

Coyne, C. A., Demian-Popescu, C., & Friend, D. (2006). Social and cultural factors influencing health in Southern West Virginia: A qualitative study. *Preventing Chronic Disease: Public Health Research, Practice, and Policy*, *3*, 1–8.

Darling, C. A., Hill, E. W., & McWey, L. M. (2004). Understanding stress and quality of life for clergy and clergy spouses. *Stress and Health: Journal of the International Society for the Investigation of Stress*, *20*(5), 261–277.

Daughtery, M. L. (1978). Serpent handling as sacrament. In J. D. Photadis (Ed.), *Religion in Appalachia: Theological, social, and psychological dimensions and correlates* (pp. 103–113). Morgantown: West Virginia University.

Davis-Smith, M. (2007). Implementing a diabetes prevention program in a rural African American church. *Journal of the National Medical Association*, *99*, 440–446.

Dillon, M., & Savage, S. (2006). Values and religion in rural America: Attitudes toward abortion and same-sex relations. *Carsey Institute*, *1*, 1–10.

Dong Pil, Y. (2006). Factors affecting subjective well-being for rural elderly individuals: The importance of spirituality, religiousness, and social support. *Journal of Religion & Spirituality in Social Work*, *25*(2), 59–75.

Farley, G. E., & Ruesink, D. C. (1997). Churches. In G. A. Goreham (Ed.), *Encyclopedia of rural America: The land and people* (pp. 102–105). Santa Barbara, CA: ABC-Clio Inc.

Fox, J., Merwin, E., & Blank, M. (1995). De facto mental health services in the rural south. *Journal of HealthCare for the Poor and Underserved*, *6*, 434–468.

Gallup, G. H. Jr. (2002). *The Gallup Poll: Public opinion 2001*. Wilmington, DE: Scholarly Resources.

Gallup Organization. (2009). *Religion*. Retrieved from http://www.gallup.com/poll/1690/Religion.aspx.

Gallup Organization. (2010). *Religion*. Retrieved from www.gallup.com/poll/145379/Religious-Americans-Lead-Healthier-Lives.aspx.

Garrison, M. E. B., Marks, L. D., Lawrence, F. C., & Braun, B. (2005). Religious beliefs, faith, community involvement and depression: A study of rural, low-income mothers. *Women & Health*, *40*(3), 51–62.

Gill, C. S., Barrio Minton, C. A., & Myers, J. E. (2010). Spirituality and religiosity: Factors affecting wellness among low-income, rural women. *Journal of Counseling and Development*, *88*, 293–302.

Glenna, L. (2003). Religion. In D. L. Brown, & L. E. Swanson (Eds.), *Challenges for rural America in the twenty-first century* (pp. 262–272). University Park, Pennsylvania: The Pennsylvania State University Press.

Guthrie, T., & Stickley, T. (2008). Spiritual experience and mental distress: A clergy perspective. *Mental Health, Religion, & Culture*, *11*(4), 387–402.

Handwerk, B. (2007). *Snake handlers hang on in Appalachian churches*. Retrieved from http://news.nationalgeographic.com/news/2003/04/0407_030407_snake handlers.html.

Hatch, J., & Lovelace, K. (1980). Involving the southern rural church and students of the health professions in health education. *Public Health Reports, 95,* 272-28.

Hill, P. C., Pargament, K. I., Hood, R. W., McCullough, M. E., Swyers, J. P., Larson, D. B., ... Zinnbaurer, B. J. (2000). Conceptualizing religion and spirituality: Points of commonality, points of departure. *Journal for the Theory of Social Behaviour, 30,* 51-77.

Holt, C. L., Schulz, E., & Wynn, T. A. (2009). Perceptions of the religion—Health connection among African Americans in the Southeastern United States: Sex, age, and urban/rural differences. *Health Education & Behavior, 36*(1), 62-80.

Hood, R. W., Hill, P. C., & Williamson, W. P. (2005). *The psychology of religious fundamentalism*. New York, NY: Guilford Press.

Hook, J. N., Worthington, E. L., Jr., Davis, D. E., Jennings, D. J., II, Gartner, A. L., & Hook, J. P. (2010). Empirically supported religious and spiritual therapies. *Journal of Clinical Psychology, 66*(1), 46-72.

Jones, L. (1994). *Appalachian values*. Ashland, KY: The Jesse Stuart Foundation.

Keefe, S. E. (2002). Religious healing in Southern Appalachian communities. In R. Celeste (Ed.), *Southern heritage on display: Public ritual and ethnic diversity within Southern regionalism* (pp. 144-166). Birmingham: University of Alabama Press.

Kirchner, J. E., Farmer, M. S., Shue, V. M., Blevins, D., & Sullivan, G. (2011). Partnering with communities to address the mental health needs of rural veterans. *The Journal of Rural Health, 27,* 416-424.

McAuley, W. J., Pecchioni, L., & Grant, J. (2000). Personal accounts of the role of God in health and illness among rural African American and white residents. *Journal of Cross Cultural Gerontology, 15,* 13-35.

McMinn, M. R., Campbell, C. D., Chaddock, T. P., Edwards, L. C., & Limb, B. R. K. B. (1998). Psychologists collaborating with clergy. *Professional Psychology: Research and Practice, 29,* 564-570.

McMinn, M. R., Runner, S. J., Fairchild, J. A., Lefler, J. D., & Suntay, R. P. (2005). Factors affecting clergy-psychologist referral patterns. *Journal of Psychology and Theology, 33,* 299-309.

Milstein, G., Manierre, A., Susman, V. L., & Bruce, M. L. (2008). Implementation of a program to improve the continuity of mental health care through Clergy Outreach and Professional Engagement (C.O.P.E.). *Professional Psychology: Research and Practice, 39*(2), 218-228.

Moreira-Almeida, A., Neto, F., & Koenig, H. G. (2006). Religiousness and mental health: A review. *Revista Brasileira de Psiquiatria, 28*(3), 242-250.

Neitz, M. J. (2005). Reflections on religion and place: Rural churches and American religion. *Journal for the Scientific Study of Religion, 44,* 243-247.

Plante, T. (2008). What do the spiritual and religious traditions offer the practicing psychologist? *Pastoral Psychology, 56*(4), 429-444.

Post, B. C., & Wade, N. G. (2009). Religion and spirituality in psychotherapy: A practice friendly review of research. *Journal of Clinical Psychology, 65,* 131-146.

Rose, E. M., Westefeld, J. S., & Ansley, T. N. (2001). Spiritual issues in counseling: Clients' beliefs and preferences. *Journal of Counseling Psychology, 48,* 61-71.

Schoenburg, N. E., Hatcher, J., Dignan, M. B., Shelton, B., Wright, S., & Dollarhide, K. F. (2009). Faith moves mountains: An Appalachian cervical cancer prevention center. *American Journal of Health Behavior, 33*, 627-638.

Smith, T. (2002). Religious diversity in America: The emergence of Muslim, Buddhists, Hindus, and others. *Journal for the Scientific Study of Religion, 41*, 577-585.

Swierenga, R. (1997). The little white church: Religion in rural America. *Agricultural History, 71*(4), 415-441.

Taylor, R., Ellison, C. G., Chatters, L. M., Levin, J. S., & Lincoln, K. D. (2000). Mental health services in faith communities: The role of clergy in black churches. *Social Work, 45*(1), 73-87.

Wang, P., Berglund, P., & Kessler, R. (2003). Patterns and correlates of contacting clergy for mental disorders in the United States. *Health Services Research, 38*(2), 647-673.

Weaver, A. J., Flannelly, L. T., Garbarino, J., Figley, C. R., & Flannelly, K. J. (2003). A systematic review of research on religion and spirituality in the Journal of Traumatic Stress: 1990-1999. *Mental Health, Religion, & Culture, 6*(3), 215-228.

Wiggins, M. I. (2009). Therapist self-awareness of spirituality. In J. D. Aten, & M. M. Leach (Eds.), *Spirituality and the therapeutic process: A comprehensive resource from intake to termination* (pp. 53-74). Washington, DC: APA Books.

Woodberry, R. D., & Smith, C. S. (1998). Fundamentalism: Conservative protestants in America. *Annual Review of Sociology, 24*, 25-56.

Worthington, E. L., Jr., & Aten, J. D. (2009). Psychotherapy with religious and spiritual clients: An introduction. *Journal of Clinical Psychology, 65*(2), 123-130.

Zinnbauer, B. J., & Pargament, K. I. (2005). Religiousness and spirituality. In R. Paloutzian, & C. Park (Eds.), *Handbook of the Psychology of Religion and Spirituality* (pp. 21-42). New York: Guildford.

7

Ethical and Professional Challenges of Mental Health Care Delivery in Rural Communities
(or "A Day in the Life of a Small Town Psychotherapist")

JAMES L. WERTH, JR.

INTRODUCTION

*A*ny discussion on rural mental health practice must include at least some mention of special ethical and legal issues that arise in these settings. Although not necessarily unique to rural areas (e.g., similar issues may arise in other small communities such as ethnic groups or the military), the concerns are different enough from what may occur in more populated areas that they must be outlined to prepare the new practitioner, or to provide a context in the event that a complaint is filed against a rural practitioner before an ethics committee or licensing board that is composed predominantly of urban members. Fortunately, the publications about ethical matters associated with rural work have expanded in recent years (e.g., Hargrove, 1986; Helbok, 2003; Helbok, Marinelli, & Walls, 2006; Schank, Helbok, Haldeman, & Gallardo, 2010; Schank & Skovholt, 2006; Werth, Hastings, & Riding-Malon, 2010). This chapter provides information on ethical and professional challenges in what, hopefully, will be a new yet engaging way.

Following is an outline of a day in the life of a fictitious small town psychotherapist named Dr. John Smith. The events in Dr. Smith's day are reflective of anecdotes that are either present in the literature or have happened to the author, his colleagues, or students. Some of the details have been changed to disguise the identities of those involved but the underlying situations are based on their stories. It would be remarkable if all these events took place on one day, but it is feasible for them to happen over the course of even just a week. After outlining the day's events, each aspect is discussed by identifying the major underlying ethical or professional issue, linking it to the American Psychological Association (APA) Ethics Code (2010) when relevant.

A DAY IN THE LIFE OF A SMALL TOWN PSYCHOTHERAPIST

Wednesday, April 14

6:00: Go for a run and see Thomas Barnes (Monday's intake) at the track; he says hello.

7:00: Return home and wait on road while Samantha Cole (a client who will be seen on Friday and who lives in the neighborhood) is walking her dog by my house; she waves.

7:45: Take younger daughter Janie, who is in third grade, to school and notice Margaret Johnson, who is the mother of Janie's best friend and was a client until we terminated recently, dropping off her daughter; she asks if I want to get coffee and chat before work (I decline).

8:00: Arrive in office and see my secretary, who is the wife of a County Sheriff's officer, who tells me that her husband arrested Randy Adams last night on a possession charge. He is a client I have been seeing for substance abuse issues and whose last session was on Monday.

8:30: Receive a subpoena for records related to a divorce/child custody case from the town attorney, who also happens to be my own attorney.

9:00: First client of the day, an intake of a young woman who appears to meet the criteria for anorexia nervosa—a condition I have never worked with before.

10:00: Next client, a complex case that I cannot seem to get a handle on and would like to conduct some psychological assessment (but I am aware that a new edition of the instrument that I have on hand has come out recently).

11:00: Third client, who is a friend of another client (and she knows the other person is seeing me too) talks about that person.

12:00: Skip lunch to take on a client who was referred by her physician, but she wants to talk about something different from what she told her physician. She does not want to sign a release for me to talk with him about the issue.

1:00: Fifth session with a client who had seemed vaguely familiar and it comes out in session that he is my second cousin who has a different last name and I have never met before.

2:00: A couple's session with my elder daughter's former 6th grade teacher and her husband; he admits to having an affair with another person who is a client I see tomorrow.

3:00: Older adult client who says she saw me having a couple of drinks at dinner on Saturday.

4:00: Third session with an 8-year-old child of a prominent businessperson and it appears as if there has been some child abuse.

5:30: I stop at the town gas station to fill my car and Bob Sanders says, "How's business? Do you have a full caseload of nuts?" but while walking to our cars after paying, he whispers, "See you next Tuesday, right?"

6:15: Attend the end of my elder daughter's softball game and during a break between innings the town physician comes over and in a normal voice asks about Ruth Markus, by name, who is the person he referred and I saw at noon today.

6:30: After the game see my elder daughter holding hands with a male adolescent client who has some conduct disorder tendencies.

6:50: Stop at market to get milk and see client from this morning; she does not acknowledge me.

7:00: Come home and over dinner my wife says we were invited to a dinner with a new friend she made at the grocery store; the friend's husband is a client.

8:00: Open mail and see an announcement of a continuing education opportunity on ethics in a city four hours away.

9:00: Get emergency call from client who is suicidal and whose support system is unwilling to take her to the emergency room because it is a 45 min drive each way.

10:30: Get to emergency room to assist ER nurse in determining disposition of client.

MAJOR ETHICAL ISSUES AND PROFESSIONAL CHALLENGES IN RURAL AREAS

Dr. Smith had quite a day. However, his experiences are not unlike what other rural practitioners experience on a regular basis. This section includes an overview of the ethical and professional issues associated with the various parts of Dr. Smith's day.

Incidental Encounters

Because Dr. Smith lives in a small community, it is not surprising that at several points during the day he has "incidental" or "extratherapeutic" encounters with clients. These are brief, unexpected interactions where the client and Dr. Smith have to make a decision about how to interact. There has been limited research on these types of experiences (Cochran, Stewart, Kiklevich, Flentje, & Wong, 2009; Pulakos, 1994; Sharkin & Birky, 1992) but the work that has been done has indicated that there may be some differences both in terms of how various clients feel about these interactions and in terms of how clients feel versus how the therapists feel. First, not unexpectedly (and as reflected in Dr. Smith's day), different clients will want varying levels of interaction with the therapist. Some do not want acknowledgement and others want a typical greeting. Complicating this situation, clients may want different degrees of interaction depending on the setting and the people they are with. In contrast to clients, therapists as a rule seem to be hesitant about any level of interaction with clients outside the confines of the office and have negative emotional reactions to these encounters.

In rural communities, these types of interactions are to be expected. It would not be a surprise to see a client exercising at the same place the therapist does or to see a client at a gas station or grocery store, especially because there may be only one of each of these types of facilities in town. Given this fact, therapists should consider including some discussion of incidental encounters in their written informed consent and then spend at least some time discussing the practicalities of what will happen when they happen to see each other in town. Although it may be tempting to try to find out from each client what one would want to have happen in these situations, this procedure would soon become unwieldy. Given the tendency for small town folks to be friendly with each other, it would seem unusual for two people to ignore each other so a baseline might be that the therapist and client would acknowledge each other as they would had they not been in counseling together. If the client wants more than this, then there would need to be some additional discussion about boundaries and the limits on the therapist's ability to talk in public because of confidentiality. The therapist also should consider processing any encounters that occur with current clients to see whether they have affected the therapeutic relationship in any way.

As a side-note, the encounter at the gas station deserves special mention. There is still some stigma associated with mental health counseling in the general public and the research indicates that this may be even more present in rural areas where the "acceptability" of having psychological issues is lower than in more urban communities (see Chapter 4 for additional discussion of this topic). Thus, the therapist should be prepared for people—clients and family members of clients as well as those uninvolved in therapy—to be dismissive of counseling in public and perhaps to hold negative attitudes of those who are receiving therapy.

Visibility of the Therapist

A related issue that rural therapists must be ready to handle is their visibility in the community (Helbok, 2003; Helbok et al., 2006; Schank et al., 2010; Schank & Skovholt, 2006). As was the case with Dr. Smith, because of the lack of available providers and the curiosity associated with the work that therapists do (even at the same time as those who see counselors may be stigmatized), the presence of a therapist may invite attention and scrutiny. This is true whether the professional grew up in the community and moved away for school but returned home to practice (is an "insider") or is new to the area (is an "outsider"). Combining this with the fact that small town mental health professionals will see people with whom they have other connections (see next subsection on multiple relationships), there is the very real possibility that the therapist's actions and the actions of the counselor's significant others will be known to clients and others in town.

In a city, it would be unusual for a client to know where the therapist lives (or if the client knew then there might be some concerns about Axis II issues) but in a rural area this would not be surprising. Clients may walk by the therapist's house without this being a sign of pathology, others may choose to make it clear that they have seen the therapist engaging in some behavior of which they disapprove, or may indicate that problems in the practitioner's family (e.g., a child or partner with behavior/addiction issues) lead to questions about the therapist's ability to counsel others. Therapists may feel as if they have to be "on" at all times, that they and their families must be role models of individual and familial functioning, and that their homes and vehicles must be show-worthy at all times. This is unrealistic and sets the stage for resentment and burnout. Therapists may therefore want to set clear boundaries with clients while also acknowledging that they and their loved ones are human too. As was mentioned above, therapists may want to process any situation where the visibility of the counselor may have been an issue for either the professional or the client.

A side-note to this point is that therapists must take their visibility into account when deciding whether and how to be active in social issues debates. Mental health professionals may have different values from their fellow rural community members and client base (Bradley, Werth, & Hastings, 2012). Thus, a therapist who might think nothing of putting a candidate's sign in one's yard or window or a bumper sticker on one's car in a city or suburban neighborhood might find that this sets them apart from their neighbors, potential referral sources, and pool of clients (Bradley et al., 2012). Many mental health professionals want to be active in social justice activities but they need to be thoughtful about these actions and aware of the potential consequences in rural areas.

Multiple Relationships

Perhaps the ethical issue that is discussed most often in the rural ethics literature is multiple relationships, and for good reason (Campbell & Gordon, 2003;
Hargrove, 1986; Helbok, 2003; Helbok et al., 2006; Schank et al., 2010; Werth
et al., 2010). As can be seen in the previous two sections, the rural environment
naturally sets the stage for counselors and past, current, and potential future
clients to have interactions on a regular basis. Thus, practitioners need to be
prepared for relationships to be present before counseling begins, to take
shape during the course of therapy, or to occur after sessions are over. Importantly, the presence of a multiple relationship is not in and of itself unethical.
The APA (2010) ethics code and the codes of other professional associations
focus on exploitation, impairment, and conflict of interest as opposed to
forbidding all extratherapeutic relationships (see APA Standard 3—Multiple
Relationships).

Current Clients
Because of the limited number of mental health providers in most rural areas, it is
impractical to refuse to see people with whom the therapist has connections.
Multiple relationships with current clients can arise in any number of ways.
For example, if the town has only one plumber, who happens to be a client of
the therapist, and the therapist has a broken pipe, then a multiple relationship
may develop over the course of the therapy. On the other hand, a relationship
may have existed earlier and then the therapeutic connection occurred, such
as if the town car dealer sold the therapist her vehicle and then 6 months later
wants to come in to deal with the stress associated with the bad economy and
poor sales. There can also be situations where there are ongoing connections,
such as if the client and therapist attend religious gatherings at the same location,
the client owns or is the cashier at the only grocery store or gas station, or if the
client is another professional in town such as a nurse or accountant.

The possible permutations are endless so it is pointless to attempt to set
hard and fast rules for what is acceptable and what is not because it is the
context that matters (Verges, 2010). Thus, it is in the best interests of the therapist and client to attempt to identify any existing or possible additional relationships that exist between them and discuss how these may affect therapy or be
affected by it. This discussion will take place ideally as part of the initial
informed consent and then be revisited again as the counseling proceeds,
after interactions occur, and when termination approaches. These types of
developments illustrate why many consider informed consent to be a
process that needs to be revisited over the course of therapy and not a
one-time event that is checked off at the beginning of counseling and then considered complete (Pomerantz, 2005).

Of course, there is the possibility of a significant multiple relationship
becoming known after a therapeutic relationship has been established. This,

combined with the lack of other providers, can make it difficult to navigate multiple relationship situations that would seem clear in other settings (e.g., seeing a family member). It is in these cases that consultation and documentation (and documentation of the consultation) become especially important. All therapists should regularly consult and use good documentation procedures, but these professional activities become more important in unusual situations (Kennedy, Vandehey, Norman, & Diekhoff, 2003). When engaging in consultation in these types of situations, the choice of the consultant will be of paramount importance. The rural provider will want to find a consultant who is familiar with small community practice and who can consider these contextual issues as opposed to being limited to an urban-centric perspective. If the consultant recommends an action and the therapist decides not to follow up because it does not seem realistic for the setting in which the counselor practices, then one is more likely to be found culpable if something goes wrong than if consultation had not been undertaken. These contextual components should be included in the written documentation that explains why the provider made such a decision and why other options were rejected.

Former Clients
When termination is planned, the possibility of posttherapy nonsexual relationships can be discussed and planned for. However, not all clients end therapy when anticipated (Younggren & Gottlieb, 2008) so the counselor may want to include the potential for posttherapy relationships in the initial informed consent discussion as well as when therapy appears to be winding down (Anderson & Kitchener, 1998). In a rural, underserved setting it is unrealistic to unequivocally state that the counselor and client will not have any posttherapy contact and it is also unwise to assume that the former client will never want or need to return to counseling again with the therapist. Thus, these realities must be considered when reviewing options for how to handle posttherapy relationships. This is especially true if the therapist and/or client has significant others and any of these individuals (including the therapist or client) may come into contact with one another. The web of relationships in small areas can be remarkably intertwined.

Among Current/Former Clients
Just as the therapist and client may have some additional connections, the same can be true among current or former clients. This brings in the additional issue of confidentiality (see APA [2010] Ethics Code Standard 4) because these clients may or may not know that one knows someone else the counselor is seeing. It is entirely feasible for the therapist to see two or more members of the same nuclear or extended family for counseling or for the counselor to see several members of the same circle of friends; in fact, these situations may arise because a current or former client refers one's family members or friends to the therapist. In these situations, the challenge is not only to be

ready for the likelihood of such interrelationships and be ready for the possibility of accidentally breaking confidentiality but also to decide how to use any extra-therapeutic information received. For example, if one client says that a male friend is drinking too much again and gives specific examples and says that she is telling you because she knows her friend is also your client, do you use this information with the male client and if so, how do you do so without breaking the confidentiality of the female client who gave you the information? What are the implications for your work and for the therapeutic relationship with both clients if you do or do not talk to the male friend?

As with many of the other examples, given the possibility of these types of situations it makes sense for the therapist to be proactive in addressing them when discussing multiple relationships and confidentiality in the initial informed consent and then returning to this discussion at relevant points in ongoing therapy. Unfortunately, at times this type of arrangement can seem forced or ridiculously unrealistic, such as when two clients who know each other ask to swap sessions and the therapist has to act with each as if she does not know the other client or when two clients see each other in the waiting room and then want to talk about each other. However, unless releases are signed or something is built into the informed consent process, therapists are ethically (and often legally or by licensure regulation) bound to protect the confidentiality of all clients.

Among the Therapist's Significant Others and Current/Former Clients or Significant Others of Current/Former Clients

Some of the most difficult and complicated situations related to multiple relationships involve interactions that are between people that are beyond the direct control of the counselor. If a rural therapist has a partner and/or children then it is extremely likely that there will be some situations where there is interaction between the current or former client or someone in that person's life and someone in the counselor's life (Schank & Skovholt, 2006; see also Woody, 1999). Because of the potential for these situations, the therapist needs to prepare one's significant others, to the extent possible, for the possibility of these events taking place. Having a plan or script in mind might be useful for situations where a current or former client self-identifies as such to a family member (e.g., "my mom doesn't talk to me about anyone she sees so I don't know anything about that" or "Rebecca and I don't talk about the people she sees") or if a complicated situation might arise (e.g., "If I bow out of something without an explanation, don't take offense and don't ask questions") (Whiting, Nicely, & Werth, 2011).

Perhaps the hardest situation involving multiple relationships and confidentiality present in the literature (e.g., Schank & Skovholt, 2006), or discussed anecdotally (e.g., Werth et al., 2011), is found when a therapist's child is dating a current or former client and the counselor knows confidential information about the boyfriend/girlfriend that leads the provider to not want the child to date this person. In such a situation, it would appear as if the professional is in a double bind in that client confidentiality is set against one's child's well-being/ parent–child relationship. There is no easy solution in the event this occurs.

Among Staff/Consultants and Clients/Former Clients

Given that in rural towns everyone seems to know everyone, and know about each other's lives, it would not be surprising for office staff to know clients and to hear about clients' lives. Training staff about confidentiality is crucial in all mental health settings (Fisher, 2009) but may require special attention in rural settings because otherwise people will be reluctant to come in for sessions. It would only take one instance where a secretary talks about a client with friends or family members for the therapist to not get any new clients for fear of loss of confidentiality. This would also set the counselor up for ethical, legal, or regulatory complaints and HIPAA fines.

On the other hand, there is also the possibility that just as the therapist may learn relevant information about clients from other clients or from community members, the same is true for office staff. As was the case earlier, the issue becomes what to do with any information obtained in this way. Being clear with staff about policies and procedures when they have information about clients would be important at both the time staff is hired and at regular intervals.

Another issue that can arise in a rural area but is unlikely to happen in a more urban setting, is when one's own consultants (e.g., an attorney) may be retained by another party and then the connections cross; suddenly, instead of being able to use the consultant, this person ends up being on the other side of the situation. If this type of event occurs, the therapist and consultant may want to discuss it among the parties so that everyone understands what has happened and how to move forward with the least disruption of relationships.

The Special Case of Barter

Although barter is included in the APA (2010) Ethics Code in Standard 6 under fees, one of the reasons this type of payment arrangement can lead to ethical problems is because it has the potential to set up a multiple relationship between the parties. The 2010 version of the APA code is more tolerant of barter but some state licensure regulations (such as in Virginia) actively discourage barter arrangements. Earlier discussions on barter (e.g., Woody, 1998) discussed the possibility of a client paying by trading goods or services for counseling sessions in a generic sense and recommended against the practice. However, in the rural literature (e.g., Schank & Skovholt, 2006), barter is acknowledged as a reality and there was some relief that the newest edition of the APA Ethics Code allows it as long as the arrangement is not clinically contraindicated and not exploitative of the client. One of the primary ways to minimize the potential for perceived or actual exploitation and to minimize the multiple relationship component is by bartering for goods that can be appraised by a neutral person (e.g., a painting by a client who is a recognized artist) as opposed to services that take place either once (e.g., painting the counselor's house) or on an ongoing basis (e.g., yard maintenance) (Schank & Skovholt, 2006; Woody, 1998). A consideration for a therapist who is willing to barter is held in the question, "How many clients will I allow to pay using barter?" A beautiful painting to place in one's office or home is nice, but it will not help pay the rent or cover staff salaries.

Confidentiality

The ethical issue of confidentiality (APA [2010] Ethics Code, Standard 4) was mentioned above in the section on multiple relationships; however, there are other ways that confidentiality can become an issue in rural communities (Hargrove, 1986; Helbok, 2003; Helbok et al., 2006; Schank et al., 2010; Werth et al., 2010). These examples are not necessarily unique to small towns but the issues they raise can be complicated by the dynamics present in rural areas. A common example of a problematic situation that may arise in a rural area is interactions with a referring provider (e.g., physician, nurse, clergy member). Given the stigma associated with psychotherapy noted earlier and elsewhere in this book (see Chapter 4), it should not be surprising that many rural residents get help for their mental health issues from the town physician, nurse, or clergy member. When these professionals believe that the matter is beyond their abilities, they may refer to the therapist. Many times the person may not follow through with the referral but there is a chance that the individual may become a client of the therapist.

In such situations, it is good practice to get a release of information signed by the client in order to be able to consult with the referring party, as well as provide information to that person so that the other professional can offer better services for the person. However, at times the client may not be willing to sign a release. This can place the therapist in a difficult situation because client confidentiality then becomes a barrier to communication with the referring party. In theory, a health care provider or religious leader should understand confidentiality and abide by it oneself. However, there are many anecdotal reports of rural therapists being approached by another professional and asked about a person who was referred. When the therapist indicates that one cannot even acknowledge whether the person came in for a session, the referring party becomes upset and indicates that, "If you will not communicate with me about mutual clients, then I will not refer anyone else to you." One way to try to handle this type of potential problem is for the therapist to be proactive with potential referring agents regarding confidentiality. By appreciating each other's perspective and coming to an agreement ahead of time, the chances of problems developing later are decreased and the therapist can refer back to the earlier discussion if the referring party seems unhappy with the lack of discussion or the need to obtain a release.

Another fairly common situation that can become complicated quickly is if the therapist suspects child abuse (Kalichman, 1999) or abuse of other individuals covered by state laws. Making a report to Child Protective Services is an unpleasant experience. The therapist may be concerned about maintaining the therapeutic relationship, whether the report will precipitate more violence against the child, or whether it is the therapist who will become the target of retaliation. Although there are ways to try to minimize the disruption to the therapeutic alliance through the use of informed consent and negotiating with clients (e.g., Stadler, 1989), the therapist can never know—for sure—what will happen after a report has been made. In rural areas, the therapist may be especially concerned that it will become known, or at least assumed, that the counselor is "the one" who made the report. This could cause problems in the future for the therapist, depending on who is accused of being an abuser and the power one (or one's supporters) may have in town. This certainly should not deter a counselor from making a report if a good faith belief exists that abuse or neglect may have occurred, but the therapist should be prepared for repercussions (e.g., by taking active measures to counteract negative effects).

Competence

The final major issue often discussed in the rural ethics literature is competence (APA [2010] Ethics Code, Standard 2). Although the topic is an umbrella to capture different areas that could be discussed separately, its base has to do with whether the provider is competent to provide services to a type of client (e.g., child or older adult) about a particular clinical issue (e.g., anorexia nervosa), given the consideration of referral options (Hargrove, 1986; Helbok, 2003; Helbok et al., 2006; Schank et al., 2010; Werth et al., 2010). A related issue is access to continuing education (CE) workshops in order to remain competent or become competent in other areas. Rural providers may have less access to CE opportunities because the workshops are often offered in major cities, causing practitioners to close their office for an entire day for a workshop that lasts only a few hours (see Johnson, Brems, Warner, & Roberts, 2006), unless a state licensing board allows all hours to be obtained in non-face-to-face ways.

Clinical Competence
One of the oft-mentioned issues with rural mental health practice is the therapist's need to practice as a generalist (Hargrove, 1986; Helbok, 2003; Helbok et al., 2006; Schank et al., 2010; Werth et al., 2010). In other words, because of the shortage of available psychotherapists, therapists need to be ready to see whoever presents at the office instead of planning to specialize in a given population or clinical issue. The therapist will be hard pressed to refer out clients with issues about which one feels less than an expert. Thus, therapists need to be ready to see children, adolescents, adults, and older adults in

individual, couples, family, and group therapy. Rural mental health practitioners need to be able to see people with a wide variety of presenting
issues, beyond the standard mood and anxiety disorders, because specialists
in topics such as eating disorders or personality disorders are unlikely to be
available nearby. One topic that has been discussed specifically is the need
to be able to treat people with substance abuse issues (Cellucci & Vik,
2001), including alcohol, illegal drugs, and prescription medication. The APA
(2010) Ethics Code has provisions for providers to obtain competence
through continued education and consultation. In such instances it would
seem appropriate to discuss the options with the client and document their
willingness to see the provider even if one has little prior experience with
the condition. Given that research indicates that the therapeutic relationship
is responsible for a significant amount of the change that occurs in counseling
(Duncan, Miller, Wampold, & Hubble, 2010), the key issue may be whether the
client and counselor can form an alliance as they work on the client's issues
together and the therapist develops competence over the course of treatment.

Assessment Competence

Just as a counselor needs to be ready to see clients in a variety of different forms
of therapy, those professionals for whom psychological assessment is part of
their scope of practice need to be prepared to provide such services using
the most current editions of instruments. However, in many rural and other
underserved areas, there may be funding and other limitations that affect
what measures are available (Turchik, Karpenko, Hammers, & McNamara,
2007). Although most agencies should have the MMPI-II by now, there may
be places that do not have the most recent edition of intelligence or other cognitive functioning or neuropsychological instruments and the cost of these
materials may be beyond the budget of many agencies. Even if the instruments
are available, staff may not have been trained in using the updated versions of
the tests. Turchik and colleagues offer ideas for how to cope with these problems. For example, if the problem is "purchasing assessment materials on a
limited budget," they suggested (among other things) that practitioners look
for less costly alternatives and for instruments that have one time licensing
fees, are in the public domain, or are free in the literature as well as comparison
shopping across sources and looking for bulk rate discounts (p. 163). If the
issue is "providing assessments with a limited number of qualified practitioners," they offered several ideas, including having psychologists focus on
assessment, hiring a psychometrician, collaborating with other clinics, and utilizing technology to its fullest (pp. 163–164).

Expansion of Responsibilities Because of Lack of Available
Referral Options

The final issue for consideration is that because there is a tremendous shortage
of psychiatrists in rural areas, other mental health providers may be called upon

to serve in additional capacities with clients who may be severely mentally ill, a danger to themselves or others, or in need of medication (see Campbell, Kearns, & Patchin, 2006). Counselors may be asked to assist the local hospitals or medical clinic with assessments and therapists may be asked for medication recommendations. Therapists need to act within their scope of practice but can be of assistance in these situations if they have the appropriate training and credentials. Thus, rural practitioners may want to ensure that they are current on psychopharmacology, common medical conditions, and risk assessment. They may want to develop collaborative arrangements or acquire privileges with medical facilities.

RECOMMENDATIONS FOR PRACTICE IN RURAL AREAS

On the basis of the material reviewed above, it should be clear that the most important aspect for a rural therapist to consider is to anticipate and plan ahead for the issues that might arise (Helbok, 2003; Helbok et al., 2006; Schank et al., 2010; Schank & Skovholt, 2006). Before seeing clients, the therapist may want to meet with as many other professionals and potential referral sources as possible, not only for introductions but to discuss how referrals might work and the limits of confidentiality. Similarly, meeting with appropriate personnel at the local medical facilities may be important in order to be proactive for emergency arrangements. In like fashion, the therapist will want to discuss potential issues that might arise with significant others so that partners, children, and other family members will be prepared when relationships intersect and confidentiality becomes an issue.

When meeting with clients, providers will want to have a thorough written informed consent form and will want to follow this up with a verbal review of highpoints. In addition to the standard information, the therapist may want to consider having an additional section that focuses on incidental encounters and multiple relationships (during and after therapy). This material can be emphasized to a greater or lesser extent at the outset of psychotherapy, depending on the circumstances. This can then be revisited, when necessary, over the course of therapy and before termination. Similarly, the written and verbal section on confidentiality may be expanded to include mention of situations that the therapist anticipates may arise. If the counselor finds oneself working with a client whose issues are beyond the therapist's proficiency, it may be worthwhile for the provider and client to have a discussion about options and then have a written and signed addendum to the standard informed consent form.

Just as all mental health professionals want to conscientiously document the course of treatment, rural providers will want to pay special attention to including information in their notes about how extratherapeutic contacts or multiple relationships were handled, when they arose, and how they were discussed with the client. If the contact was with a former client, it may be worthwhile to add a note to that person's file with similar information. At times it may be useful to have clients co-sign notes about these incidents. In a similar manner, if barter is used as a form of payment, there should be a separate contract defining the arrangement and, if possible, a neutral third party should be involved to witness the agreement and/or to provide an objective appraisal of the value of goods/services that are included in the arrangement (of course, the client should sign a release to allow the therapist to talk to this person about the situation). All these situations are examples of times when consultation would be in order.

In conclusion, although the focus of this chapter has been on ethical and professional challenges of practice in rural areas, this review would remain incomplete if the benefits of working in small communities were not mentioned (see also Schank & Skovholt, 2006). Many of the things that were mentioned as challenges can be flipped over and seen as advantages to rural practice—knowing lots of people in the client's support system and being able to talk directly with other professionals involved with clients may be a rarity in more urban or suburban areas. Not having much competition and therefore having some negotiating power may be seen as a benefit of rural practice. Many people find the amenities of rural living to be enjoyable, such as lower cost of living, opportunities for owning land, often better air quality, slower pace of life, often beautiful views, increased safety, a sense of making a definite contribution to the quality of life of others and the entire community, the opportunity for loan repayment, and fresher food.

Rural life and practice may not appeal to everyone but for those counselors who are prepared and planful, the benefits of this lifestyle can outweigh the challenges. The material in this chapter may help therapists be ready for the special issues that can arise in rural work and therefore reduce stress and enhance enjoyment.

REFERENCES

American Psychological Association. (2010). *Ethical principles of psychologists and code of conduct* (2002, Amended June 1, 2010). See http://www.apa.org/ethics/code/index.aspx

Anderson, S. A., & Kitchener, K. S. (1998). Nonsexual posttherapy relationships: A conceptual framework to assess ethical risks. *Professional Psychology: Research and Practice, 29,* 91–99.

Bradley, J. M., Werth, J. L. Jr., & Hastings, S. L. (2012). Social justice advocacy in rural communities: Practical issues and implications. *The Counseling Psychologist, 40,* 363–384.

Campbell, C. D., & Gordon, M. C. (2003). Acknowledging the inevitable: Understanding multiple relationships in rural practice. *Professional Psychology: Research and Practice, 34,* 430–434.

Campbell, C. D., Kearns, L. A., & Patchin, S. (2006). Psychological needs and resources as perceived by rural and urban psychologists. *Professional Psychology: Research and Practice, 37*, 45–50.

Cellucci, T., & Vik, P. (2001). Training for substance abuse treatment among psychologists in a rural state. *Professional Psychology: Research and Practice, 32*, 248–252.

Cochran, B. N., Stewart, A. J., Kiklevich, A. M., Flentje, A., & Wong, C. C. (2009). The impact of extratherapeutic encounters: Individual reactions to both hypothetical and actual incidental contact with the therapist. *Professional Psychology: Research and Practice, 40*, 510–517.

Duncan, B. L., Miller, S. D., Wampold, B. E., & Hubble, M. A. (2010). *The heart and soul of change: Delivering what works in therapy* (2nd ed.). Washington, DC: American Psychological Association.

Fisher, M. A. (2009). Ethics-based training for nonclinical staff in mental health settings. *Professional Psychology: Research and Practice, 40*, 459–466.

Hargrove, D. S. (1986). Ethical issues in rural mental health practice. *Professional Psychology: Research and Practice, 17*, 20–23.

Helbok, C. M. (2003). The practice of psychology in rural communities: Potential ethical dilemmas. *Ethics and Behavior, 13*, 367–384.

Helbok, C. M., Marinelli, R. P., & Walls, R. T. (2006). National survey of ethical practices across rural and urban communities. *Professional Psychology: Research and Practice, 37*, 36–44.

Johnson, M. E., Brems, C., Warner, T. D., & Roberts, L. W. (2006). The need for continuing education in ethics as reported by rural and urban mental health care providers. *Professional Psychology: Research and Practice, 37*, 183–189.

Kalichman, S. C. (1999). *Mandated reporting of suspected child abuse: Ethics, law and policy* (2nd ed.). Washington, DC: American Psychological Association.

Kennedy, P. F., Vandehey, M., Norman, W. B., & Diekhoff, G. M. (2003). Recommendations for risk-management practices. *Professional Psychology: Research and Practice, 34*, 309–311.

Pomerantz, A. M. (2005). Increasingly informed consent: Discussing distinct aspects of psychotherapy at different points in time. *Ethics & Behavior, 15*, 351–360.

Pulakos, J. (1994). Incidental encounters between therapists and clients: The client's perspective. *Professional Psychology: Research and Practice, 25*, 300–303.

Schank, J. A., Helbok, C. A., Haldeman, D. C., & Gallardo, M. E. (2010). Challenges and benefits of ethical small-community practice. *Professional Psychology: Research and Practice, 41*, 502–510.

Schank, J. A., & Skovholt, T. M. (2006). *Ethical practice in small communities*. Washington, DC: American Psychological Association.

Sharkin, B. S., & Birky, I. (1992). Incidental encounters between therapists and their clients. *Professional Psychology: Research and Practice, 23*, 326–328.

Stadler, H. A. (1989). Balancing ethical responsibilities: Reporting child abuse and neglect. *The Counseling Psychologist, 17*, 102–110.

Turchik, J. A., Karpenko, V., Hammers, D., & McNamara, J. R. (2007). Practical and ethical assessment issues in rural, impoverished, and managed care settings. *Professional Psychology: Research and Practice, 38*, 158–168.

Verges, A. (2010). Integrating contextual issues in ethical decision making. *Ethics & Behavior, 20,* 497–507.

Werth, J. L., Jr., Hastings, S. L., & Riding-Malon, R. (2010). Ethical challenges of practicing in rural areas. *Journal of Clinical Psychology: In Session, 66,* 537–548.

Whiting, E. L., Nicely, Z. K., & Werth, J. L., Jr. (2011, Fall). The ethics of rural practice: Focus on confidentiality. *The Virginia Psychologist,* pp. 9–11.

Woody, R. H. (1998). Bartering for psychological services. *Professional Psychology: Research and Practice, 29,* 174–178.

Woody, R. H. (1999). Domestic violations of confidentiality. *Professional Psychology: Research and Practice, 30,* 607–610.

Younggren, J. N., & Gottlieb, M. C. (2008). Termination and abandonment: History, risk, and risk management. *Professional Psychology: Research and Practice, 39,* 498–504.

8

Rural Mental Health Practitioners: Their Own Mental Health Needs

DAVID S. HARGROVE AND LISA CURTIN

INTRODUCTION

A person who provides a service is often perceived as an ideal for admiration, regard, and emulation increasing the likelihood of our consulting these persons with dilemmas of life. Hairdressers are expected to be exceptionally well coiffed and stylish, nurses are thought to be healthy role models for personal health practices, and psychological therapists are expected to live well-balanced, healthy, contented, productive lives. Expectations for high standards of behavior typically accompany public perceptions of professional persons. These, at least in part, are the reasons for professional codes of ethics that are designed to protect the public on one hand and to protect the professional person on the other.

Even without the sometimes unrealistic expectations of individuals and the public, mental health professionals are vulnerable to physical, emotional, social, and spiritual malady. The vulnerability comes from both the individual professional and from the environment in which the professional practices. Rural mental health providers are particularly vulnerable, as discussed herein.

The goal of this chapter is to address the situation of mental health practitioners in rural settings. The uniqueness of practicing mental health disciplines in rural environments has been well documented since the 1970s (Hargrove, 1982, 1986; Hargrove & Howe, 1981; Keller & Murray, 1982; Mohatt, Bradley, Adams, & Morris, 2005). Knowledge of the characteristics of rural practice emerged as training programs in psychology, social work, nursing, and psychiatry attended to the lack of human resources in underserved areas (Hargrove & Howe, 1981). Dating back to 1963, the National Institutes of Mental Health has focused on service provision to rural communities through the Community Mental Health Centers Act. In line with the Act, teachers and researchers have attempted to develop ways to best prepare future practitioners. As educators in these fields developed interest in rural practice, efforts to identify the precise nature and characteristics of rural communities mounted from academic and governmental institutions; today many training programs focus on developing future rural mental health practitioners. While research into the mental health needs of rural populations and the training needs of those intending to engage in rural practice has become more common, research has not focused extensively on how practicing in a rural area impacts the person of the therapist.

This chapter focuses on the self-care of the rural mental health professional. Rural mental health professionals are vulnerable to the same (and perhaps more) stresses as mental health professionals in other environments. Because of the nature of the rural community, coping with these stresses is difficult and sometimes seems impossible. Much of the early literature emphasized the procedural difficulties of practicing in rural communities, and the emotional/social difficulties were largely not discussed. However, it is known that there are psychological, physical, ethical, and social peculiarities of practicing in rural communities. Sometimes these peculiarities are sufficient to drive individuals and families from the rural community and, perhaps, away from practice altogether.

Below, the research is summarized on mental health providers' distress, impairment, and burnout, specifying how some of the well-known characteristics of rural communities may relate to the psychological and physical well-being of the rural practitioner. The literature review is followed by a summary of Bowen Family Systems Theory and the rationale for its use to think about practice in the rural environment. Third, a case study of a psychologist is used as an example of predicaments that are likely to occur in rural communities. The overall goal is to suggest procedures for mental health practitioners in rural areas to identify and respond to problematic situations in their own lives, in an effort to improve personal well-being and ethical and effective professional practice.

PROVIDER DISTRESS, IMPAIRMENT, AND BURNOUT

Self-report surveys indicate, overall, that psychotherapists are a fairly healthy group of professionals who report personal and professional satisfaction (Mahoney, 1997; Stevanovic & Rupert, 2004; Thoreson, Miller, & Krauskopf, 1989). For example, Thoreson et al. (1989) found that the majority of doctoral-level psychologists reported satisfaction with their personal relationships, reported their work as interesting, felt useful, and exercised regularly. More recently, Stevanovic and Rupert (2004) found that 94% of surveyed psychologists affiliated with a state psychological association reported at least minimal satisfaction with their job. Specifically, these psychologists reported feeling satisfied with helping clients grow, professional independence, and cognitive stimulation.

However, mental health professionals are not immune to personal and professional distress and impairment. Despite the absence of universal definitions of distress and impairment, both put mental health professionals at risk of compromised personal well-being, as well as impaired professional practice that can leave the therapist vulnerable to ethical or legal transgressions and sanctions. In general, psychotherapist "distress" involves the experience of stress that impacts well-being and functioning. "Impairment" is further along the spectrum, and typically involves an inability to practice the profession in a manner consistent with standards of practice due to personal stressors, mental illness, or substance use (American Psychological Association [APA], 2006).

On anonymous self-report surveys, psychotherapists most frequently report marital and relationship problems, depression, and alcohol misuse (Deutsch, 1985; Thoreson et al., 1989). In addition, psychotherapists report problems with loneliness (Mahoney, 1997; Thoreson et al., 1989), and, although less common, some practitioners report current or past suicidal ideation or behavior (Deutsch, 1985; Gilroy, Carroll, & Murra, 2002). Depression is fairly consistently reported as a current or historical problem among therapists. In 1986, Deutsch reported a depression rate of 57% among surveyed therapists; that rate remained stable in Gilroy et al.'s (2002) independent survey of counseling psychologists that found a rate of 62% for current or past depression.

Personal and work-related stressors are not necessarily independent of each other. For example, Gray-Stanley et al. (2010) found work stress positively related with symptoms of depression among professionals serving adults with intellectual and developmental disabilities. Although the studies reviewed here suffer from methodological problems such as self-reported responses to broad survey questions, return rates of approximately 50%, and, in some cases, homogeneous professional groups, they repeatedly suggest that mental health providers experience personal distress.

Of particular concern is the finding that professionals may continue to work despite the potential for impaired professional functioning. For example, among a national sample of psychologists in the United States, 36.7% reported that personal and professional stressors impacted the quality of services they provided, and nearly 5% reported that such stressors resulted in their providing inadequate client care (Guy, Poelstra, & Stark, 1989). Although the majority (70%) reported actively addressing personal distress, most frequently seeking individual or family therapy, many continued to practice regardless. However, access to therapy for practitioners in rural areas is typically not available as they may be the only practitioner in their area.

Professional burnout involves elements of distress and professional impairment. Burnout among health providers is generally assessed using the Maslach Burnout Inventory (MBI; Maslach, Jackson, & Leiter, 1996). Using this measure, burnout is defined as a combination of emotional exhaustion (e.g., overwhelmed by work responsibilities), depersonalization (e.g., distancing self from work; cynical attitudes about clients), and a low sense of personal and professional accomplishment (e.g., sense of incompetence). In one study, psychologists scored in the middle range of burnout on the emotional exhaustion and depersonalization scales of the MBI, but on average reported a positive sense of professional accomplishment (Rupert & Morgan, 2005). Stevanovic and Rupert (2004) found a sample of psychologists rated economic uncertainty, perception of responsibility for clients, time pressure, and uncontrollable constraints on services as their greatest sources of stress; as discussed further in this chapter, each of these factors can disproportionately burden mental health providers in rural areas.

In a meta-analysis of individual and environmental factors in relation to burnout among mental health professionals, Lim et al. (2010) found age and work setting related most consistently and robustly with burnout. Specifically, younger age related to greater work-related emotional exhaustion, higher levels of depersonalization, and lower professional accomplishment. Agency settings, as opposed to private practice settings, reliably related to higher levels of emotional exhaustion and depersonalization. Not surprisingly, a greater number of hours worked related to more emotional exhaustion. In addition, moderate relationships were noted between higher levels of education and emotional exhaustion, and female professionals scored lower on depersonalization compared to male professionals. Rupert and Morgan (2005) found similarly higher rates of emotional exhaustion among group and agency psychologists compared to solo practicing psychologists, and solo and group psychologists reported higher accomplishment than psychologists working in agency settings.

High rates of attrition and turnover suggest relatively higher rates of burnout among behavioral health workers, both professional and paraprofessional, who serve rural communities (DeStefano, Clark, Potter, & Gavin, 2004; Kee, Johnson, & Hunt, 2002). Two surveys of rural mental health providers found that the majority of respondents endorsed moderate–to-high levels of burnout, suggesting that rural environments may increase risk of professionals' stress (DeStefano et al., 2004; DeStefano, Clark, Gavin, & Potter, 2005).

Indeed, some of the characteristics of living and working in a rural community may enhance the vulnerability of mental health practitioners to psychological, physical, ethical, or spiritual difficulties. Given the relatively small size of rural communities, mental health services are often not readily available. Frequently, a practitioner is the only mental health service provider available, likely increasing perceptions of responsibility and decreasing perceptions of control and choice. Although isolative work conditions are common among all mental health professionals given the importance of client confidentiality (O'Connor, 2001), rural mental health providers often work in even greater isolation (Mohatt et al., 2005) with less access to consultation, supervision, and referral networks. Indeed, Kee et al. (2002) found that burnout among rural mental health practitioners was predicted by a lack of contact with other professionals—a common situation in underserved rural areas, many of which are recognized mental health professional shortage areas. In addition, the rural mental health provider, as a function of working and living in an environment characterized by fewer people and potentially more intense personal relationships (Hargrove, 1986), may have a more difficult time maintaining boundaries between personal and professional life. As a result, the rural mental health providers' personal problems will likely be more public and potentially be judged more harshly than in larger communities.

Cultural factors may also enhance some of the challenges to providing and receiving mental health care in the rural environment. Stigma, a major barrier to seeking mental health care regardless of locale, is acute in the rural community because of the smaller population and general knowledge of people's personal lives (Mohatt et al., 2005; see Chapter 4 for further discussion). Many mental health providers move to rural areas for their jobs and may be considered as outsiders who need to earn the trust of the community before successfully establishing a practice. This unspecified mandate may be experienced as an additional stressor, personally, professionally, and financially, for the mental health provider and one's family.

In addition to personal vulnerabilities such as a personal trauma history (Baird & Kracen, 2006), unique role responsibilities and environmental variables may help explain distress, impairment, and burnout among some mental health practitioners. For example, O'Connor (2001) suggests that practicing psychologists assume many complex roles, alternate responsibilities frequently throughout the day, and engage in emotionally tiring, sensitive, and often isolative work, potentially increasing the risk for distress, impairment, or burnout. Indeed, Rupert and Morgan (2005) found that emotional exhaustion as an indicator of burnout related to a greater number of working hours, less perceived control over work responsibilities, more time spent on paperwork and other administrative tasks, seeing fewer clients who paid out of pocket and more clients under a managed care system, and managing more negative client behaviors (e.g., aggression). Given the realities of rural practice, many of these indicators are more common in rural areas. On the other hand, DeStefano et al. (2005) found that a supportive work environment (e.g., supervisor support) as well as involvement in decision-making and innovation predicted job satisfaction among a large sample of mental health professional and paraprofessionals serving rural communities. Wilcoxon (1989) also found that depersonalization-related burnout among mental health providers in rural areas was lowest when coupled with greater supervisor support and structure. Given the frequent isolation of rural mental health practitioners, such supervisory support may not be readily available. However, technology can increase access to supervision (Wood, Miller, & Hargrove, 2005), and rural practice can offer opportunities to consult with other professionals.

PREVENTION, DETECTION, AND INTERVENTION: IMPORTANCE OF SELF-CARE

Self-care is often recommended for mental health providers (Barnett, Baker, Elman, & Schoener, 2007; Norcross, 2008). Studies of well-functioning psychologists suggest that use of a variety of self-care activities may prevent distress, impairment, and burnout. Coster and Schwebel (1997) define well-functioning as "the enduring quality in one's professional functioning over time and in the face of professional and personal stressors" (p. 5), essentially the opposite of professional impairment. They conducted two studies, one interview based with well-functioning psychologists identified by peers, and one survey of attributions for well-functioning with a random sample of licensed psychologists. Both studies suggest that well-functioning psychologists are self-aware and self-monitor, seek and utilize personal and professional sources of support, know their personal values, and use a variety of strategies to maintain a balance between their personal and professional life (e.g., exercise, vacations).

Kramen-Kahn and Hansen (1998) surveyed licensed therapists (e.g., social workers, marriage and family therapists, psychologists) and found that use of a variety of "career sustaining behaviors" (CSBs) related positively with endorsement of work-related rewards and negatively with work-related stress. The most frequently reported CSBs included maintaining a sense of humor, viewing clients as interesting, participating in renewing and relaxing leisure activities, and consulting with peers. Similarly, Stevanovic and Rupert (2004) surveyed members of a state psychological association and found that more satisfied psychologists reported using more CSBs; spending time with family, balancing personal and professional life, and maintaining a sense of humor were rated as most important. In addition, findings suggest that female providers report higher levels of work-related rewards, greater endorsement of CSBs, and greater use of relational-education strategies (e.g., peer support, supervision) than male providers (Kramen-Kahn & Hansen, 1998; Stevanovic & Rupert, 2004).

Thus, self-care appears as important for therapists as for their clients. Given the unique emotional stressors associated with clinical work, particularly within rural settings, self-care may be especially important for mental health providers to function well professionally and personally. Barnett et al. (2007) remind practitioners that self-care should be considered essential to the delivery of services and to prevent potential ethical violations. For example, Principle A of the ethics code of the American Psychological Association (APA) states "Psychologists strive to be aware of the possible effect of their own physical and mental health on their ability to help those with whom they work" (APA, 2002, p. 1062). Similarly, the American Association for Marriage and Family Therapy (AAMFT, 2001) code of ethics states "Marriage and family therapists seek appropriate professional assistance for their personal problems or conflicts that may impair work performance or clinical judgment" (para. 29).

Self-reported self-care relates to general well-being among mental health professionals (Richards, Campenni, & Muse-Burke, 2010), and, in turn, may prevent or help address distress and potential impairment among mental health providers. Ideally, preventive self-care includes adequate sleep, regular exercise, a healthy diet, a quality personal and professional support system, use of a wide variety of coping strategies including regular engagement in leisure, and balance between personal and professional life. These suggestions are consistent with those reported by well-functioning psychologists (Coster & Schwebel, 1997), and career sustaining behaviors reported by practitioners (Kramen-Kahn & Hansen, 1998; Stevanovic & Rupert, 2004). Integration of the importance of self-care and resources to support self-care during training may serve an institutional preventative function (Smith & Moss, 2009). Unfortunately, many of these strategies are more difficult for providers in rural areas where anonymity is limited and income generated from services is not as high.

In addition to prevention of distress, impairment, and burnout, the mental health professional ideally engages in routine self-monitoring (Norcross, 2008). For example, mental health providers frequently find themselves impatient and frustrated with clients or disinterested in their clients' problems (Mahoney, 1997) which may suggest burnout and a need to increase self-care strategies. Mental health providers, especially those functioning in rural environments, must vigilantly attend to their personal levels of distress and potential impairment as well as to how decisions they make in their personal lives may impact their professional relationships. Rural practitioners have less easy access to peer consultation, support, and supervision, potentially limiting assistance with self-monitoring of personal and professional functioning. A history of personal psychotherapy or current psychotherapy may increase therapist self-awareness (Pope & Tabachnick, 1994), but again these services are not readily available to therapists practicing in rural settings.

Finally, when self-care and personal monitoring prove insufficient, distress can evolve into impairment or burnout and require more active intervention. Typically, intervention will take the form of personally pursued psychotherapy, a colleague assistance program, or professional sanctions. Most mental health professionals, approximately 75%, have pursued personal psychotherapy at some point in their lives, and many, nearly 50%, report returning for further psychotherapy (Norcross, 2005). O'Connor (2001) suggests that fear of stigma or sanctions (likely amplified in rural settings) may prevent psychotherapists from seeking professional assistance, making it important that help-seeking among professionals is not punitive.

Bowen's theory (discussed below) affirms the central importance of the self in the context of larger systems including both nuclear and extended families and other social groups of which a person might be a part. Thus, the principles of Bowen's theory present a relevant context for mental health practice in the rural community because of the emphasis on the importance of an individual's awareness of self in the midst of a system of relationships, and its emphasis on understanding emotional illness as a maladaptive response to environmental conditions.

BOWEN FAMILY SYSTEMS THEORY

Bowen Theory is a broad systems theory that consists of eight interlocking concepts: the family as an emotional system, differentiation of self, triangles, emotional cutoff, sibling position, family projection process, multigenerational transmission of anxiety, and emotional process in society (Bowen, 1978). The family as an *emotional system* containing reciprocally influential relationships is central to the theory. Thus, the family is the level of analysis for thinking about the functioning of the human system and the individuals who comprise it. If symptomatic behavior is present (e.g., individual panic attacks), the clinician looks to the system of which the person is a part, not merely to the person who is experiencing the anxiety, for an understanding of the level of functioning. For example, when stress occurs within a couple in an intimate relationship it typically is expressed in a number of predictable ways. First, there is distance between the two individuals. Second, one of the individuals becomes dysfunctional, physically, psychologically, and/or socially. Third, one person overfunctions, while the other person, in turn, underfunctions. Fourth, the anxiety may be projected onto a child, if there is one. Typically, more than one of these mechanisms is brought into play in the family in response to stress.

Differentiation of self is the way that an individual manages oneself emotionally, cognitively, and behaviorally in systems of which one is a part. Persons who react emotionally to anxious stimuli or cannot connect with others in the system function at lower levels and are vulnerable to symptomatic processes. Higher levels of functioning are associated with a balance of emotional and cognitive responsiveness.

Triangles form in systems to respond to stress. Two human beings are able to manage an intense one-to-one relationship as long as there is minimal stress. When the stress reaches a tipping point, however, a third person is brought into the relationship system to distribute the anxiety. Bowen considers triangles as neither good nor bad; they simply exist as a part of relationship systems. The important factor is how one manages oneself in the triangle.

Through the *family projection process* a parent or parents project their own anxiety onto one or more children who, in turn, may underfunction or poorly develop. A simple example of this process is the "Little League dad" whose own frustrated athletic ambitions are poured into a child, creating stress for the child to perform at higher levels, potentially resulting in a lack of confidence and enjoyment of the game.

The *multigenerational transmission of anxiety* underscores the importance of emotional process in extended families. Individuals acquire automatic behaviors that constitute the emotional process in their families that are difficult to change without diligent work. The family projection process goes through multiple generations. In the nuclear family, one child typically is the primary object and functions less well than the others, who are not as involved with the parents' projection. Children who are freer from the family emotional process typically reach higher levels of differentiation than the parents (Bowen, 1978).

Emotional cutoff is a way that people manage the transition from one generation to another. It is a "process of separation, isolation, withdrawal, running away, or denying the importance of the parental family" (Bowen, 1978, p. 379). Cutoff often comes in the midst of heavily fused relationships with the parents, reflecting unresolved attachment that leads to discomfort and results in emotional cutoff. Rather than reduce the intensity of the relationship, cutoff merely creates emotional and physical distance.

Bowen relied upon Toman (1962) for the construct of *sibling position* as one of the constructs of the theory. The importance of Toman's ideas of birth order and sibling position is that each child in the same family has a "different" set of parents; each child's experience of parents is unique.

The constructs of Bowen Theory have also been utilized to understand the activity of larger *social groups*, including congregations, clubs, businesses, and other aggregations of human beings. Similarly, the constructs of Bowen Theory can be used to understand and manage oneself as well as a multitude of relationships in the tightly woven rural environment. The case study and interpretation that follow depict some common personal and professional situations involving complex relationships in a small, fairly public rural community that may be understood via the application of Bowen Theory.

CASE STUDY

Background

Elijah Winrod, PhD, maintained a solo private clinical psychology practice for 15 years in Ruralton, a small rural community approximately 125 miles from a small city, Metrocity, of 130,000 inhabitants. Having grown up in another part of the state, Dr. Winrod agreed to establish a practice in Ruralton as a part of an agreement with the state mental health agency in exchange for payment for his graduate training at the state university. He was particularly interested in the location because it was on the other side of the state from the community in which he was raised. His relationship with his extended family was strained and contact with them was infrequent. On completion of his internship in a state psychiatric hospital, he was welcomed into Ruralton by many in the community who had unsuccessfully sought to have a community mental health center established. At 29 years of age, he opened an office for the general practice of psychology, and established relationships with practitioners and agencies in the community. After approximately 18 months, his practice was meagerly surviving, drawing clients from a three-county area who traveled to Ruralton to seek his services.

Across the years, Elijah's practice grew in number but not income. He saw more *pro bono* patients because of the difficulties collecting from many third-party payers and because of the extensive poverty in the area. He experienced increasing difficulty turning people away, particularly when he knew (simply from living in the community) that they suffered from health and mental health problems that could be managed with some intervention. He was acutely aware that he was the only available mental health provider.

Elijah was married to Joyce for 18 years. Joyce worked part-time in the community as a computer programmer and was the mother of their two children, 17 and 15, both of whom attended the public schools in the community. Joyce was raised in suburban Metrocity where her parents, her three siblings, and their families still lived. Her father was a retired minister; he and Joyce's mother actively volunteered in their community and visited as often as possible. Joyce always assumed she and Elijah would only temporarily move to Ruralton to fulfill his loan repayment. Prior to the past year, she experienced some difficulty integrating into community groups and activities as she was often uncomfortable interacting with other members who disclosed that they were seeing Elijah professionally. Throughout their years in Ruralton, Joyce urged Elijah to consider a move to Metrocity. However, Joyce's recent involvement in their church offset her desire to leave.

During the last year, Elijah became disinterested and impatient with some of his clients who appeared not to want to change their behavior and resolve their problems. Joyce also pointed out that his alcohol consumption increased, and that he was impatient with her and their children. Elijah excused his behavior in light of the difficulties at his office, particularly dealing with third-party payers and other administrative responsibilities, and working many hours a week with a number of challenging clients. Without agreeing with Joyce's observations or the recommendation of his physician who noted concern over a pattern of increases in his blood pressure, cholesterol, and fatigue, he decided that time away from work could prove relaxing and might appease Joyce and his physician.

Living in the rural area of the state that offered ample opportunity for hunting, fishing, and other outdoor activities, Elijah purchased a shotgun, ammunition, and fishing gear. He registered for a gun safety course and a boating course, hoping to meet other men who were interested in hunting and fishing. The courses, however, were sparsely attended and both had current or former clients in them thereby limiting Elijah's level of comfort and ability to form personal relationships. For about a month, Elijah experienced some enjoyment from solitary fishing and hunting, and some decrease in his alcohol consumption and marital tension. He also attempted to spend more time with his children, but they often wanted to invite their friends, many of whom were connected with families Elijah currently or historically saw professionally. After a certain point of time, he began to believe he could not escape his professional stressors, he felt angry with his wife and children for having relationships with his clients and colleagues, and the loneliness that he felt at the office and at home followed him into the woods and waters. His nightly drinking returned to previous levels and his relationship with Joyce fell back to being distant and tense.

In the meantime, Joyce became much more involved in their church. She joined the choir and assumed responsibility for the entire educational program of the church, which threw her into constant contact with the minister, the Rev. Whimsey. Eventually, she spent considerable time at home doing administrative work for the educational program and time during the week in meetings with the minister and other church leaders.

As he struggled with both himself and the environment in which he worked, Elijah became much more aware of the importance of the networks of relationships in which he and virtually all his patients were embedded. The reality of the importance of these systems of relationships struck him when he realized that he was uncomfortable with the relationship between Rev. Whimsey and Joyce. Rev. Whimsey frequently referred individuals to Elijah and had an informal relationship with Elijah in which they discussed ways in which psychology and psychotherapy were relevant to his work as a minister. Elijah resented the time Joyce spent assisting Rev. Whimsey and the church especially because she did not assist him with administrative work at his practice. He was also aware that Joyce was feeling more satisfied with her life as Elijah was experiencing less personal and professional satisfaction.

Elijah realized that he blamed others for his problems, and sought solitary ways of resolving his personal and professional difficulties with loneliness, isolation, decreased sense of competence and relationships. Having studied community psychology in graduate school, it occurred to him that the systems in which he was involved influenced his own functioning. This led him to the belief that these networks were important aspects of the clinical processes in which he was involved, so he sought additional training at a regional family training institute to gain skills in family psychotherapy and family systems thinking. Elijah believed that the problems of the person he was seeing must be, at least in part, related to the relationships in which the person was involved. Systems training helped him make some sense of the people he was seeing as well as of his own role in the system. He earned continuing education credit for his training and it put him in touch with a number of other people with similar professional and personal experiences.

The training experience with the family institute included quarterly didactic and experiential sessions as well as monthly telephone contact with a trainer. After a few months, Elijah wanted a more intense supervision experience, perhaps personal psychotherapy. At Elijah's request, his supervisor agreed to see him face to face on a bi-weekly basis although Elijah had to take an entire day off to make the two-hour-each-way trip for their meetings.

Interpretation of Case Study

Bowen Theory provides a framework to understand Elijah's experience of fatigue, interpersonal tension, and lack of enthusiasm in both his personal and professional lives. The realization that his functioning is influenced by both dimensions, which are highly interdependent in the rural environment, is an important one that prompts him to seek consultation and psychotherapy. Since he was in a cutoff position with his own family and Joyce was fused with her family, the ground for marital and intrapersonal conflict was fertile.

The triangle with Rev. Whimsey and Joyce was reminiscent of Elijah's relationship with her father and Joyce, in which Elijah was on the outside position. This increased Elijah's sense of loneliness, already salient as a solo practitioner in a rural community, and drove him toward solitary solutions to the difficulties. Until he realized the role that he played in the triangles, he was quick to externalize the problems and blame his wife, the minister, his father-in-law, and even his clients for his discomfort, especially given his own recent doubts about pursuing a career in such an isolated community.

As Elijah became more familiar with Bowen Theory through instruction and supplementary coaching, he gained a sense of self that enabled him to take responsibility for his own behavior and his contribution to the problems that he was experiencing. With this realization, he was able to see Joyce's relationship with the minister as an expression of the emotional process that involved her father. He tried to understand that the anxiety in his family was the fault of no one, but was inherent in the blending of families with different emotional processes. Joyce's fusion with her family, counterbalanced by his cutoff from his family, created an anxious marriage, in which he and Joyce tried to find fulfillment in the other and blamed the other for dissatisfaction. Across time, Elijah realized that Joyce's relationship with Rev. Whimsey was an expression of the triangle that was a part of the multigenerational transfer of anxiety in their family. His ultimate lack of alarm at this relationship provided Joyce the space to come to her own understanding of the relationship, allowing her to manage it appropriately. The management of anxiety in triangles with an appreciation of the multigenerational transmission of emotional process provides an example of how Bowen Theory offers an interpretive perspective of this case. It is equally important to be aware of the myriad relationships in the community that intersect with the mental health provider and his family and therefore influence his functioning.

The literature on mental health practitioners further inform Elijah's situation. First, he was more vulnerable to personal distress, impairment, and burnout as a function of the number of hours worked, lack of supervision or peer consultation, isolated working conditions, heavy reliance on third-party payers, and related administrative tasks. In addition, being a rural "generalist," Elijah did not believe that he had control over the clientele that he served or the hours that he worked. On the other hand, his being an experienced private practitioner likely buffered him from even greater professional burnout. Feeling isolated and overwhelmed by his work responsibilities, his self-care was limited until he detected impatience in his personal and professional relationships, his wife pointed out his increased alcohol consumption, and his physician noted physical symptoms. At that time he sought relief in solitary leisure activities that, although important relative to self-care, were not satisfactory in the long run. He subsequently utilized an opportunity for coaching at a family institute that resulted in some personal psychotherapy. The coaching experience enabled Elijah to access both personal and professional support outside of the community in which he lived, and to realize that attention to personal and professional relationships, including within his own community, was necessary to effect change at both levels.

CONCLUSION

It is important that professional persons practicing in rural environments realize the vulnerability to which they are subject. The isolation, limited number of relationships, and lack of resources enhance vulnerability for distress and potential impairment or burnout. Preventive self-care in the form of regular exercise, a healthy diet and sleep schedule, engagement in leisure activities, and personal and professional support systems may buffer the rural practitioner's distress. Clearly, stress and distress cannot always be prevented; thus, mental health professionals, especially those functioning in greater isolation, must vigilantly attend to possible signs of increased anxiety or other indicators of distress or impairment. Finally, a willingness to seek assistance when stress is high is an important third step in the process of managing oneself personally and professionally in the rural community. In rural communities, however, a mental health provider may need to travel lengthy distances to access help or utilize technology to supplement access to services and supervisory support.

A concentrated effort toward self-care of a mental health professional in a rural community is essential for good, healthy, and ethical practice. Bowen Theory provides a framework for the development and maintenance of boundaries in a dynamic system of relationships that is consistent with the demands of rural practice and living. The multiple, interconnected relationships can be a complex array of political, social, personal, and economic forces that influence the lives of people who live and work there. Self-care, of course, must be designed for each individual in each family living in each community. Bowen Theory offers a structure to guide the realization and strategy for healthy self-care among mental health practitioners in a rural environment.

REFERENCES

American Association for Marriage and Family Therapy. (2001). *Association for marriage and family therapy code of ethics.* Retrieved from http://www.aamft.org/resources/LRM_Plan/Ethics/ethicscode2001.asp

American Psychological Association. (2002). Ethical principles of psychologists and code of conduct. *American Psychologist, 57*, 1060–1073.

American Psychological Association. (2006). Advancing colleague assistance in professional psychology. *CAP Monograph.* Retrieved from http://www.apa.org/practice/resources/assistance/monograph.pdf

Baird, K., & Kracen, A. C. (2006). Vicarious traumatization and secondary traumatic stress: A research synthesis. *Counseling Psychology Quarterly, 19*, 181–188.

Barnett, J. E., Baker, E. K., Elman, N. S., & Schoener, G. R. (2007). In pursuit of wellness: The self-care imperative. *Professional Psychology: Research and Practice, 38*, 603–607.

Bowen, M. (1978). *Family therapy in clinical practice.* New York: Aronson.

Coster, J. S., & Schwebel, M. (1997). Well-functioning in professional psychologists. *Professional Psychology: Research and Practice, 28*(1), 3–13.

DeStefano, T. J., Clark, H., Potter, T. W. L., & Gavin, M. (2004). Assessment of burnout among rural mental health staff. *Rural Mental Health, 30*, 18–24.

DeStefano, T. J., Clark, H., Gavin, M., & Potter, T. (2005). The relationship between work environment factors and job satisfaction among rural behavioral health professionals. *Journal of Rural Mental Health, 30*, 18–24.

Deutsch, C. J. (1985). A survey of therapists' personal problems and treatment. *Professional Psychology: Research and Practice, 16*, 305–315.

Gilroy, P. J., Carroll, L., & Murra, J. (2002). A preliminary survey of counseling psychologists' personal experiences with depression and treatment. *Professional Psychology: Research and Practice, 33*, 402–407.

Gray-Stanley, J. A., Muramatsu, N., Heller, T., Hughes, A., Johnson, T. P., & Ramirez-Valles, J. (2010). Work stress and depression among direct support professionals: The role of work support and locus of control. *Journal of Intellectual Disability Research, 54*, 749–761.

Guy, J. D., Poelstra, P. L., & Stark, M. J. (1989). Personal distress and therapeutic effectiveness: National survey of psychologists practicing psychotherapy. *Professional Psychology: Research and Practice, 20*, 48–50.

Hargrove, D. S. (1982). The rural psychologist as generalist: A challenge for professional identity. *Professional Psychology, 13*(2), 302–308.

Hargrove, D. S. (1986). Ethical issues in rural mental health practice. *Professional Psychology: Research and Practice, 17*, 20–23.

Hargrove, D. S., & Howe, H. E. (1981). Training in rural mental health delivery: A response to prioritized needs. *Professional Psychology, 12*(6), 722–731.

Kee, J., Johnson, D., & Hunt, P. (2002). Burnout and social support in rural mental health. *Journal of Rural Community Psychology.* Retrieved from http://www.marshall.edu/jrcp/sp2002/Kee.htm

Keller, P., & Murray, J. D. (1982). *Handbook of rural community mental health.* New York: Human Sciences Press.

Kramen-Kahn, B., & Hansen, N. D. (1998). Rafting the rapids: Occupational hazards, rewards and coping strategies of psychotherapists. *Professional Psychology: Research and Practice, 29,* 130–134.

Lim, N., Kim, E. K., Kim, H., Yang, E., & Lee, S. M. (2010). Individual and work-related factors influencing burnout of mental health professionals: A meta-analysis. *Journal of Employment Counseling, 47,* 86–96.

Mahoney, M. J. (1997). Psychotherapists' personal problems and self-care patterns. *Professional Psychology: Research and Practice, 28,* 14–16.

Maslach, C., Jackson, S. E., & Leiter, M. P. (1996). *Maslach burnout inventory manual* (3rd ed.). Palo Alto, CA: Consulting Psychologists Press.

Mohatt, D. F., Bradley, M. M., Adams, S. J., & Morris, C. D. (2005). *Mental health and rural America: 1994–2005.* Washington, DC: U.S. Department of Health and Human Services.

Norcross, J. C. (2005). The psychotherapist's own psychotherapy: Educating and developing psychologists. *American Psychologist, 8,* 840–850.

Norcross, J. C. (2008). Psychotherapist self-care: Practitioner-tested, research-informed strategies. *Professional Psychology: Research and Practice, 31,* 710–713.

O'Connor, M. F. (2001). On the etiology and effective management of professional distress and impairment among psychologists. *Professional Psychology: Research and Practice, 32,* 345–350.

Pope, K. S., & Tabachnick, B. G. (1994). Therapists as patients: A national survey of psychologists' experiences, problems, and beliefs. *Professional Psychology: Research and Practice, 25,* 247–258.

Richards, K. C., Campenni, C. E., & Muse-Burke, J. L. (2010). Self-care and well-being in mental health professionals: The mediating effects of self-awareness and mindfulness. *Journal of Mental Health Counseling, 32,* 247–264.

Rupert, P. A., & Morgan, D. J. (2005). Work setting and burnout among professional psychologists. *Professional Psychology: Research and Practice, 5,* 544–550.

Smith, P. L., & Moss, S. B. (2009). Psychologist impairment: What is it, how can it be prevented, and what can be done to address it? *Clinical Psychology Science and Practice, 16,* 1–15.

Stevanovic, P., & Rupert, P. A. (2004). Career-sustaining behaviors, satisfactions, and stressors of professional psychologists. *Psychotherapy: Theory, Research, Practice, and Training, 3,* 301–309.

Thoreson, R. W., Miller, M., & Krauskopf, C. J. (1989). The distressed psychologist: Prevalence and treatment considerations. *Professional Psychology: Research and Practice, 20,* 153–158.

Toman, W. (1962). *Family constellation: Its effects on personality and social behavior* (3rd ed.). New York: Springer.

Wilcoxon, S. A. (1989). Leadership behavior and therapist burnout: A study of rural agency settings. *Journal of Rural Community Psychology.* Retrieved from http://www.marshall.edu/jrcp/v102.pdf

Wood, J. A., Miller, T. W., & Hargrove, D. S. (2005). Clinical supervision in rural settings: A telehealth model. *Professional Psychology: Research and Practice, 36,* 173–179.

II

Models of Service Delivery

9

Integrated Care in Rural Areas

DAVID LAMBERT AND JOHN A. GALE

INTRODUCTION

*O*ver the past decade, there has been a substantial push within our health care system to integrate physical and mental health care. One impetus for integration is that the traditional separation of general health and mental health services may hinder a holistic medical approach necessary to treat effectively what are often comorbid health problems. Another impetus is that there are simply not enough mental health clinicians to treat all the persons with a mental health problem or illness. In addition, many individuals prefer receiving mental health care in a primary care setting, for reasons presented below. In fact, more persons with a mental health problem or illness are treated by a primary care provider than by a specialty mental health care provider (Regier, Goldberg, & Taube, 1978; Regier et al., 1993).

Efforts to integrate primary and mental health care came early to rural America. There was simply no choice—more than 80% of psychiatrists and PhD psychologists reside in urban areas and this distribution has remained essentially unchanged for decades (New Freedom Commission on Mental Health, 2003). There is rich experience to draw on in designing and sustaining integrated programs in rural areas. This same experience suggests that there are also significant and persistent barriers to rural integration. Successful rural integrated programs are increasing, but they often require adapting to the local infrastructure and community context and understanding the changing policy environment.

This chapter is presented in six sections. Following this overview, the next section presents the background for integration including definitions, models, barriers, and evidence from the general integration literature. The third section describes the history of integration in rural areas. The fourth section takes a closer look at current and best practices of integrating care in rural areas and highlights several exemplary programs. The penultimate section takes a look at the road ahead for integrating care in rural areas, including an analysis of current policy initiatives—parity, person-centered medical homes, and health care reform—that will inevitably affect this road. The final section presents resources for finding out more about integrating care in rural areas.

BACKGROUND

There is widespread support for the "idea" of integration—people's physical and mental health problems should be coordinated and not treated separately or in isolation from each other. Seminal reports have endorsed the importance of integration, including the Surgeon General's Report on Mental Health (U.S. Department of Health and Human Services, 1999), The President's New Freedom Commission on Mental Health (2003), and Institute of Medicine's (2006) *Improving the Quality of Health Care for Mental and Substance-Use Conditions*. Comprehensive health care policy initiatives—such as the Bureau of Primary Health Care's New Access Initiative (2003) expanding the role and reach of community health centers (Proser & Cox, 2004) and current development and promotion of the patient-centered medical home—include an important place for integration.

Despite widespread support for the idea of integration, there is less agreement about what integration means, how it should work, and what it has accomplished. Below is presented the current state of discussion and understanding of definitions, specific integrated care models, and evidence for integrated care. Several comprehensive reviews dealing with these issues are available in the published literature.

Definition of Integration

A number of definitions of integration are found within the literature, usually reflecting the specific clinical settings and health care providers being studied or described. In their review of this literature, the federal Agency for Healthcare Research and Quality (AHRQ) posits a simple but robust definition of integration (Butler et al., 2008, p. 9): "Integrated care occurs when mental health specialty and general medical care providers work together to address both the physical and mental health needs of their patients." The AHRQ paper notes that integration can work in two ways: integrating specialty mental health care into primary care or integrating primary care into specialty mental health care. AHRQ further emphasizes that it is important to consider at least two dimensions: integration of providers and integration of processes of care. Making a similar distinction, Gale and Lambert (2008) note that it is important to move beyond the question of *where* care is provided and by whom to the question of *how* care is provided. It is important to move beyond the *structure* of integration to the *function* of integration. This distinction is particularly important in understanding and improving integrated care in rural areas.

Models of Integration

A number of different approaches and models of integration have been developed. An important foundational model for much of this work is the Four Quadrant Clinical Integration Model, first introduced in 1998 to depict treatment options for persons with co-occurring mental health and substance abuse disorders (National Association of State Mental Health Program Directors, 1998). The model characterizes clients by the severity of their mental health/substance abuse problems and severity of their physical health problems to determine the most appropriate treatment setting. In 2003, the National Council for Community Behavioral Healthcare issued a paper that argued that integration had become "stuck" at the policy idea level and required support at the policy, training, and clinical levels to move forward (Mauer, 2003). The Report adapted the Four Quadrant Model to classify the level of integration and clinical competencies needed to treat persons with differing behavioral health (BH) and physical health (PH) complexity. The resulting four quadrants are: (1) low BH, low PH; (2) high BH, low PH; (3) low BH, high PH; and (4) high BH, high PH. The Four Quadrant Model continues to be adapted and used in policy discussions, including the rationale and need to include behavioral health in the patient-centered medical home (Mauer, 2009).

As mentioned above, depictions of integration models have evolved from the question of *where* care is provided (general health care or specialty health care) to *how* care is provided. Schemes such as Wagner's Chronic Care Model (Wagner, 1998), anchored by a care manager, and Strosahl's model (Strosahl, 1998), in which mid-level behavioral health specialists help engage primary care patients, have gathered significant support. In general, there is a preference within the literature for more highly integrated models. However, this preference tacitly assumes that sufficient infrastructure and resources are available to support full integration. This is often not the case in many urban areas and is rarely the case in rural areas. Doherty, McDaniel, and Baird (1996) capture these issues in a five-level classification of integration: (1) separate systems and facilities, (2) basic collaboration from a distance, (3) basic collaboration on site, (4) close collaboration in a partially integrated system, and (5) fully integrated system. This model allows for practices to adapt the level of integration most suitable to their resources and needs and to move to higher levels of integration as need and resources allow.

Barriers to Integration

Efforts to develop and to sustain integrated programs face substantial barriers that are well documented and described in the literature (Butler et al., 2008; Institute of Medicine, 2005; Lambert & Hartley, 1998). Gale and Lambert (2009) summarize this literature in terms of five levels:

National and system-level barriers include the limited supply of specialty behavioral health providers and their mal-distribution relative to need; the separation of funding streams for general and behavioral health care services; and the lack of parity between coverage for general medical and behavioral health conditions.

Regulatory barriers include state-level licensure laws governing the requirements for a professional title; the scope of practice (specific activities persons meeting these requirements are permitted to perform); and facility licensure governing the provision of services by behavioral health agencies.

Reimbursement barriers include lack of reimbursement for integrative and preventive services; variation in reimbursement rules across third-party payers; different coding and billing classifications by setting and payer, and mental health carve-outs (in which payment and management of mental health care is separated from physical health care).

Practice and cultural barriers between primary and mental health practice include different practice styles, culture, language, and administration. Differences include methods used to reach a diagnosis, lengths and content of typical visits; the use of separate patient records; and approaches to charting, record keeping, and communication with other providers. The lack of integration of information technology, both within and across practices, compounds these barriers.

Patient-level barriers include poor access to behavioral health services; limitations on coverage and reimbursement by third-party payers; impact of high-deductibles and co-pays on use of services; complexity of authorization and utilization review; and patient perception of stigma in receiving behavioral health care.

Evidence for Integration

In their evidentiary review of the integration literature, AHRQ identified 33 clinical trials of integrated programs that fit their screening criteria and differentiated them according to level of provider integration and level of processes of care (Butler et al., 2008). Integrated care programs tended to have positive outcomes for symptom severity, treatment response, and remission compared to usual care. However, there was wide variation in levels of provider integration and integrated processes of care, but this variation was not related to outcome. This led the authors to characterize the evidence on the effectiveness on integrated care as being a choice of viewing the glass as half empty or half full, cautioning that "while there is much to be optimistic about there is also little to suggest adherence to strict orthodoxy in defining and adhering to what an effective integrated care program might be" (Butler et al., 2008; p. 6).

INTEGRATED CARE IN RURAL AREAS

Efforts to integrate care in rural areas extend back over 40 years and can be traced to major Federal initiatives to expand access to health care. Legislation creating community and migrant health centers in 1967 required these entities to offer basic mental health services (Geiger, 1984). During the late 1970s and early 1980s, programs such as the Rural Health Initiative, the Health Underserved Rural Areas grants, the Rural Mental Health Demonstration Program, and the Linkage Initiative Program provided incentives to link primary care and mental health in rural areas. The creation in 1989 of Federally Qualified Health Centers that could be reimbursed on a cost basis by Medicare and Medicaid introduced additional resources to linking care in rural areas. However, by the early 1990s, it was not clear as to what extent there were sustained integrated care programs in rural areas. Evaluations of the earlier demonstration programs suggested that while they were initially effective, the programs and their services did not last once their funding ended. It was also not clear as to what extent Federally Qualified Health Centers were able to provide mental health services in rural areas. To better understand the scope and nature of integrated care in rural areas, the Maine Rural Health Research Center conducted a national survey of 53 primary care programs in rural areas that provided or coordinated mental health care (Bird, Lambert, Hartley, Coburn, & Beeson, 1998). They found that rural primary care providers used four different strategies or models to integrate care:

- *Diversification*: care provided on-site directly with a Center's own mental health staff.
- *Linkage/co-location*: care provided on-site by a non-Center staff health worker.
- *Referral*: care provided off-site by non-Center staff under a formal agreement.
- *Enhancement*: primary care practitioners are trained to provide mental health care on-site.

At the time the survey was conducted, rural Community Health Centers and other primary care providers had relatively limited information to help them develop and provide mental health services. In the ensuing decade, a variety of screening tools and guidelines were developed for identifying mental health problems and linking and integrating care. In 2004, the National Rural Health Association asked the Maine Rural Health Research Center to revisit their earlier study and to assess whether rural primary care providers were using similar or different approaches to integrating care than a decade earlier and to assess what challenges rural providers faced in integrating care. To examine these issues, the Maine Rural Health Research Center conducted case studies of community health centers in Colorado, Montana, New Hampshire, North Carolina, Pennsylvania, and South Dakota (Lambert & Gale, 2006).

The case studies found that rural community health centers were more likely than 10 years before to provide mental health care using staff employed by the health centers (diversification model). The authors described two key components of care delivered in these settings—integrative activities and direct care services—that create a synergy which contributes to the success of integrated programs. Integrative activities were usually performed by the mental health clinician and include patient screening and engagement, consulting with primary care staff (in formal meetings and "hallway consults"), "warm handoffs" to introduce patients to the mental health clinicians, and responding to patient and staff questions. Warm handoffs are particularly useful to enhance the trust and rapport developed between the primary care provider and the patient and to improve the likelihood that the patient will follow through with mental health treatment. Integrative activities help to reduce demands on primary care staff and allow them to see more patients, but are usually not directly reimbursable services.

Direct care services include medication management by the primary care physician and counseling and therapy provided by the mental health (licensed counselor) staff using appropriate behavioral health codes. Direct services, when delivered by an appropriately licensed clinician, as defined by state law and/or third-party payer policies, are usually reimbursable by third-party payers.

Five of the six centers used a standardized screening tool for depression with most patients (usually the PHQ-9) as a screening mechanism for identifying depression. The PHQ-9 is the nine question depression module of the Patient Health Questionnaire, a self-administered diagnostic tool containing five modules covering anxiety, somatoform, alcohol, and eating disorders developed by Robert L. Spitzer, MD, Janet B.W. Williams, DSW, and Kurt Kroenke, MD. Medication management and obtaining psychiatric consultations to support the primary care providers in prescribing psychotropic medications remained an ongoing challenge for most centers. Depression is the most common mental health condition identified and treated in rural primary care centers and many primary care clinicians are comfortable in prescribing front-line antidepressants. The challenge emerges when these medications are not effective or comorbidities are present without a readily accessible mental health specialist with whom to consult. A confounding problem is the increased complexity and severity of mental health problems of patients turning to rural primary care providers for care. Two factors have contributed to this trend: (1) decreased funding for specialty mental health care in nearly every state; and (2) specialty mental health providers and agencies, unlike community health centers, are not funded to be safety-net providers (i.e., to serve low-income, uninsured, and under-insured clients).

The study found that rural community health centers were more likely to provide mental health care than a decade earlier, which was consistent with policy expectations. As the authors observe, the question facing rural CHCs had largely shifted from *whether* to *how* to provide mental health care (Lambert & Gale, 2006: p. 21): "The primary questions rural CHCs face are how to treat these problems in an acute care setting with very limited options for psychiatric consultation and referral and how to improve the functioning of their clinical team. CHCs must determine how many patients and what conditions they can treat."

CURRENT AND BEST PRACTICES IN RURAL INTEGRATION

There is no single best way to integrate care in rural areas (Gale & Lambert, 2006; Lambert & Gale; 2006; Lambert & Hartley, 1998). Rather, a variety of approaches can and do work. What seems to be important is that providers first understand what their goals are and prioritize them. Is their goal to expand access to mental health services for all persons in their community or to those whom they are already treating for physical health conditions (i.e., current patients of their practice)? What behavioral health conditions will the persons whom they will treat have? How severe and complex are these conditions likely to be? Given these considerations, what role and function do they envision for their primary care staff and how will they work with behavioral health clinicians? What resources for referral and/or consultation are available in the community? How will the program be reimbursed? Are resources available to support nonreimbursable services, typically the integrative component of the program? When rural providers understand their integration goals, it is possible to start modestly and evolve and expand with experience.

CASE STUDIES OF INTEGRATED CARE IN RURAL COMMUNITIES

This section reviews the experience and lessons learned by four rural primary care providers who have successfully integrated care. One rural federally qualified health center (FQHC), Community Health Partners in Livingston, Montana, strategically chose to add mental health services incrementally.

Another FQHC, the Open Door Community Health Centers in northwest California, added tele-mental health to enhance its integration approach. The DIAMOND (Depression Improvement Across Minnesota Offering a New Direction) Program, a collaborative initiative involving third-party payers, the Minnesota Department of Human Services, and providers, developed an integrated model and reimbursement mechanisms to treat Medicaid beneficiaries with depression. The fourth program, Cherokee Health Care System in eastern Tennessee, is a well-resourced and organized care system that integrates community health and community mental health centers and is widely touted as a model of rural mental health and primary care integration. These rural providers have been selected because they vary in size, approach, and funding, yet have all been successful. Their variety of approaches and funding illustrates a key point of this chapter: providers should choose models and approaches for which there is evidence and that fit their needs, experience, and resources.

Community Health Partners (CHP) is a small network of FQHCs in south-central Montana (Lambert & Gale, 2006). The primary site was established in Livingston in 1997 and a second site was opened in Bozeman in 2002. The population served by CHP includes a significant percentage of persons in poverty as well as high-income persons attracted to the state's natural resources. Specialty mental health services were not readily available to CHP's clients, prompting CHP in the early 2000s to develop mental health services.

CHP choose to adopt Kirk Strosahl's model of integration. In this model, primary care providers screen for behavioral health problems during patient exams (Strosahl, 1998). If the screen is positive, the patient is encouraged to meet that day with an on-site clinical counselor, who tries to engage the patient in treatment. During this brief initial behavioral health encounter (15–30 min), the counselor undertakes an initial assessment and begins the development of a treatment plan. The PHQ-9 is administered to screen more fully for depression and to assess functionality. Motivational interviewing is used to encourage the patient to identify stressors and additional counseling visits are scheduled as necessary. To accommodate "same day referrals," the counselor leaves half of her daily schedule open.

The Strosahl model fits well with CHP's strategic needs and organizational culture that includes a relatively young, highly motivated staff. The counselor provides an important consulting resource to the primary care staff in addition to her direct service responsibilities (Lambert & Gale, 2006). A psychiatrist is available on-site one afternoon a month for consultation. Approximately 60% of CHP's funding is supported by its Section 330 federal grant, 10% by Medicaid, 10% by private insurance, and 20% by private pay patients and other grants. Section 330 of the Public Health Service Act defines federal grant funding opportunities for organizations to provide care to underserved populations. Types of organizations that may receive 330 grants include: FQHCs/Community Health Centers, Migrant Health Centers, Health Care for the Homeless Programs, and Public Housing Primary Care Programs.

Open Door Community Health Centers (Open Door) has nine sites and a mobile dental unit serving primarily low-income persons over a very large rural area in northwest California including Humboldt and Del Norte Counties and portions of Trinity and Siskiyou Counties in Northwest California (California HealthCare Foundation, 2010; Duclos, Hook, & Rodriguez, 2010). Starting in 1971 as a small local clinic staffed largely by volunteers, Open Door has expanded its staff services and locations over the last four decades. Today its staff includes 37 full-time equivalent (FTE) medical staff, nine FTE dental staff, and nine FTE behavioral health practitioners and offers a wide array of services including family practice, pediatrics, women's health, prenatal and birth, family planning, geriatrics, dental care, urgent care, mental and behavioral health, STD testing and counseling, HIV/AIDS care, alternative medicine, health education, and smoking cessation. Open Door earned Federally Qualified Health Center (FQHC) status in 1999, making it eligible for Section 330 grant funding to support care for the uninsured as well as enhanced Medicare and Medi-Cal (California's Medicaid program) reimbursement.

Although Open Door found it difficult to recruit and retain specialist providers, it was able to hire a psychiatrist in 2004 to rotate among several clinic locations. While this hire enhanced the Center's ability to provide behavioral health services, the significant travel demands of up to several hours a day (also known as "windshield time" among providers) led the psychiatrist to leave Open Door after a year. Excessive travel demands were experienced by Open Door's patients as well. A 2005 survey conducted by Open Door found that its patients, on average, traveled 558 miles and 12 hours to see a specialist (Duclos et al., 2010).

These issues lead the Open Door to expand its current use of telehealth to provide specialty services to remote locations. Open Door first used telehealth in the late 1990s (working with the California Telemedicine and eHealth Center and sponsored by Blue Cross of California) to provide specialty consultation using a large computer screen, a video camera, and keyboard. The heaviest demand was for dermatology and psychiatry. To provide tele-mental health services, Open Door worked with a group of psychiatrists in Santa Rosa (200 miles south of the Center). Limited telehealth reimbursement ultimately limited the use of these psychiatrists and the service despite the relatively high demand for psychiatric services by Open Door's patients.

To enhance its telehealth services, Open Door opened the Telehealth and Visiting Specialist Center (TVSC) in 2006. TVSC is housed in its own building with significantly improved equipment (a Polycom VSX 5000 video conferencing unit) supported by foundation funding. TVSC enabled Open Door to centralize (and thus spread) the costs related to its telehealth programs, including connectivity, training, support staff, and equipment.

Open Door also received funding from the Health Resources Services Administration (HRSA) to expand the scope of its services, including those now provided through the TVSC. This allowed Open Door to charge a higher reimbursement that included the costs of the TVSC computer. In addition to providing services to its own clients through the TVSC, Open Door contracts to provide specialty services using telehealth to other organizations across California, thus working as both a "hub" as well as a "spoke" of telehealth services. In 2009, Open Door provided nearly 1,000 telehealth visits including 158 pediatric, 132 psychiatric, and 40 pediatric behavioral health visits (California HealthCare Foundation, 2010).

Open Door's experience suggests that telehealth can be used effectively to complement existing on-site mental health to persons spread over a very large rural area. However, Open Door's experience also suggests that the service must be large enough to incorporate other health services (in addition to mental health) in order to spread the costs of staff, equipment, and space across a wider array of services.

In 2003, the Minnesota Council of Health plans and the Minnesota Department of Human Services created the Minnesota Mental Health Action Group (MMHAG) to promote public–private partnerships and initiatives to improve access to quality mental health services. In 2007, the Governor's Mental Health Initiative built on the work of the MMHAG to: (1) develop a comprehensive mental health benefit for proven treatment across public and private plans; (2) integrate mental health and physical health services; and (3) make significant investments in mental health infrastructure (Minnesota Department of Human Services, 2007). Work on integration focused on developing integrated service networks that would receive reimbursement for providing integrated care under a "preferred integrated network" status. This effort resulted in the *DIAMOND Initiative* (Depression Improvement Across Minnesota Offering a New Direction) which was created in 2008. Under the DIAMOND initiative, ten primary care clinics across the state screen adult primary care patients for depression (using the PHQ-9) using a care management model. The integrative care management service is provided by a care manager for which the clinics receive a periodic depression care fee payment from the participating third-party payers. Support for the care manager is not time limited as it was under earlier demonstrations and the specific payment details are negotiated between each health plan and medical clinic. Minnesota is developing a bonus program to pay primary care physicians for providing quality depression care under a pilot program involving a coalition of the state's 40 largest employers (Mental Health Weekly, 2008).

Minnesota has taken a strategic path to integrating primary and behavioral health care that started with facilitating discussions among key players and later evolved to implementing focused regulatory and reimbursement changes. Noteworthy from a policy perspective are the development and continued use of viable public–private partnerships. Noteworthy from a practice perspective is the decision to reimburse for the integrative services provided by care managers. These services are not usually considered reimbursable services by many third-party payers. If they are covered, it is usually paid for as part of a demonstration project, which has proved to be a barrier to maintaining integration over time.

Cherokee Health Systems (CHS) spans 22 sites in 15 eastern Tennessee counties and is a frequently cited example of the integration of primary and behavioral health care in a rural setting (Cherokee Health Systems, 2010; Takach, Purington, & Osius, 2010). The agency started as a single site mental health center in 1960 and changed its name in 1973 to the Cherokee Guidance Center to de-stigmatize mental illness. School-based psychology services were established in 1970 and outreach to primary care began in 1980. CHS's involvement in primary care increased in 1984 when it established its first primary care clinic. In 1989, CHS was designated as the mental health carve-out provider in eastern Tennessee by HealthSource, a behavioral health management company that contracted with third-party payers to manage mental health benefits. In 1994, CHS was designated as the Behavioral Health Organization under the mental health program component of TennCare, Tennessee's Medicaid care program established under a Medicaid Waiver. CHS continued to add clinical services and locations, assisted by a series of Health Resources and Services Administration grants including: a 2002 Rural Health Outreach grant (to provide outreach and services to the growing Hispanic population in Grainger, Hamblen, and Jefferson Counties) and a 2003 Bureau of Primary Health Care (BPHC) grant to support the evolution of a number of sites into comprehensive community health centers (Cherokee Health Systems, 2010). In 2005, CHS received BPHC designation as a migrant health center. In 2009, the Tennessee Legislature and Board of Pharmacy approved Cherokee to operate a tele-pharmacy program at two locations (Takach et al., 2010).

Twelve of CHS's 22 sites are fully integrated with a licensed behavioral health specialist embedded within each primary care team through the use of a shared electronic health record. Primary care providers conduct the initial physical assessments which include screening for behavioral health issues. For appropriate patients, the primary care providers do "warm hand-offs" to the behavioral health consultants who provide brief targeted interventions and arrange for follow-up services as needed. Visits with the behavioral health consultants typically last between 15 and 25 minutes instead of the 45 to 50 minute visits that are common in traditional mental health settings. These consultants routinely see patients for a limited duration of time (one to three visits) instead of five or more visits as in traditional settings. This practice improves the behavioral health consultants' productivity and improves access to care. A psychiatrist is available for consultation either by telephone or telehealth technology. CHS also participates in the 340B Drug Pricing Program which provides access to reduced-price psychiatric medications for patients.

RURAL INTEGRATION IN A CHANGING POLICY ENVIRONMENT: THE ROAD AHEAD

As this chapter is written, a number of national trends and policy initiatives are likely to influence access to rural mental health care in the years ahead. While these trends and initiatives will evolve and change over time, they will almost certainly increase the demand for integrated behavioral and physical health care. In this last section, emerging trends and initiatives are described and suggestions are made for next steps that rural providers should consider in developing integrated services.

State Fiscal Pressures

As a result of the economic downturn, nearly all states were experiencing significant budget shortfalls and fiscal distress in 2010 (Rosenberg, 2010). In response, most states significantly reduced their general fund obligations, including funds committed to the state Medicaid match. Currently, state Medicaid programs are supported by a match of state and federal funds. Medicaid financing rules require states to spend their own funds to receive a federal financial match for Medicaid services. Each state dollar draws down an equal or higher number of federal dollars. As a result, many states have decreased reimbursement to community mental health providers and have increased or renewed the use of managed care programs to control state Medicaid spending for mental health services. This has contributed to a significant downsizing and consolidation of community mental health systems and reduced the supply of mental health clinicians and access to their services. As access to care in community mental health systems has declined, more persons with mental health and emotional issues have turned to integrated behavioral health programs for care. These persons are likely to have more serious and complex needs than in the past and there are fewer specialty mental health providers to consult with primary care providers.

At the same time that fiscal pressures constrain availability of specialty mental health services, the Paul Wellstone and Pete Domenici Mental Health Parity and Addiction Equity Act of 2008 (Public Law 110-343, Division C, Section 511, 2008, October 3) and the Patient Protection and Affordable Care Act (ACA) (Public Law 111-148, 2010, March 23) have increased legal and regulatory pressure to expand access to mental health care and for insurers to provide benefits equivalent to those provided for physical health services. Providers and service systems are being asked to do more with less. As previously noted, this is likely to result in more persons with more complex and severe mental health conditions seeking care through primary care providers. While this trend is not new, efforts to control specialty mental health spending in combination with expansion of access to services under parity legislation is likely to the accelerate the demand on primary care providers.

Another trend likely to increase the demand for service integration is the increasing policy focus on development of patient-centered medical homes (PCMHs). The basic concept is that all patients, but particularly those with chronic and complicated conditions, should have a primary medical home where their medical conditions and health can be managed and coordinated. At the core of the PCMH model is care management and support for the patient and an increased role for patients to direct their care in partnership with interdisciplinary teams of providers, typically directed by a physician. A number of states including Maine and North Carolina have implemented medical home pilot programs that call for the increased integration of behavioral and physical health services in their pilot sites (Gale & Lambert, 2009; Levis, 2006).

The ACA also included an option and resources for state Medicaid programs to provide chronic disease management to targeted Medicaid beneficiaries through health homes. States choosing this option must describe in their State Plan Amendments how the behavioral health needs of health home beneficiaries will be met. An important question is to what extent behavioral health will be included and integrated within medical homes, within Medicaid and elsewhere. The case for including behavioral health in medical homes is compelling; however, medical homes may very well run into the same workforce and financial barriers in including behavioral health that other programs and initiatives have (Gale & Lambert, 2009).

Another trend is the promotion by the specialty mental health sector of integrating primary care into behavioral health sites (sometimes referred to as "reverse integration"). The case for this is compelling on clinical grounds. Persons with a serious mental illness die, on average, 25 years younger than persons without a serious mental illness (National Association of State Mental Health Program Directors, 2006), suffer from higher rates of chronic illnesses, and routinely do not receive recommended courses of primary and preventive care; in addition, routine physical health screening is often not conducted in behavioral health settings (even if medications are being prescribed). To address this gap, the National Council for Community Behavioral Healthcare (NCCBH) has recommended that behavioral health providers assure regular physical health screening and tracking at the time of psychiatric visits for persons receiving psychotropic medications, including blood pressure, glucose and lipid levels, and body mass index (Mauer, 2009). The NCCBH currently serves as the Coordinating Center for the Substance Abuse and Mental Health Services Administration's Primary Care-Mental Health Initiative which promotes integration of behavioral health into primary care settings and integration of primary care into behavioral health settings. Until recently, the vast majority of integration efforts have involved the former rather than the latter despite the compelling need for both.

The Road Ahead

Earlier, much of the impetus and energy behind integration originated at the policy level, particularly the development and promotion of different models. While the policy level will remain very important, integration will ultimately succeed or fail at the clinical level. Changes occurring at the clinical level are unlikely to go away, regardless of the specific path that health care reform or patient-centered medical homes take.

Primary care clinicians will increasingly be asked to screen for a range of behavioral health problems and to treat or refer those patients as necessary. Given the shortage of specialty mental health services in rural areas, this is a role that will heavily affect rural primary care providers. In addition to direct care services, mid-level behavioral health providers will increasingly assume the role of a care manager for a range of behavioral and physical health issues. As described in the discussions of Community Health Partners in Montana and the Cherokee Health Systems in Tennessee, behavioral health specialists will be called on to see a greater number of patients but for shorter periods of time. They will also be asked to maintain the flexibility to see and engage patients as the need arises and to consult with the primary care team. Integrative skills will be as important as direct service clinical skills. While it is hoped that reimbursement policies will change to help support this new role, it is not clear as to whether reimbursement levels will be adequate to support this expanded behavioral health role.

PRACTICAL STEPS TO GETTING STARTED

Given this picture, how might rural primary care and behavioral health providers begin to undertake the development of integrated care programs? First, they should decide what their goals are and prioritize them. Do they want to expand access to mental health services within the general community or address the needs of patients within their clinics and settings? Are they focused on integrating services within their clinic (i.e., vertical integration) or improving the integration of services across practices within the community (i.e., horizontal integration)? Do they want to provide direct care or consultative services for primary care practitioners? Is their major focus on increasing the productivity of primary care providers or improving the coordination of care?

Next, providers should determine the best way to achieve each goal within the context of their practice settings and available resources. Recall that the evidence indicates that integrated care achieved positive outcomes but that improvements in outcomes did not increase as levels of provider integration or integrated process of care increased (Butler et al., 2008). This suggests that no single model of care integration is right for all settings. It is often best to view integration at the provider level as a "work in progress" by starting simply. This would involve assessing the practice's current readiness for integration and implementing an appropriate model of integration that is consistent with the clinic's capacity, resources, and patient needs. With experience, clinics can move further along the continuum of integration, as appropriate.

It is important to understand the functional elements of integration: clinical, administrative, and structural aspects of the care process can be managed to improve access, quality, patient and provider satisfaction, and efficiency. These structural components are important considerations as they drive how care is delivered and coordinated, how the patient is served, how information is shared, and where patients access the service. From a clinical standpoint, the functional issues that must be considered include the extent to which the practice and all providers: use a shared medical/health record; share clinical decision making; engage in regular communications in staff and clinical meetings; use common treatment plans and models; use critical pathways or practice guidelines; and refer patients between the services within the clinic. From an administrative/structural standpoint, the key issues are where the behavioral health services are located; the extent to which the behavioral health service is fully integrated into the clinic (i.e., the service is owned by the clinic and the behavioral health staff are employees of the practice) or a subcontracted service in which space is provided to external behavioral health staff to care for patients; the extent to which medical records, billing, and scheduling are shared by all services; and the extent to which the risk for the success of the service is shared by all parties.

It is also important for providers to avoid unnecessary competition for scarce resources within their organizations and communities. Unless a new provider is recruited to the community, expansion of services through hiring of clinicians in one setting will come at the expense of other clinics or agencies. At the very least, this may negatively impact on the relationship between agencies and existing referral patterns and service capacity.

It is very important to be clear about what services are being offered and how they fit the needs of patients. Is the service designed to expand access to traditional mental health services to address the needs of patients with episodic or chronic depression, anxiety, or mood disorders? Will the service target the needs of specific populations such as the elderly and/or children? Will the service target the behavioral health issues of individuals with chronic illnesses such as diabetes, obesity, and hypertension? These different types of behavioral health services are not fully interchangeable from the perspective of providers, patients, and third-party payers.

It is also very important to review and understand mental health reimbursement policies across the range of third-party payers covering the practice's patient populations. Procedure and diagnostic coding expertise is a skill that can heavily influence the success of an integrated service. The primary categories of procedure codes that may be used in integrated settings include:

- Evaluation and management codes used for the delivery of office, inpatient, and nursing home services to new and existing patients;
- Health and behavioral assessment codes used for the delivery of services provided to patients not diagnosed with a psychiatric problem, but whose cognitive, emotional, social, or behavioral functioning affect prevention, treatment, or management of a physical health problem; and
- Psychiatric codes used for the delivery of specific psychiatric services including initial psychological diagnostic interview exams, medication management, individual or group psychotherapy, and so on.

Third-party payers have different policies regarding which types of clinical providers can use each of these codes. It is important to check with individual programs and insurance carriers to verity their billing policies prior to developing specific services. It is also important to understand the managed care requirements (e.g., prior authorization, limits on number of visits) implemented by third-party carriers as this will influence levels of coverage and how services can be delivered. Providers can use this information to develop and implement an integrated service that best meets the needs of their practice and patients.

Developing integrated physical and behavioral health services can be a significant undertaking for providers, particularly in rural areas, as reflected in the examples provided in this chapter. Despite the challenges, it can also be a rewarding activity that improves the range and quality of services provided to patients and can enhance the satisfaction of providers practicing in rural integrated settings. Finally, evidence suggests that integration improves patient satisfaction which enhances patient loyalty and retention.

REFERENCES

Bird, D., Lambert, D., Hartley, D., Coburn, A., & Beeson, P. (1998). Integrating primary care and mental health in rural America: A policy review. *Administration and Policy in Mental Health, 25*(3), 287–308.

Bureau of Primary Health Care. (2003). *Program information notice 2003-03: Opportunities for health centers to expand/improve access to mental health and substance abuse, oral health, pharmacy services, and quality management services during fiscal year 2003.* Retrieved from http://ftp.hrsa.gov/bphc/docs/2003pins/2003-03.pdf

Butler, M., Kane, R., McAlpine, D., Kathol, R., Fu, S., Hagedorn, H., & Wilt, T. (2008). *Integration of mental health/substance abuse and primary care No. 173* (AHRQ Publication No. 09-E003). Rockville, MD: Agency for Healthcare Research and Quality.

California HealthCare Foundation. (2010). *Chronicling an entry into telehealth: Open door community health centers.* Retrieved from http://www.chcf.org/~/media/ MEDIA%20LIBRARY%20Files/PDF/O/PDF%20OpenDoorTelehealth.pdf

Cherokee Health Systems. (2010). *History of Cherokee health systems.* Retrieved from http://www.cherokeehealth.com/index.php?page=About-Us-Timeline

Doherty, W., McDaniel, S., & Baird, M. (1996). Five levels of primary care/behavioral health care collaboration. *Behavioral Healthcare Tomorrow, 5,* 25–27.

Duclos, C., Hook, J., & Rodriguez, M. (2010). *Telehealth in community clinics: Three case studies in implementation.* Retrieved from California HealthCare Foundation website: http://www.chcf.org/~/media/MEDIA%20LIBRARY%20Files/PDF/T/ PDF%20TelehealthClinicCaseStudies.pdf

Gale, J., & Lambert, D. (2006). Mental health care in rural communities: The once and future role of primary care. *North Carolina Medical Journal, 67*(1), 66–70.

Gale, J., & Lambert, D. (2008). *Maine barriers to integration study: Environmental scan.* Portland, MN: University of Southern Maine, Muskie School of Public Service.

Gale, J., & Lambert, D. (2009). *Maine barriers to integration study: The view from Maine on the barriers to integrated care and recommendations for moving forward.* Portland, MN: University of Southern Maine, Muskie School of Public Service.

Geiger, H. (1984). Community health centers: Health care as an instrument of social change. In V. W., Sidel, & R. Sidel (Eds.), *Reforming medicine: Lessons of the last quarter century* (pp. 11–32). New York: Pantheon Books.

Institute of Medicine, Committee on Crossing the Quality Chasm. (2005). *Quality through collaboration: The future of rural health: Quality Chasm Series.* Washington, DC: National Academies Press.

Institute of Medicine, Committee on Crossing the Quality Chasm: Adaptation to Mental Health and Addictive Disorders. (2006). *Improving the quality of health care for mental and substance-use conditions: Quality Chasm Series.* Washington, DC: National Academies Press.

Lambert, D., & Gale, J. (2006). *Integrating primary care and mental health services in rural community health centers.* Kansas City and Washington, DC: National Rural Health Association.

Lambert, D., & Hartley, D. (1998). Linking primary care and mental health: Where have we been? Where are we going? *Psychiatric Services, 49*(7), 965–967.

Levis, D. (2006). Piloting mental health integration in the community care of North Carolina program. *North Carolina Medical Journal, 67,* 68–70.

Mauer, B. (2003). *Behavioral health/primary care integration, models, competencies, and infrastructure: Background paper.* Rockville, MD: National Council for Community Behavioral Healthcare.

Mauer, B. (2009). *Behavioral health/primary care integration and the person-centered health care home.* Rockville, MD: National Council for Community Behavioral Healthcare.

Mental Health Weekly. (2008, June). Minnesota doctors will be eligible for bonuses tied to depression care. *Mental Health Weekly, 18*(22), 1–9.

Minnesota Department of Human Services. (2007). *Governor's mental health initiative: Fast facts. 2007 Legislative session.* St. Paul, MN: Minnesota Department of Human Services. Retrieved from http://www/mhcsn.net/DHS.pdf

National Association of State Mental Health Program Directors and National Association of State Alcohol and Drug Abuse Directors. (1998). *National dialogue on co-occurring mental health and substance abuse disorders.* Alexandria, VA: Author.

National Association of State Mental Health Program Directors and National Association of State Alcohol and Drug Abuse Directors. (2006). *Morbidity and mortality in people with serious mental illness.* Alexandria, VA: Author.

New Freedom Commission on Mental Health. (2003). *Achieving the promise: Transforming mental health care in America. Final Report.* (DHHS Pub. No. SMA-03-3832). Rockville, MD: U.S. Department of Health and Human Services.

Proser, M., & Cox, L. (2004, September). *Health centers' role in addressing the behavioral health needs of the medically underserved* (Special Topics Issue Brief No. 8). Washington, DC: National Association of Community Health Centers, Inc.

Public Law 110-343, Division C, Section 511: Paul Wellstone and Pete Domenici Mental Health Parity and Addiction Equity Act of 2008. (122 Stat. 3765, Division C, Section 511; 2008, October 3). Retrieved from http://www.gpo.gov/fdsys/pkg/PLAW-110 publ343/pdf/PLAW-110publ343.pdf

Public Law 111-148: Patient Protection, Affordable Care Act. (124 Stat. 119; 2010, March 23). Retrieved from http://www.gpo.gov/fdsys/pkg/PLAW-111publ148/pdf/PLAW-111publ148.pdf

Regier, D., Goldberg, I., & Taube, C. (1978). The de facto US mental health services system: A public health perspective. *Archives of General Psychiatry. 35*, 685-693.

Regier, D., Narrow, W., Rae, D., Manderscheid, R., Locke, B., & Goodwin, F. (1993). The de facto US mental health and addictive disorders service system: Epidemiologic catchment area prospective 1-year prevalence rates of disorders and services. *Archive of General Psychiatry, 50*, 85-94.

Rosenberg, L. (2010). Healthcare reform—Let's get down to business! *National Council Magazine, 2*, 6. Retrieved from http://www.thenationalcouncil.org/galleries/business-practice%20files/Mauer.pdf

Strosahl, K. (1998). Integrating behavioral health and primary care services: The Primary Mental Health Model. In: A. Blount (Ed.), *Integrated primary care: The future of medical and social mental health collaboration* (pp. 139-166). New York, NY: W.W. Norton & Company.

Takach, M., Purington, K., & Osius, E., (2010). *A tale of two systems: A look at state efforts to integrate primary care and behavioral health in safety net settings.* Portland, MN: National Academy for State Health Policy.

U.S. Department of Health and Human Services, National Institute of Mental Health. (1999). *Mental health: A report of the Surgeon General.* Rockville, MD: Author.

Wagner, E. (1998). Chronic disease management: What will it take to improve care for chronic illness? *Effective Clinical Practice, 1*, 2-4.

10

Technological Innovations in Rural Mental Health Service Delivery

SARAH E. VELASQUEZ, ANGELA BANITT DUNCAN, AND
EVE-LYNN NELSON

INTRODUCTION

*I*n many rural communities, mental health services are limited or nonexistent, with the majority of federally designated mental health professional shortage areas located in nonmetropolitan areas (Office of Shortage Designation, 2011). As discussed in Chapter 1, there are significant geographical and cultural challenges to seeking mental health services in rural areas. Technologies provide promising strategies to bridge this access gap to quality mental health services in rural communities (Institute of Medicine, 2004).

Technological advances make it possible for clients to interact with mental health specialists from almost any place in the world, anytime night or day, both in real and asynchronous time. This expanded access brings unique benefits and challenges in providing mental health services. In an American Psychological Association survey, psychologists indicated that they are increasingly using telephones and e-mail to provide services including psychotherapy, counseling, consulting, and supervision. According to the survey, over 60% of respondents used telephone contact with clients weekly (APA Center for Workforce Studies, 2010). E-mail use more than tripled among practicing psychologists between 2000 and 2008, with approximately 10% of providers using it weekly or more in 2008. Psychologists' use of videoconferencing, while still limited, increased from 2% to 10% during that same time period (APA Center for Workforce Studies, 2010).

In a comprehensive review, Hailey, Roine, and Ohinmaa (2008) found that the majority of evidence for the successful use of technology for mental health intervention, especially telephone and Internet technologies, was in the areas of child psychiatry, depression, dementia, schizophrenia, posttraumatic stress disorder (PTSD), panic disorder, substance abuse, eating disorders, preventing suicide, and cessation of smoking, with less evidence for obsessive-compulsive disorder (OCD), and minimal evidence for other mental health conditions. This chapter describes current telemental health service delivery approaches across the lifespan, specifically highlighting the following technologies: telephone, videoconferencing, mobile devices, computer-based assessment, and web/Internet. With so many new technologies emerging for mental health intervention, it is difficult to address all innovations. Because of this challenge, representative technologies within mental health service delivery have been chosen with the hope that lessons learned will be applicable across technologies. The research findings related to each technology are summarized with descriptions of advantages and challenges for implementation in rural settings.

TELEPHONE

Telephone technology was one of the earliest technologies to bridge the access gap in rural communities, and almost 90% of psychologists use the telephone at least monthly to provide direct services (APA Center for Workforce Studies, 2010). For direct mental health service delivery, telephone delivery has been shown promising for preventing suicide, diagnosing mental illness, reducing substance use, treating depression, and serving rural primary care (Baca, Alverson, Manuel, & Blackwell, 2007; Bischof et al., 2008; Bombardier et al., 2009; Brown, Saunders, Bobula, Mundt, & Koch, 2007; Mohr, Hart, & Marmar, 2006). Direct psychological care is variably defined, depending on the treatment context. More intensive interventions often include scheduled, repeated, evidence-based therapy delivered on a one-to-one basis by trained therapists who are supervised to ensure treatment fidelity. Each telephone call is typically aimed at 30 to 45 minutes in duration. Add-on components, such as letters or postcards, are also commonly used as reminders of upcoming visits or summarizations of the previous session's content.

One of the most studied telephone interventions is for the treatment of depression. Most protocols have delivered telephone psychotherapy as an adjunct to pharmacotherapy, with reduced cost and high treatment adherence (Ludman, Simon, Tutty, & VonKorff, 2007). In one of the largest randomized telephone-delivered trials delivered to 600 depressed primary care patients, Simon, Ludman, Tutty, Operskalski, and Von Korff (2004) found that a program combining telephone care management and brief, structured psychotherapy significantly improved outcomes for primary care patients initiating antidepressant treatment. The researchers underscored that the telephone format allowed therapists to use detailed agendas and checklists during therapy sessions, thus increasing consistency and treatment quality across patients. The researchers elaborate that while telephone programs may sacrifice the richness of traditional in-person therapy, the intervention helped engage patients who might not be reached by traditional in-person treatment. The telephone sessions eliminated travel and waiting time and allowed more flexible scheduling, factors critical in working with rural populations. Simon et al. (2004) summarize that telephone intervention may be particularly valuable within rural settings where access to psychotherapists is more limited, travel burdens are high, and the stigma attached to visiting a mental health provider may be greater.

Recently, cognitive-behavioral telephone therapy has been evaluated as a stand-alone treatment for depression. Tutty, Spangler, Poppleton, and Simon (2010) implemented a 10-session series of telephone-delivered cognitive-behavioral therapy (CBT)-based psychoeducation and motivational interviewing for 30 nonpsychotic adults. The intervention resulted in a 50% reduction of depressive symptoms for at least half of the participants, with 77% of participants completing more than eight telephone sessions, and 69% stating they were "very satisfied" with the treatment at 6-month follow-up. In addition, the cost of each telephone call was less than half of the cost of traditional face-to-face office visits. Mohr and his research team found promising early results with a similar telephone-delivered intervention with veterans (Mohr et al., 2006), although nonsignificant results were reported with a refractory population seen in community-based outpatient clinics (Mohr, Carmody, Erickson, Jin, & Leader, 2011).

In addition to depression intervention, Leach and Christensen (2006) summarize findings from telephone-based interventions across mental health diagnoses. They found that cognitive-behavioral therapy was the most widely used and adaptable to telephone delivery given the structured homework tasks, workbooks, and diaries. This approach may be most beneficial to rural settings as it allows for monitoring of progress and a basis for feedback. Similar to many telephone intervention studies, patients receiving telephone counseling for alcohol problems cited convenience, accessibility, control, and freedom to talk as major benefits (Reese, Conoley, & Brossart, 2006).

There may also be unique benefits with telephone delivery in some conditions. For example, Lovell et al. (2006) found that using the telephone for delivery of CBT for OCD yields the same outcomes as face-to-face encounters, but with less time required. In addition to direct service delivery, telephone technologies are also used to promote adherence to behavioral and mental health interventions. For instance, telephone calls have helped to increase adherence to continuing care plans following release from residential substance abuse treatment programs (Hubbard et al., 2007).

In addition to the direct mental health service interventions described above, telephone technology also supports consultative mental health service. Rural primary care providers are at the front lines in providing mental health services but face many challenges with time, mental health specialization, and other barriers to addressing mental health concerns. One innovative approach links rural-based primary care providers with metropolitan-based mental health specialists by telephone (Hilty, Yellowlees, Cobb, Neufeld, & Bourgeois, 2006; Sarvet, Gold, & Straus, 2011). The technology allows provider-to-provider consultation to support evidence-supported diagnosis and treatment of rural patients and has been used successfully in several states. The Massachusetts Child Psychiatry Access Project (MCPAP) is an excellent example of this provider-to-provider model and responds to mental health questions related to more than 6,000 youth/year (Sarvet et al., 2011). The state-supported initiative links rural primary care providers with regional child psychiatry teams offering consultation, care coordination, and educational programming. The program addresses a wide array of questions including assessment, treatment planning, psychiatric medications, resource navigation, and referral to face-to-face psychiatric care when needed. Consistent with medical home goals, the consultative model encourages collaborative care among the local primary care leader and the regional mental health team.

TELEVIDEO INTERVENTIONS

Televideo services allow the mental health provider to meet with the patient using real-time videoconferencing. Most commonly, the goal is to approximate face-to-face mental health intervention. As Richardson, Frueh, Grubaugh, Egede, and Elhai (2009) summarize, "the multisensory output and real-time quality of videoconferencing make it an attractive alternative to other technologies that access a narrower range of sensory modalities when assessing or intervening in mental health settings" (p. 323). Mental health interventions are among the most common applications of telemedicine specialties, particularly with psychiatry and a growing number of therapies. Consensus telemental health guidelines—drawn from numerous demonstration projects, programmatic evaluations, and a small but growing research base—suggest that televideo services are well received by providers and patients across the lifespan and varied diagnoses, with high ratings on measures of satisfaction, acceptance, and rapport (Grady et al., 2011). Early studies also suggest that the intervention is cost-effective. Evaluation and treatment over televideo have shown to be promising both with psychiatric and psychological interventions (Hilty, Yellowlees, Sonik, Derlet, & Hendren, 2009; Nelson, Bui, & Velasquez, 2011; Pesamaa et al., 2004).

Diagnostic efficacy studies have shown good reliability between most diagnoses over televideo and face-to-face with both children and adults, particularly when well-validated assessment tools are used (Ciemins, Holloway, Coon, McClosky-Armstrong, & Min, 2009; Grady et al., 2011; Richardson et al., 2009; Shore, Brooks, Savin, Manson, & Libby, 2007). In addition, a growing body of research suggests that televideo services are comparable to face-to-face services both in quality of care and patient/provider satisfaction in telepsychiatry and telepsychology (Grady et al., 2011; Myers, Palmer, & Geyer, 2011; Nelson & Bui, 2010; Van Allen, Davis, & Lassen, 2011). Advantages noted with the technology include reduced travel time and associated expense, reduced absence from work, fewer missed school days, reduced worry of stigma, shortened waiting time, and hastened treatment (Hilty et al., 2009; Paing et al., 2009). For providers, the acceptance of telehealth services has been largely driven by patient satisfaction (Hilty et al., 2009; Van Allen et al., 2011).

There is increasing evidence from randomized trials that videoconferencing-delivered interventions yield similar results as face-to-face encounters (De Las Cuevas, Arredondo, Cabrera, Sulzenbacher, & Meise, 2006; Garcia-Lizana & Munoz-Mayorga, 2010; Ruskin et al., 2004). For PTSD, cognitive behavioral interventions delivered face-to-face and over videoconferencing were effective in improving overall functioning (Frueh et al., 2007; Germain, Marchand, Bouchard, Drouin, & Guay, 2009). Bouchard et al. (2004) found that patients with panic disorder and agoraphobia who were treated via tele-video were just as likely to improve as patients who received face-to-face therapy. O'Reilly et al. (2007) found no difference between randomized face-to-face or videoconferencing consultations/brief follow-ups for patients with mixed psychiatric diagnoses. There have been clinical improvements in depression and/or anxiety with the use of CBT for rural clients (Griffiths, Blignault, & Yellowlees, 2006; Shepherd et al., 2006). Similarly, in a telemedicine-based collaborative care setting, antidepressants can be managed successfully via televideo (Fortney et al., 2006). Finally, telemedicine interventions have been successfully used to promote adherence to treatment regimens for patients with mental health concerns (Frangou, Sachpazidis, Stassinakis, & Sakas, 2005). While these results are promising, further research is needed to evaluate the efficacy and effectiveness of telemental health interventions across diagnoses and service settings (Myers et al., 2011; Richardson et al., 2009).

Videoconferencing interventions have become more feasible with the decreased equipment costs and expanded connectivity in urban and rural communities. Advantages include reduced travel times and cost, decreased lost work or school time, shortened wait times, and a heightened sense of personal control (Richardson et al., 2009). A strong benefit of the communication technology is the ability to link systems of care. This has been most discussed in relation to school-based telemedicine sites, which link the child, family, school personnel, and mental health specialist, but has great potential to increase communication with local primary care providers, other local patient providers, and patient advocates. The increased communication facilitates increased evaluation input as well as a team approach to implement and tailor treatment recommendations (Nelson & Bui, 2010).

Common barriers to televideo interventions include coordinator and provider concerns about proficiency with the videoconferencing technology. Consensus guidelines advise clear protocols and ongoing training to increase

confidence with using the technology (Grady et al., 2011). In addition, therapists must think creatively to adapt the session needs to the videoconferencing
setting, such as faxing handouts or supplying books to the rural site ahead of
the session (Shepherd et al., 2006). In addition, a comprehensive multidisciplinary approach across family needs is challenging in rural areas due to
limited or no referral options across health specialists (Office of Shortage Designation, 2011; Mohatt, Adams, Bradley, & Morris, 2006).

For mental health professionals, a major advantage of videoconferencing
is expanding services to high need rural populations without having to be
away from competing clinical responsibilities. There may be initial concerns
about developing a relationship with the distant site, defining expectations
for both the mental health professional and the telemedicine coordinator,
and engaging in new telemedicine roles. Initial onsite visits with the distant
site can help build a strong relationship and develop clear expectations
across parties.

MOBILE INTERVENTIONS

Mobile devices include personal digital assistant (PDA) devices and cellular
telephones. With the majority of today's devices including Internet access, use
in health and mental health applications is growing. There are several uses of
mobile technologies; however, they have been mostly used for self-monitoring
of target symptoms. Targeted mental health symptoms including depression
and anxiety can be monitored while patients go about their everyday business.
In the past, paper diaries were used for such monitoring, but there are many
challenges with consistent and long-term use of the traditional paper format.
Self-monitoring is most effective when it is maximally convenient and takes
place in real time to reduce recall bias and increase accuracy (Piasecki,
Hufford, Solhan, & Trull, 2007). Mobile devices meet this need as they are
immediately available and integrated in the individual's everyday activities.
Termed Ecological Momentary Assessment, or EMA, mobile phone monitoring
"captures the film rather than a snapshot of daily life reality of patients" (Myin-
Germeys et al., 2009, p. 1533).

Mobile devices have been established in behavioral health areas including
managing migraines, enhancing physical activity, ceasing smoking, and controlling weight (Proudfoot et al., 2010). While use with mental health problems is
more recent, mobile technologies have been used successfully to monitor
symptoms associated with anxiety, depression, psychosis, personality disorders, and substance abuse (Depp et al., 2010; Ebner-Priemer & Trull, 2009;
Heron & Smyth, 2010; Myin-Germeys et al., 2009).

Proudfoot et al. (2010) completed an extensive community survey in
Australia concerning community perception of mobile devices for symptom
monitoring and found very positive community attitudes toward use of the

technology, with the caveat that security features must first be assured. Respondents indicated a desire for feedback on monitoring information and for receiving self-help suggestions from such a mobile phone program. Advantages noted with mobile technologies include: assessing thoughts, feelings, and behaviors in real-time; monitoring clinical and context-specific changes; integrating psychological, physiological, and behavioral data; allowing real-time integrative feedback; and increasing external validity (Ebner-Priemer & Trull, 2009). However, some researchers in this area may question whether consistent and frequent real-time self-monitoring is healthy for patient engagement. Broderick and Vikingstad (2008) found that about 10% of individuals with a depressed mood became even more depressed post-EMA, compared to the 20% who reported improvements in depression symptoms upon completion of intensive EMA. Therefore, mental health professionals may ask patients about their experience with self-monitoring and address any emergent concerns resulting from self-monitoring. Mobile symptom monitoring tools have not been used as extensively as initially anticipated in mental health interventions (Piasecki et al., 2007). Major barriers to adopting mobile electronic tools may include the time-intensive process of learning and implementing the technology, a high cost of devices, a shortage of reimbursement from managed care, and limited research to date concerning clinical benefits (Piasecki et al., 2007; Trull & Ebner-Priemer, 2009).

To date, most mobile applications for mental health have focused on symptom monitoring. Early research supports text messaging via mobile devices as a strategy to increase adherence to behavioral modifications (Cole-Lewis & Kershaw, 2010; Fjeldsoe, Marshall, & Miller, 2009; Krishna, Boren, & Balas, 2009; Wei, Hollin, & Kachnowski, 2011). Furber et al. (2011) report a novel intervention providing clients with direct mobile phone access to their therapist in a youth outreach mental health service. They audited the text message content and found that it was a safe, practical way of maintaining contact and coordinating meetings.

COMPUTER-BASED TECHNOLOGIES

The use of computer-based technologies to assist in assessment and treatment of mental health disorders is increasing, particularly in communities with limited access to care such as rural settings. Computer-based assessment—sometimes called computer-assisted interviewing—is the computerized administration of measures to assess behavioral or mental health conditions (Bertollo, Alexander, Shinn, & Aybar, 2007). This type of assessment is mentioned for use in primary care facilities, jails, shelters, and job centers. Similarly, computer-based therapy is the use of a computer to assist in the treatment of mental health conditions, most often using Internet or web-based approaches. This type of mental health intervention can be used in mental health facilities, homes, schools, hospitals, and community resource centers (Cavanagh & Shapiro, 2004; Titov, Andrews, & Sachdev, 2010). Finally, web-based social media strategies are included within the computer-based section as another means of interaction and therapy for mental health issues.

Computer-Based Assessment

Computer-based assessment has been used across mental health conditions including anxiety, depression, suicidal feelings, and addiction (Emmelkamp, 2005). One study explored the use and satisfaction of electronic waiting room screening questionnaires to address problem behaviors—such as depression, substance abuse, and suicidal thoughts—and determined that the previsit assessment facilitated greater time toward addressing the problem behaviors during the billed visit (Chisolm, Gardner, Julian, & Kelleher, 2008). Researchers have also indicated that computer-based assessment dramatically reduces therapist time (Chisolm et al., 2008; Stuhlmiller & Tolchard, 2009). In addition, 60% of patients described themselves as "highly satisfied" with the program, with girls and older youths more satisfied than others (Chisolm et al., 2008). Similarly, another study assessed the satisfaction of patients using a handheld computer for assessment versus the conventional use of pen and paper, which resulted in most patients preferring the handheld computer as it was easier to use than the traditional method (Goldstein et al., 2010).

Other benefits have been associated with computer-based assessment. These include immediate scoring, availability of various languages, audio and visual presentation of questions, and accessibility (Bertollo et al., 2007; Cartreine, Ahern, & Locke, 2010; Stuhlmiller & Tolchard, 2009). This method of assessment or information collection can be beneficial to rural practices that might have limited staff for data entry. Rural practitioners without local access to mental health facilities may find this type of assessment beneficial for screening for mental health conditions as it partially counteracts the lack of access (Emmelkamp, 2005). The possibility of audio and visual presentation of questions may make this type of assessment available to those with special needs, such as the deaf and blind. There has also been some evidence that people are more likely to disclose private information about themselves to a computer rather than in face-to-face situations (Chisolm et al., 2008; Emmelkamp, 2005).

A major disincentive to using computerized assessment in rural areas is the lack of available treatment resources when mental health concerns are identified. This includes a lack of availability of providers trained to treat specific mental health conditions as well as a lack of availability of providers across language needs. Concerns about the equivalency of computer assessment to traditional methods have been expressed (Emmelkamp, 2005).

However, studies comparing computer-based and pencil and paper versions of assessments have demonstrated that computer-based assessments are equivalent (Emmelkamp, 2005; Goldstein et al., 2010); in addition, handheld computerized assessments also eliminate errors with data entry (Chisolm et al., 2008; Goldstein et al., 2010). Other concerns include the expense and the availability of computers to all patients (Stuhlmiller & Tolchard, 2009); however, new cost-friendly and widely available technologies, such as handheld tablets, may close this gap (Goldstein et al., 2010).

Computer-Based Therapy

There is a vast array of computer-based therapies. Early computer-based therapies used less interactive, computer-centered approaches, while most current applications use web-based, interactive materials. Computer-based therapies have been particularly used with cognitive-behavioral strategies for anxiety and depression (Khanna & Kendall, 2008), but have also been used across other mental health conditions including PTSD, phobias, OCD, and panic (Cavanagh & Shapiro, 2004; Klein et al., 2009). Web-based strategies are also promising with smoking cessation and alcohol treatments (Bewick et al., 2008; Bock, Graham, Whiteley, & Stoddard, 2008). Although web-based strategies are just beginning to be used with children and adolescents, web-based CBT shows encouraging results in youth with depression symptoms as well as other behavioral concerns (Calear & Christensen, 2010; Cuijpers, van Straten, & Andersson, 2008; Richardson, Stallard, & Velleman, 2010; Stinson, Wilson, Gill, Yamada, & Holt, 2009).

Computer-based therapies are diverse in format, with some programs self-guided and others therapist-guided. Some programs focus on psychoeducation and support components and some programs approximate elements of face-to-face mental health service delivery. Some newer applications integrate videochat with web-based content (Maheu & McMenamin, 2010). For example, Carlbring et al. (2005) demonstrated that a 10-module web-based CBT, combined with minimal therapy E-mails, was equivalent to the same content delivered in 10 individual weekly sessions for panic disorder, with results remaining equivalent at a 1-year follow-up. Another 10-week web-based bibliotherapy self-help program, along with short weekly telephone calls, was effective at treating panic disorder with or without agoraphobia (Carlbring et al., 2006). Shandley et al. (2008) found that a web-based program for panic disorder, Panic Online, was effective both when self-guided and when supported by a general practitioner or psychologist. For registered users completing a freely available 12-week CBT-based web program for panic disorder and agoraphobia, there were significant reductions in self-reported frequency and severity of panic attacks (Farvolden, Denisoff, Selby, Bagby, & Rudy, 2005). The same was true for those completing only three sessions of the program.

Overall, web-based CBT for panic has been shown effective; however, there are significant concerns with specific studies. For instance, Farvolden et al. (2005) only had 12 users (1%) complete the entire 12-week protocol, and Shandley et al. (2008) found a higher attrition rate for the group receiving support from a general practitioner compared to a psychologist. To date, web-based intervention studies have been focused on efficacy within controlled research studies. Studies on the horizon will investigate the effectiveness of web-based intervention in rural communities.

Overall, Internet-based interventions can improve mental health symptoms and have effect sizes comparable to similar face-to-face interventions, especially for those without access to traditional care (Garcia-Lizana & Munoz-Mayorga, 2010). In terms of web-based intervention, the majority of treatment studies conducted have been based on cognitive-behavioral therapy to treat depression, anxiety, and other mental health problems (Andersson, 2009). The versatile nature of web-based CBT makes it particularly amenable to broad use as it not only presents text, but also presents films, audio files, self-assessments, and discussion groups to facilitate patient learning and strengthen treatment effect (Andersson, 2009). Newer studies suggest that mental health providers can enhance their assessment and treatment of patients by integrating web-based applications into their methods of care (Cucciare, Weingardt, & Humphreys, 2009). The National Institute for Health and Clinical Excellence (2006) summarized findings across web-based CBT programs and concluded that the rate of clinical improvement with these programs was similar to more traditional treatment. However, the presence of a live therapist in addition to web-based treatment resulted in greater clinical improvements than web-based CBT alone (Andersson et al., 2005).

While CBT is the most commonly studied intervention noted, broader Internet-based applications for depression and anxiety include both self-help forums and clinical interventions. Compared to a control group, 20% of patients receiving either self-help forums or clinical intervention showed an improvement in depression scores at the end of 16 weeks, and there were no differences in adherence between the intervention groups (Clarke et al., 2005). Across both CBT and non-CBT therapy strategies, Ybarra and Eaton (2005) report evidence for the positive impact of mental health interventions across therapist-led and self-guided web-based approaches; they also call for the need for more research in this area. Meyer et al. (2009) found that an intervention based on multiple psychological theories significantly reduced symptoms of depression and improved social function. Other researchers (van Straten, Cuijpers, & Smits, 2008) found a problem-solving intervention effective for reducing depression and anxiety while improving quality of life.

Nonadherence to online treatment components and dropouts are challenges across computer-based therapies. Batterham, Neil, Bennett, Griffiths, and Christensen (2008) found that better adherence to a cognitive-behavior website was predicted by higher depression and/or anxiety severity, a greater level of dysfunctional thinking, younger age, higher education, being female, and being referred to the site by a mental health professional. In addition, those who experienced some benefit from the site were more likely to complete subsequent modules. Christensen, Griffiths, and Farrer (2009) reviewed the adherence rates of 16 randomized controlled trials of web-based interventions for depression and anxiety, and found that patients followed the treatment plan 43% to 90% of the time. Several reasons for dropout were reported with the most salient being time constraints, perceived lack of treatment effectiveness, lack of motivation, and improvement in condition (Christensen et al., 2009). Different strategies are used to increase adherence and decrease drop-out. For example, Neil, Batterham, Christensen, Bennett, and Griffiths (2009) found that adolescents randomized to a school setting accessed three times more online modules than adolescents in the community-delivered sample.

While gaps in access to the Internet, or the "digital divide," have decreased over the last decade, barriers remain, with almost one quarter of households not including an Internet user (Department of Commerce, 2010). The Department of Commerce report "Exploring the Digital Nation Home Broadband Internet Adoption in the United States" found that gaps continue to be more pronounced in rural areas. The elderly and poor constitute a large percentage of nonusers (Benight, Ruzek, & Waldrep, 2008). In addition, those in rural areas tend to use the Internet less than individuals living in urban settings, largely due to disparities in education, income, and broadband availability (Hale, Cotten, Drentea, & Goldner, 2010). Different strategies have been utilized to increase overall Internet access to health-related interventions in rural areas, including encouraging access at public venues including libraries and schools (Institute of Medicine, 2004; Mohatt et al., 2006).

Computer-assisted therapies may have the potential to create social isolation rather than encourage interaction (Battles & Wiener, 2002). There is some evidence indicating that individuals who are socially anxious may prefer online interactive technologies over face-to-face encounters in their daily life (Bonetti, Campbell, & Gilmore, 2010; Caplan, 2007). This could help explain why several computer-assisted therapies for social phobia are successful, but evidence is lacking regarding the translation of skills learned with online treatment to adaptive face-to-face interactions (Andersson et al., 2006; Titov, Gibson, Andrews, & McEvoy, 2009). Others express concern about the potential for web-based therapies worsening psychological disorders (Mihajlovic, Hinic, Damjanovic, Gajic, & Dukic-Dejanovic, 2008). Additionally, therapists hypothesize about the potential negative impact on the provider–patient relationship (Khanna & Kendall, 2008), although there is little information about this outcome in practice. Possible breaches of privacy have also been a concern; however, a search for literature on hacking or client identity mismanagement has not resulted in any evidence of a problem (Khanna & Kendall, 2008; Stuhlmiller & Tolchard, 2009).

On the other hand, 80% of American Internet users, amounting to about 113 million adults, have searched the Internet for information on several health topics, showing that the Internet is widely used for health-related applications (Fox, 2006). Web-based programs can also gather information faster and at a higher quantity than traditional assessments or treatments (Emmelkamp, 2005). Overall, Internet users have reported satisfaction with web-based mental health interventions and would recommend them to others (Meyer et al., 2009; National Institute for Health and Clinical Excellence, 2006; Titov et al., 2010). Significantly, the computer-based therapies have the potential to reach rural areas that would otherwise be without access to *any* mental health services (Farrell & McKinnon, 2003), and overall results to date have been comparable to face-to-face interventions. Other factors supporting the use of web-based applications include cost savings, convenience, easier dissemination, increased privacy, patient customization, improved standardization, multimedia inclusion, regular monitoring (Khanna & Kendall, 2008), and reduced isolation and stigma (Griffiths, Lindenmeyer, Powell, Lowe, & Thorogood, 2006). As with onsite therapy approaches, computer-based mental health interventions will be a better fit for some patients than others. Researchers call for increased theory-driven investigations and more rigorous methodologies in the field (Postel, de Haan, & De Jong 2008; Ritterband, Thorndike, Cox, Kovatchev, & Gonder-Frederick, 2009). More research is needed to understand the best "fit" of computer-based strategy with particular patient diagnoses and individual characteristics. This includes a consideration of therapy format (e.g., all online or supplement with online; self-guided or therapist guided, etc.), technology type (e.g., asynchronous versus real-time interaction), therapy length, and other components.

There are clearly some barriers to initiating computer-based therapy, as only about a third of patients will try computer-based CBT (Waller & Gilbody, 2009). Reasons for this lack of uptake could be due to a lower education level, a perception that the program is too demanding or fast paced, visual impairment, older age, and lack of time (Waller & Gilbody, 2009). However, Stulmiller and Tolchard (2009) state that when patient demographics are known, computer-based CBT is widely used by those of lower socioeconomic status. Patient safety may also explain a slow uptake of computer-assisted therapies, but some computer-based CBT programs have built-in mechanisms to alert providers of suicidal or homicidal ideation (Stuhlmiller & Tolchard, 2009). However, this does not address the existence of misguided and potentially harmful websites that can lead patients astray. For instance, Ipser, Dewing, and Stein (2007) found poor to moderate level quality for the content of anxiety disorder websites. Griffiths, Farrer, and Christensen (2007) advocate for increased provider involvement in selecting and referring patients to websites that are appropriate to their needs. However, the overall content quality of websites is lacking, and it is suggested that academic or specialized institutions create more evidence-based, comprehensive websites for patient use (Nemoto et al., 2007).

Residents in rural areas tend to be older, less educated, and of lower socioeconomic status—characteristics associated with less participation in overall online activity (Boase, 2010). Further, because these characteristics are common, rural social networks are likely to be homogenous, significantly impacting on the uptake of computer-assisted technology (Boase, 2010). These barriers to adoption should be considered when implementing computer-based therapies in rural communities in order to determine creative dissemination strategies, such as including local opinion leaders within outreach efforts.

SOCIAL MEDIA TOOLS

Social media and Web 2.0/3.0 technologies are described as "second generation medicine" and are anticipated to affect health by communication and collaboration among and between health care consumers, caregivers, patients, health professionals, and biomedical researchers (Eysenbach, 2008). In general and related to health, online social networking applications (e.g., Facebook, Twitter, YouTube, and many others) are one of the fastest-growing mechanisms to share personal and professional information. Chou et al. (2009) outline potential benefits associated with the technology, although research across health areas is in its infancy. First, the Internet-based social networks may increase perceived social support. Second, with the increase of user-generated content, the technology has the potential to generate patient/consumer-centered information sharing. Third, the technology has potential to disseminate public health behavioral interventions such as smoking cessation and dietary interventions. In addition to these benefits, indirect negative health impacts of social media have also been identified. First, the participatory nature of social media entails an open forum for information exchange, therefore increasing the possibility of wide dissemination of noncredible, and potentially erroneous, health information. Second, there are concerns of a "double divide," in which individuals without Internet access miss several avenues for health information.

Online social networking is becoming a popular form of communication and learning about health conditions, as well as its emergence as a marketing tool (Lukes, 2010). Because of this phenomenon, many mental health facilities are reaching out to patients using these networks. Facebook, the most popular and second most visited general social networking site in the world, has attracted many mental health facilities and organizations that are trying to reach out to possible patients or families of patients (Lukes, 2010). A general search on Facebook for "mental health" results in hundreds of pages and groups associated with mental health causes. Some are local facilities reaching out to their patients, while others are national organizations promoting education and awareness about mental health. As an example, organizations such as the American Psychological Association support a Facebook page providing news, research, tools, and discussions about mental health.

Although social networking can be a way for patients to find information and connect with others with similar conditions, the technology can have negative effects (Battles & Wiener, 2002). Some clinicians have expressed concern over the lack of face-to-face interaction associated with online networking. Others have suggested that increased time on social networking sites may be similar to an addiction. Studies on the effects of social networking on well-being have indicated that sites like Facebook can lower the self-esteem of users, which can be counterproductive to mental health treatment (Kalpidou, Costin, & Morris, 2010). Pediatrics leaders suggest that overuse of social media may precipitate depression (O'Keeffe, Clarke-Pearson, & Council, 2011). Sites may also be misused for cyberbullying, sexting, and other negative purposes, particularly among adolescents and young adults (Valkenburg & Peter, 2011). Because of the relative newness of these technologies, their use in rural areas has not been well investigated; however, they present additional opportunities for innovation in mental health service delivery.

TECHNOLOGY IMPLEMENTATION WITH MENTAL HEALTH INTERVENTIONS

The extensive technologies available to support mental health services across geographies bring exciting new potential to deliver high-quality mental health services. With these new opportunities come cautions in making sure that mental health providers continue to focus on the safety and well-being of patients (Paing et al., 2009). While technology-focused consensus guidelines and professional parameters provide direction, it is important to refer to overall best practices within mental health when introducing technologies (Grady et al., 2011; Myers & Cain, 2008). For example, the American Psychological Association advises that psychologists "... take reasonable steps to ensure the competence of their work and to protect clients/patients, students, supervisees, research participants, organizational clients, and others from harm" (American Psychological Association, 2002, Standard 2: Competence) and this guidance remains paramount when integrating technology into practice.

Technology-focused guidelines encourage transparency concerning the purpose of the technology related to mental health intervention. Questions to consider include: (1) is the technology meant to augment onsite therapy strategies or to replace them? and (2) is the technology meant to be a direct clinical service approach or a support strategy? Mental health professionals considering technologies in practice are encouraged to outline risks and benefits of the particular technology with the client. Risks/benefits may be readdressed over time in the context of the therapeutic relationship. In relation to mental health evaluation and treatment using technology, it may be useful to acknowledge the early state of the science of technologies in practice. Legal counsel can assist mental health professionals and organizations in developing such consent. Optimally, the mental health professional may outline treatment options both with and apart from the technology in order to allow choice. This is difficult when there are few other options available, as is frequently the case in rural settings.

Mental health professionals utilizing technology in practice must consider associated licensing and credentialing requirements, most notably when utilizing videoconferencing technology to approximate face-to-face, billable services. With these technologies, detailed and continuously updated telehealth protocols are encouraged. This includes backup plans with the local telemedicine coordinator in the event the patient reports suicidal, homicidal, abuse, or other safety concerns. As in traditional settings, expectations concerning therapist coverage should be outlined within the informed consent. In addition to the safety plans, the informed consent delineates who the patient is to contact with crisis needs. Practically, the mental health professional orients the family on what to expect when utilizing the technology, and discusses back-up plans if the technology fails. Consent documents may outline the expected role of both the mental health professional and the client. As in the traditional clinic setting, it is important to socialize clients and families to the mental health system and client rights as well as responsibilities.

New technologies also bring new challenges related to ensuring confidential treatment. Confidentiality/security risks relate both to the technology itself as well as the treatment setting. For example, with videoconferencing treatments, the therapist should describe the encryption procedures specific to the technology as well as procedures related to loss of therapist direct control over the physical environment. It is important to discuss with the patient who will have access to the information generated and potential confidentiality risks when utilizing the particular technology in the office, at home, or in other settings. When providing mental health services over technology, professionals should consider proficiency with the technology as well as with the target population, including competencies with rural patients. Ideally, mental health professionals will have mentors and receive ongoing training and peer support when with the technology-supported approach.

CONCLUSION

The research base, as well as national consensus guidelines, continues to move the telehealth field forward but much work remains as rural access gaps continue to grow. The technologies reviewed are used for different intervention purposes and each has unique strengths and weaknesses. With decreased technology costs and increased connectivity across geographies, we may see integrative practice in which several technologies are combined to deliver a strong intervention (Mohr, 2009). With such integration comes the potential for new paradigms of care that leverage the unique strengths offered by telecommunication technologies.

The recent Health Information Technology for Economic and Clinical Health Act (HITECH) legislation has the potential to positively impact other mental health technology approaches (HITECH, 2009). The HITECH legislation, which was signed into law in February 2009, provides $20 billion-plus in financial rewards to health care professionals for their "meaningful use" of health information technology, such as e-health record and computerized physician order entry systems. While the details of implementation are emerging, it is anticipated that the technological infrastructure for secure electronic exchange of data will complement other technology uses, such as telemedicine (American Telemedicine Association, 2006). The training and support in technology use (e.g., health information technologies regional extension centers) are also anticipated to encourage a technology-friendly environment that may facilitate adoption of the technology interventions reviewed in this chapter, particularly in primary care settings. Important gaps are still in the process of being addressed, with mental health and related professionals not included in the original HITECH legislation, but introduced in subsequent bills (McGee, 2010). In addition, leading federal agencies such as the Substance Abuse and Mental Health Services Administration (SAMHSA) include health information technology as a priority (SAMHSA, 2010).

Across the technologies described, mental health professionals and patients work together to select the technology that will best meet the client and family preferences, the developmental and diagnostic considerations, the personnel and other resources at the distant site, and the mental health professional's comfort (Myers & Cain, 2008). Challenges remain in training new and practicing mental health professionals in use of technologies and translating the technologies into existing mental health service delivery business models. The technology lessons learned to date, especially the importance of communication across client/family, mental health professional, rural support staff, and outreach community, remain important in order to deliver safe, high quality care. The next vista is to develop approaches to match empirically supported treatments with technology delivery systems and tailor these strategies to best fit the individual patients within their unique rural community (Institute of Medicine, 2004).

REFERENCES

American Psychological Association. (2002). *American Psychological Association ethical principles of psychologists and code of conduct.* Retrieved from http://www.apa.org/ethics/code/index.aspx

American Telemedicine Association. (2006). *Telemedicine, telehealth, and health information technology: An ATA issue paper.* Retrieved from http://www.americantelemed.org/files/public/policy/HIT_Paper.pdf

Andersson, G. (2009). Using the Internet to provide cognitive behaviour therapy. *Behaviour Research and Therapy, 47*(3), 175–180. doi: 10.1016/j.brat.2009.01.010

Andersson, G., Bergstrom, J., Hollandare, F., Carlbring, P., Kaldo, V., & Ekselius, L. (2005). Internet-based self-help for depression: Randomised controlled trial. *The British Journal of Psychiatry, 187,* 456–461. doi: 10.1192/bjp.187.5.456

Andersson, G., Carlbring, P., Holmstrom, A., Sparthan, E., Furmark, T., Nilsson-Ihrfelt, E., . . . Ekselius, L. (2006). Internet-based self-help with therapist feedback and *in vivo* group exposure for social phobia: A randomized controlled trial. *Journal of Consulting and Clinical Psychology, 74,* 677–686. doi: 10.1037/0022-006x.74.4.677

APA Center for Workforce Studies. (2010). Telepsychology is on the rise. *Monitor, 41*(3), 11.

Baca, C. T., Alverson, D. C., Manuel, J. K., & Blackwell, G. L. (2007). Telecounseling in rural areas for alcohol problems. *Alcoholism Treatment Quarterly, 25*(4), 31–45. doi: 10.1300/J020v25n04_03

Batterham, P. J., Neil, A. L., Bennett, K., Griffiths, K. M., & Christensen, H. (2008). Predictors of adherence among community users of a cognitive behavior therapy website. *Journal of Patient Preferance and Adherence, 2,* 97–105.

Battles, H. B., & Wiener, L. S. (2002). Starbright World: Effects of an electronic network on the social environment of children with life-threatening illnesses. *Children's Health Care, 31*(1), 47–68.

Benight, C. C., Ruzek, J. I., & Waldrep, E. (2008). Internet interventions for traumatic stress: A review and theoretically based example. *Journal of Traumatic Stress, 21*(6), 513–520. doi: 10.1002/jts.20371

Bertollo, D. N., Alexander, M. J., Shinn, M., & Aybar, J. B. (2007). An audio computer-assisted self-interviewing system for research and screening in public mental health settings. *Psychiatric Services, 58*(6), 743–745.

Bewick, B. M., Trusler, K., Barkham, M., Hill, A. J., Cahill, J., & Mulhern, B. (2008). The effectiveness of web-based interventions designed to decrease alcohol consumption—A systematic review. *Preventive Medicine, 47*(1), 17–26. doi: 10.1016/j.ypmed.2008.01.005

Bischof, G., Grothues, J. M., Reinhardt, S., Meyer, C., John, U., & Rumpf, H. J. (2008). Evaluation of a telephone-based stepped care intervention for alcohol-related disorders: A randomized controlled trial. *Drug and Alcohol Dependence, 93*(3), 244–251. doi: 10.1016/j.drugalcdep.2007.10.003

Boase, J. (2010). Consequence of rural networks for high-speed internet adoption and email use. *American Behavioral Scientist, 53*(9), 1257–1267.

Bock, B. C., Graham, A. L., Whiteley, J. A., & Stoddard, J. L. (2008). A review of web-assisted tobacco interventions (WATIs). *Journal of Medical Internet Research, 10*(5), e39. doi: 10.2196/jmir.989

Bombardier, C. H., Bell, K. R., Temkin, N. R., Fann, J. R., Hoffman, J., & Dikmen, S. (2009). The efficacy of a scheduled telephone intervention for ameliorating depressive symptoms during the first year after traumatic brain injury. *Journal of Head Trauma and Rehabilitation, 24*(4), 230–238. doi: 10.1097/HTR.0b013e3181ad65f0

Bonetti, L., Campbell, M. A., & Gilmore, L. (2010). The relationship of loneliness and social anxiety with children's and adolescents' online communication. *Cyberpsychology, Behavior, and Social Networking, 13*, 279–285. Retrieved from: http://www.liebertpub.com/products/product.aspx?pid=10

Bouchard, S., Paquin, B., Payeur, R., Allard, M., Rivard, V., Fournier, T., ... Lapierre, J. (2004). Delivering cognitive-behavior therapy for panic disorder with agoraphobia in videoconference. *Journal of Telemedicine and e-Health, 10*, 13–25.

Broderick, J. E., & Vikingstad, G. (2008). Frequent assessment of negative symptoms does not induce depressed mood. *Journal of Clinical Psychology in Medical Settings, 15*, 296–300.

Brown, R. L., Saunders, L. A., Bobula, J. A., Mundt, M. P., & Koch, P. E. (2007). Randomized-controlled trial of a telephone and mail intervention for alcohol use disorders: Three-month drinking outcomes. *Alcohol Clinical and Experimental Research, 31*(8), 1372–1379. doi: 10.1111/j.1530-0277.2007.00430.x

Calear, A. L., & Christensen, H. (2010). Review of internet-based prevention and treatment programs for anxiety and depression in children and adolescents. *Medical Journal of Australia, 192*(Suppl 11), S12–S14.

Caplan, E. (2007). Relations among loneliness, social anxiety, and problematic internet use. *Cyberpsychology and Behavior, 10*, 234–242. doi: 10.1089/cpb.2006.9963

Carlbring, P., Bohman, S., Brunt, S., Buhrman, M., Westling, B. E., Ekselius, L., & Andersson, G. (2006). Remote treatment of panic disorder: A randomized trial of internet-based cognitive-behavior therapy supplemented with telephone calls. *American Journal of Psychiatry, 163*, 2119–2125. doi: 10.1176/appi.ajp.163.12.2119

Carlbring, P., Nilsson-Ihrfelt, E., Waara, J., Kollenstam, C., Buhrman, M., Kaldo, V. et al. (2005). Treatment of panic disorder: Live therapy vs. self-help via the internet. *Behaviour Research and Therapy, 43*, 1321–1333. doi: 10.1016/j.brat.2004.10.002

Cartreine, J. A., Ahern, D. K., & Locke, S. E. (2010). A roadmap to computer-based psychotherapy in the United States. *Harvard Review of Psychiatry, 18*(2), 80–95.

Cavanagh, K., & Shapiro, D. A. (2004). Computer treatment for common mental health problems. *Journal of Clinical Psychology, 60*(3), 239–251. doi: 10.1002/jclp.10261

Chisolm, D. J., Gardner, W., Julian, T., & Kelleher, K. J. (2008). Adolescent satisfaction with computer-assisted behavioural risk screening in primary care. *Child and Adolescent Mental Health, 13*(4), 163–168.

Christensen, H., Griffiths, K. M., & Farrer, L. (2009). Adherence in internet interventions for anxiety and depression. *Journal of Medical Internet Research, 11*(2), e13. doi: 10.2196/jmir.1194

Chou, W. S., Hunt, Y. M., Beckjord, E. B., Moser, R. P., & Hesse, B. W. (2009). Social media use in the United States: Implications for health communication. *Journal of Medical Internet Research, 11*(4), e48.

Ciemins, E. L., Holloway, B., Coon, P. J., McClosky-Armstrong, T., & Min, S. J. (2009). Telemedicine and the mini-mental state examination: Assessment from a distance. *Journal of Telemedicine and e-Health, 15*(5), 476–478. doi: 10.1089/tmj.2008.0144

Clarke, G., Eubanks, D., Reid, E., Kelleher, C., O'Connor, E., DeBar, L. L., ... Gullion, C. (2005). Overcoming depression on the internet (ODIN) (2): A randomized trial of a self-help depression skills program with reminders. *Journal of Medical Internet Research, 7*(2), e16. doi: 10.2196/jmir.7.2.e16

Cole-Lewis, H., & Kershaw, T. (2010). Text messaging as a tool for behavioral change in disease prevention and management. *Epidemiologic Reviews, 32*, 56–69.

Cucciare, M. A., Weingardt, K. R., & Humphreys, K. (2009). How Internet technology can improve the quality of care for substance use disorders. *Current Drug Abuse Reviews, 2*(3), 256–262.

Cuijpers, P., van Straten, A., & Andersson, G. (2008). Internet-administered cognitive behavior therapy for health problems: A systematic review. *Journal of Behavioral Medicine, 31*, 169–177. doi: 10.1007/s10865-007-9144-1

De Las Cuevas, C., Arredondo, M. T., Cabrera, M. F., Sulzenbacher, H., & Meise, U. (2006). Randomized clinical trial of telepsychiatry through videoconference versus face-to-face conventional psychiatric treatment. *Journal of Telemedicine and e-Health, 12*(3), 341–350. doi: 10.1089/tmj.2006.12.341

Department of Commerce, Economics and Statistics Administration. (2010). *Exploring the digital nation: Home broadband internet adoption in the United States.* Retrieved from http://www.esa.doc.gov/Reports/exploring-digital-nation-home-broadband-internet-adoption-united-states

Depp, C. A., Mausbach, B., Granholm, E., Cardenas, V., Ben-Zeev, D., Patterson, T. L., . . . Jeste, D. V. (2010). Mobile interventions for severe mental illness: Design and preliminary data from three approaches. *Journal of Nervous and Mental Disease, 198*(10), 715–721. doi: 10.1097/NMD.0b013e3181f49ea3

Ebner-Priemer, U. W., & Trull, T. J. (2009). Ecological momentary assessment of mood disorders and mood dysregulation. *Psychological Assessment, 21*(4), 463–475. doi: 10.1037/a0017075

Emmelkamp, P. M. (2005). Technological innovations in clinical assessment and psychotherapy. *Psychotherapy and Psychosomatics, 74*(6), 336–343.

Eysenbach, G. (2008). Medicine 2.0: Social networking, collaboration, participations, apomediation, and openness. *Journal of Medical Internet Research, 10*(3), e22.

Farrell, S. P., & McKinnon, C. R. (2003). Technology and rural mental health. *Archives of Psychiatric Nursing, 17*(1), 20–26. doi: 10.1053/apnu.2003.4

Farvolden, P., Denisoff, E., Selby, P., Bagby, R. M., & Rudy, L. (2005). Usage and longitudinal effectiveness of a web-based self-help cognitive behavioral therapy program for panic disorder. *Journal of Medical Internet Research, 7*(1), e7. doi: 10.2196/jmir.7.1.e7

Fjeldsoe, B. S., Marshall, A. L., & Miller, Y. D. (2009). Behavior change interventions delivered by mobile telephone short-message service. *American Journal of Preventive Medicine, 36*, 165–173. doi: 10.1016/j.amepre.2008.09.040

Fortney, J. C., Pyne, J. M., Edlund, M. J., Robinson, D. E., Mittal, D., & Henderson, K. L. (2006). Design and implementation of the telemedicine-enhanced antidepressant management study. *General Hospital Psychiatry, 28*(1), 18–26.

Fox, S. (2006, October). Most internet users start at a search engine when looking for health information online. *Pew Research Center's Internet & American Life Project.* Retrieved from http://www.pewinternet.org/Press-Releases/2006/Most-internet-users-start-at-a-search-engine-when-looking-for-health-information-online.aspx

Frangou, S., Sachpazidis, I., Stassinakis, A., & Sakas, G. (2005). Telemonitoring of medication adherence in patients with schizophrenia. *Journal of Telemedicine and e-Health, 11*(6), 675–683.

Frueh, B. C., Monnier, J., Grubaugh, A. L., Elhai, J. D., Yim, E., & Knapp, R. (2007). Therapist adherence and competence with manualized cognitive-behavioral therapy for PTSD delivered via videoconferencing technology. *Behavior Modification, 31*(6), 856–866. doi: 10.1177/0145445507302125

Furber, G. V., Crago, A. E., Meehan, K., Sheppard, T. D., Hooper, K, Abbot, D. T., . . . Skene, C. (2011). How adolescents use SMS (short message service) to micro-coordinate contact with youth mental health outreach services. *Journal of Adolescent Health, 48*(1), 113–115.

Garcia-Lizana, F., & Munoz-Mayorga, I. (2010). Telemedicine for depression: A systematic review. *Perspectives in Psychiatric Care, 46*(2), 119–126. doi: 10.1111/j.1744-6163.2010.00247.x

Germain, V., Marchand, A., Bouchard, S., Drouin, M. S., & Guay, S. (2009). Effectiveness of cognitive behavioural therapy administered by videoconference for posttraumatic stress disorder. *Cognitive Behaviour Therapy, 38*(1), 42–53. doi: 10.1080/16506070802473494

Goldstein, L. A., Connolly Gibbons, M. B., Thompson, S. M., Scott, K., Heintz, L., Green, P., . . . Crits-Christoph, P. (2010). Outcome assessment via handheld computer in community mental health: Consumer satisfaction and reliability. *Journal of Behavioral Health Services & Research, 38*(3), 414–423.

Grady, B., Myers, K. M., Nelson, E. L., Belz, N., Bennett, L., Carnahan, L., . . . Voyles, D. (2011). Evidence-based practice for telemental health. *Telemedicine Journal & e-Health. 17*(2), 131–148.

Griffiths, L., Blignault, I., & Yellowlees, P. (2006). Telemedicine as a means of delivering cognitive-behavioural therapy to rural and remote mental health clients. *Journal of Telemedicine and Telecare, 12*(3), 136–140.

Griffiths, K., Farrer, L., & Christensen, H. (2007). Clickety-click: E-mental health train on track. *Australasian Psychiatry, 15*(2), 100–108.

Griffiths, F., Lindenmeyer, A., Powell, J., Lowe, P., & Thorogood, M. (2006). Why are health care interventions delivered over the internet? A systematic review of the published literature. *Journal of Medical Internet Research, 8*(2), e10. doi: 10.2196/jmir.8.2.e10

Hailey, D., Roine, R., & Ohinmaa, A. (2008). The effectiveness of telemental health applications: A review. *The Canadian Journal of Psychiatry, 53*(11), 769–778.

Hale, T. M., Cotten, S. R., Drentea, P., & Goldner, M. (2010). Rural–urban differences in general and health-related Internet use. *American Behavioral Scientist, 53*(9), 1304–1325. doi: 10.1177/0002764210361685

Health Information Technology for Economic and Clinical Health Act. (2009). *HIPAA and HITECH.* Retrieved from http://www.hipaasurvivalguide.com/hitech-act-text.php

Heron, K. E., & Smyth, J. M. (2010). Ecological momentary interventions: Incorporating mobile technology into psychosocial and health behaviour treatments. *British Journal of Health Psychology, 15*, 1–39. doi: 10.1348/135910709X466063

Hilty, D. M., Yellowlees, P. M., Cobb, H. C., Neufeld, J. D., & Bourgeois, J. A. (2006). Use of secure email and telephone: Psychiatric consultations to accelerate rural health service delivery. *Telemedicine and E-health, 12*, 490–495. doi: 10.1089/tmj.2006.12.490

Hilty, D. M., Yellowlees, P. M., Sonik, P., Derlet, M., & Hendren, R. L. (2009). Rural child and adolescent telepsychiatry: Successes and struggles. *Pediatric Annals, 38*(4), 228–232.

Hubbard, R. L., Leimberger, J. D., Haynes, L., Patkar, A. A., Holter, J., Liepman, M. R., ... Hasson, A. (2007). Telephone enhancement of long-term engagement (TELE) in continuing care for substance abuse treatment: A NIDA clinical trials network (CTN) study. *American Journal on Addictions, 16*(6), 495–502. doi: 10.1080/10550490701641678

Institute of Medicine, Committee on the Future of Rural Health Care. (2004). *Quality through collaboration: The future of rural mental health.* Washington, DC: National Academies Press.

Ipser, J. C., Dewing, S., & Stein, D. J. (2007). A systematic review of the quality of information on the treatment of anxiety disorders on the internet. *Current Psychiatry Reports, 9*, 303–309.

Kalpidou, M., Costin, D., & Morris, J. (2010). The relationship between facebook and the well-being of undergraduate college students. *Cyberpsychology, Behavior, and Social Networking.* Advance online publication. doi: 10.1089/cyber.2010.0061

Khanna, M. S., & Kendall, P. C. (2008). Computer-assisted CBT for child anxiety the Coping Cat CD-ROM. *Cognitive and Behavioral Practice, 15*, 159–165.

Klein, B., Mitchell, J., Gilson, K., Shandley, K., Austin, D., Kiropoulos, L., ... Cannard, G. (2009). A therapist-assisted internet-based CBT intervention for posttraumatic stress disorder: Preliminary results. *Cognitive Bahviour Therapy, 38*(2), 121–131.

Krishna, S., Boren, S. A., & Balas, E. A. (2009). Healthcare via cell phones: A systematic review. *Journal of Telemedicine and e-Health, 15*, 231–240. doi: 10.1089/tmj.2008.0099

Leach, L. S., & Christensen, H. (2006). A systematic review of telephone-based interventions for mental disorders. *Journal of Telemedicine and Telecare, 12*(3), 122–129. doi: 10.1258/135763306776738558

Lovell, K., Cox, D., Haddock, G., Jones, C., Raines, D., Garvey, R., & ... Hadley, S. (2006). Telephone administered cognitive-behaviour therapy for treatment of obsessive-compulsive disorder: Randomized controlled non-inferiority trial. *British Medical Journal, 333*, 883–887.

Ludman, E., Simon, G. E., Tutty, S., & VonKorff, M. (2007). A randomized trial of telephone psychotherapy and pharmacotherapy for depression: Continuation and durability effects. *Journal of Consulting and Clinical Psychology, 5*, 257–266.

Lukes, C. A. (2010). Social media. *AAOHN Journal, 58*(10), 415–417. doi: 10.3928/08910162-20100928-02

Maheu, M. M., & McMenamin, J. (2010, August). *Legal, ethical & reimbursement solutions for the immediate implementation of telehealth & telepsychology in defined settings.* Presented at the 118th American Psychological Association Annual Convention, Division 31, San Diego, CA.

McGee, M. K. (2010, April). Bill extends HITECH to mental health. *InformationWeek: Health Care.* Retrieved from http://www.informationweek.com/news/healthcare/EMR/showArticle.jhtml?articleID = 2

Meyer, B., Berger, T., Caspar, F., Beevers, C. G., Andersson, G., & Weiss, M. (2009). Effectiveness of a novel integrative online treatment for depression (Deprexis): Randomized controlled trial. *Journal of Medical Internet Research, 11*(2), e15. doi: 10.2196/jmir.1151

Mihajlovic, G., Hinic, D., Damjanovic, A., Gajic, T., & Dukic-Dejanovic, S. (2008). Excessive internet use and depressive disorders. *Psychiatria Danubina, 20*(1), 6-15.

Mohatt, D., Adams, S. J., Bradley, M. M., & Morris, C. A. (2006). *Mental health and rural America: 1994-2005.* U.S. Department of Health and Human Services, Health Resources and Services Administration, Office of Rural Health Policy. Retrieved from ftp://ftp.hrsa.gov/ruralhealth/RuralMentalHealth.pdf

Mohr, D. C. (2009). Telemental health: Reflections on how to move the field forward. *Clinical Psychology Science and Practice, 16*(3), 343-347. doi: 10.1111/ j.1468-2850.2009.01172.x

Mohr, D. C., Carmody, T., Erickson, L., Jin, L., & Leader, J. (2011). Telephone-administered cognitive behavioral therapy for veterans served by community-based outpatient clinics. *Journal of Consulting and Clinical Psychology, 79*(2), 261-265.

Mohr, D. C., Hart, S. L., & Marmar, C. (2006). Telephone administered cognitive-behavioral therapy for the treatment of depression in a rural primary care clinic. *Cognitive Therapy and Research, 30*(1), 29-37. doi: 10.1007/s10608-006-9006-0

Myers, K., & Cain, S. (2008). Practice parameter for telepsychiatry with children and adolescents. *Journal of the American Academy of Child and Adolescent Psychiatry, 47*(12), 1468-1483.

Myers, K. M., Palmer, N. B., & Geyer, J. R. (2011). Research in child and adolsecent telemental health. *Child and Adolescent Psychiatric Clinics of North America, 20,* 155-171. doi: 10.1016/j.chc.2010.08.007

Myin-Germeys, I., Oorschot, M., Collip, D., Lataster, J., Delespaul, P., & van Os, J. (2009). Experience sampling research in psychopathology: Opening the black box of daily life. *Psycholgical Medicine, 39*(9), 1533-1547. doi: 10.1017/s0033291708 004947

National Institute for Health and Clinical Excellence. (2006). *Computerised cognitive behaviour therapy for depression and anxiety: Review of Technology Appraisal 51.* London: Author.

Neil, A. L., Batterham, P., Christensen, H., Bennett, K., & Griffiths, K. M. (2009). Predictors of adherence by adolescents to a cognitive behavior therapy website in school and community-based settings. *Journal Medical Internet Research, 11*(1), e6. doi: 10.2196/jmir.1050

Nelson, E. L., & Bui, T. (2010). Rural telepsychology services for children and adolescents. *Journal of Clinical Psychology, 66*(5), 490-501.

Nelson, E. L., Bui, T. N., & Velasquez, S. E. (2011). Telepsychology: Research and practice overview. *Child and Adolescent Psychiatric Clinics of North America, 20*(1), 67-79.

Nemoto, K., Tachikawa, H., Sodeyama, N., Endo, G., Hashimoto, K., Mizukami, K. et al. (2007). Quality of internet information referring to mental health and mental disorders in Japan. *Psychiatry and Clinical Neurosciences, 61*(3), 243-248.

Office of Shortage Designation, Bureau of Health Professions Health Resources and Services Administration (HRSA), U.S. Department of Health & Human Services. (2011). *Health Professional Shortage Areas (HPSA): Metropolitan/Non-Metropolitan Classification as of February 11, 2011.* Retrieved from http://ersrs.hrsa.gov/ ReportServer?/HGDW_Reports/BCD_HPSA/BCD_HPSA_SCR50_Smry&rs:Format=HTML3.2

O'Keeffe, G. S., Clarke-Pearson, K. & Council on Communications and Media. (2011). The impact of social media on children, adolescents, and families. *Pediatrics, 127,* 800-804.

O'Reilly, R., Bishop, J., Maddox, K., Hutchinson, L., Fisman, M., & Takhar, J. (2007). Is telepsychiatry equivalent to face-to-face psychiatry? Results from a randomized controlled equivalence trial. *Psychiatric Services, 58,* 836–843.

Paing, W. W., Weller, R. A., Welsh, B., Foster, T., Birnkrant, J. M., & Weller, E. B. (2009). Telemedicine in children and adolescents. *Current Psychiatry Reports, 11*(2), 114–119.

Pesamaa, L., Ebeling, H., Kuusimakil, M. L., Winblad, I., Isohanni, M., & Moilanen, I. (2004). Videoconferencing in child and adolescent telepsychiatry: A systematic review of the literature. *Journal of Telemedicine and Telecare, 10,* 187–192. doi: 10.1258/1357633041424458

Piasecki, T. M., Hufford, M. R., Solhan, M., & Trull, T. J. (2007). Assessing clients in their natural environments with electronic diaries: Rationale, benefits, limitations, and barriers. *Psychological Assessment, 19*(1), 25–43. doi: 10.1037/1040-3590.19.1.25

Postel, M. G., de Haan, H. A., & De Jong, C. A. (2008). E-therapy for mental health problems: A systematic review. *Telemedicine Journal of E-Health, 14*(7), 707–714. doi: 10.1089/tmj.2007.0111

Proudfoot, J., Parker, G., Hadzi Pavlovic, D., Manicavasagar, V., Adler, E., & Whitton, A. (2010). Community attitudes to the appropriation of mobile phones for monitoring and managing depression, anxiety, and stress. *Journal of Medical Internet Research, 12*(5), e64.

Reese, R. J., Conoley, C. W., & Brossart, D. F. (2006). The attractiveness of telephone counseling: An empirical investigation of client perceptions. *Journal of Counseling and Development, 84*(1), 54–60.

Richardson, L. K., Frueh, B. C., Grubaugh, A. L., Egede, L., & Elhai, J. D. (2009). Current directions in videoconferencing tele-mental health research. *Clinical Psychology, 16*(3), 323–338. doi: 10.1111/j.1468-2850.2009.01170.x

Richardson, T., Stallard, P., & Velleman, S. (2010). Computerised cognitive behavioral therapy for the prevention and treatment of depression and anxiety in children and adolescents: A systematic review. *Clinical Child and Family Psychology Review, 13,* 275–290.

Ritterband, L. M., Thorndike, F. P., Cox, D. J., Kovatchev, B. P., & Gonder-Frederick, L. A. (2009). A behavior change model for internet interventions. *Annals of Behavioral Medicine, 38*(1), 18–27. doi: 10.1007/s12160-009-9133-4

Ruskin, P. E., Silver-Aylaian, M., Kling, M. A., Reed, S. A., Bradham, D. D., Hebel, J. R., . . . Hauser, P. (2004). Treatment outcomes in depression: Comparison of remote treatment through telepsychiatry to in-person treatment. *American Journal of Psychiatry, 161,* 1471–1476.

Sarvet, B., Gold, J., & Straus, J. (2011). Bridging the divide between child psychiatry and primary care: The use of telephone consultation within a population-based collaborative system. *Child & Adolescent Psychiatric Clinics of North America, 20,* 41–53.

Shandley, K., Austin, D. W., Klein, B., Pier, C., Schattner, P., Pierce, D. et al. (2008). Therapist-assisted, Internet-based treatment for panic disorder: Can general practitioners achieve comparable patient outcomes to psychologists? *Journal Medical Internet Research, 10*(2), e14. doi: 10.2196/jmir.1033

Shepherd, L., Goldstein, D., Whitford, H., Thewes, B., Brummell, V., & Hicks, M. (2006). The utility of videoconferencing to provide innovative delivery of psychological treatment for rural cancer patients: Results of a pilot study. *Journal of Pain and Symptom Management, 32,* 453–461. doi: 10.1016/j.jpainsymman.2006.05.018

Shore, J. H., Brooks, E., Savin, D. M., Manson, S. M., & Libby, A. M. (2007). An economic evaluation of telehealth data collection with rural populations. *Psychiatric Services*, *58*(6), 830–835. doi: 10.1176/appi.ps.58.6.830

Simon, G. E., Ludman, E. J., Tutty, S., Operskalski, B., & Von Korff, M. (2004). Telephone psychotherapy and telephone care management for primary care patients starting antidepressant treatment: A randomized controlled trial. *JAMA*, *292*(8), 935–942.

Stinson, J., Wilson, R., Gill, N., Yamada, J., & Holt, J. (2009). A systematic review of internet-based self-management interventions for youth with health conditions. *Journal of Pediatric Psychology*, *34*, 495–510. doi: 10.1093/jpepsy/jsn115

Stuhlmiller, C., & Tolchard, B. (2009). Computer-assisted CBT for depression & anxiety: Increasing accessibility to evidence-based mental health treatment. *Journal of Psychosocial Nursing & Mental Health Services*, *47*(7), 32–39.

Substance Abuse and Mental Health Services Administration. (2010). *SAMHSA's Eight Strategic Initiatives*. Retrieved from http://www.samhsa.gov/about/strategy.aspx

Titov, N., Andrews, G., & Sachdev, P. (2010). Computer-delivered cognitive behavioural therapy: Effective and getting ready for dissemination. *F1000 Med Rep*, *14*(2), 49. doi: 10.3410/M2-49

Titov, N., Gibson, M., Andrews, G., & McEvoy, P. (2009). Internet treatment for social phobia reduces comorbidity. *The Australian and New Zealand Journal of Psychiatry*, *43*, 754–759. doi: 10.1080/00048670903001992

Trull, T. J., & Ebner-Priemer, U. W. (2009). Using experience sampling methods/ecological momentary assessment (ESM/EMA) in clinical assessment and clinical research: Introduction to the special section. *Psychological Assessment*, *21*(4), 457–462. doi: 10.1037/a0017653

Tutty, S., Spangler, D. L., Poppleton, L. E., & Simon, G. E. (2010). Evaluating the effectiveness of cognitive-behavioral teletherapy in depressed adults. *Behavior Therapy*, *41*(2), 229–236.

Valkenburg, P. M., & Peter, J. (2011). Online communication among adolescents: An integrated model of its attraction, opportunities, and risks. *Journal of Adolescent Health*, *48*(2), 121–127.

Van Allen, J., Davis, A. M., & Lassen, S. (2011). The use of telemedicine in pediatric psychology: Research review and current applications. *Child and Adolescent Psychiatric Clinics of North America*, *20*(1), 55–66. doi: 10.1016/j.chc.2010.09.003

van Straten, A., Cuijpers, P., & Smits, N. (2008). Effectiveness of a web-based self-help intervention for symptoms of depression, anxiety, and stress: Randomized controlled trial. *Journal of Medical Internet Research*, *10*(1), e7. doi: 10.2196/jmir.954

Waller, R., & Gilbody, S. (2009). Barriers to the uptake of computerized cognitive behavioural therapy: A systematic review of the quantitative and qualitative evidence. *Psychological Medicine*, *39*(5), 705–712.

Wei, J., Hollin, I., & Kachnowski, S. (2011). A review of the use of mobile phone text messaging in clinical and healthy behavioral interventions. *Journal of Telemedicine & Telecare*, *17*, 41–48.

Ybarra, M. L., & Eaton, W. W. (2005). Internet-based mental health interventions. *Mental Health Services Research*, *7*(2), 75–87.

11

School- and Home-Based Interventions in Rural Communities

ANGELA M. WAGUESPACK, CARMEN BROUSSARD, AND
KRISTIN GUILFOU

INTRODUCTION

*R*esponding to the unmet mental health needs of children and adolescents is one of the most difficult challenges faced by policy makers, mental health providers, families, and educational stakeholders today. According to the National Survey of Children's Health, as many as 11% of children aged 2–17 have an emotional, behavioral, or developmental condition (Child and Adolescent Health Measurement Initiative, 2007) and only about 50% of children with mental health needs receive treatment (Merikangas et al., 2010). The prevalence of mental health disorders among children and adolescents in rural areas has been shown to parallel that of youth in urban areas (Costello, Gordon, Keeler, & Angold, 2001), and there is a higher proportion of disabilities among rural children when compared with youth living in other settings (Beebe-Frankenberger, 2008). These statistics, coupled with the fact that providing mental health services is often more challenging in rural communities, make delivering home and school interventions in rural settings a difficult endeavor. Limited access to even basic health care (Bidwell, 2001), as well as multiple barriers to the provision of mental health services (Sawyer, Gale, & Lambert, 2006), are identified factors which impact on service delivery. Further, many authors conclude that the current focus of mental health centered only on those with identified mental health problems is not sufficient to address the needs of rural communities. Expansion of prevention efforts to promote wellness and early identification and intervention with at-risk youth should be a priority as well (Heflinger & Christens, 2006).

This chapter provides a review of the literature with regard to home and school interventions implemented in rural settings. Drawing from this research

173

base, as well as that of the public health and response to intervention models discussed extensively in the mental health and education literature, a multi-tiered service delivery model which incorporates both prevention and intervention for rural youth is proposed. A focus on wellness and prevention for the entire school community, in conjunction with a problem-solving approach that incorporates evidence-based interventions delivered effectively and efficiently at secondary and tertiary levels are key aspects of the proposed model. Finally, an ecological perspective which emphasizes strong family school partnerships, interagency collaboration, and involvement of all key systems in a child's life is central to the model as well. A case example designed to illustrate key aspects of this model of service delivery for home school interventions in rural communities is also provided.

THE SCHOOL AS THE HUB OF SERVICE DELIVERY

In a position statement regarding the importance of school mental health services, the National Association of School Psychologists (NASP, 2008) argues that the logical point of entry for addressing mental health and social and emotional competence of youth is the schools. In fact, several studies provide evidence that access to physical and mental health care through school-based health centers is enhanced for youth in both urban and rural communities, and the use of these centers is becoming more mainstream in U.S. society (Brown & Bolen, 2003).

In developing a model which capitalizes on strengthening existing family, school, and community resources, the school should serve as the center of service provision and coordination of outside services for several reasons. Given data regarding the limited number of service providers in rural settings, it is important to note that a national survey of over 80,000 public schools in the United States revealed that 97% of schools have some form of mental health specialist available to them on a regular basis (Foster et al., 2005). Further, almost 50% of children with emotional disorders who receive any form of treatment do so *exclusively* in the schools (NASP, 2008).

Schools in rural areas are often seen as a hub of activity for the community and a key setting for establishing programs for youth that address mental health and social competency (Macgarvey, 2005). Additionally, schools are likely closer to the home than the nearest mental health agency and school providers are available where the children are, thereby relieving the family of the burden of transporting children to service agencies. Further, in rural communities, children's needs are well known to educators, and school staff members possess an understanding of the range of services available and are able to select an agency that will meet an identified need in the event that appropriate services cannot be provided by school personnel (Esveld & Boody, 1997). In schools or districts where level of need is great, it may be cost efficient to hire mental health professionals for one or more schools. Also, there are existing funding sources that may be utilized to provide for mental health prevention and intervention, such as billing for mental health services through the state Child Health Insurance Program (CHIP) or utilizing staff to provide related services through Individuals with Disabilities Education Act (IDEA) funds (Maag & Katsiyannis, 2010).

USE OF PROBLEM-SOLVING AND A MULTITIERED SYSTEM OF SERVICE DELIVERY

Home and school interventions as part of a comprehensive model of mental health service provision within the context of a public health perspective has been discussed extensively in the research literature and is beyond the scope of this chapter (see, e.g., Adelman & Taylor, 2010; Nastasi, 2004). Researchers have suggested that the mental health needs of children and adolescents in the 21st century are simply too great to tackle on a child-by-child basis (Short, 2003). Research on comprehensive mental health programming for children and adolescents has demonstrated multiple positive outcomes, as well as direction regarding necessary program elements (Nastasi & Varjas, 2008). When using a public health framework, the premise is that by promoting wellness and resiliency in the overall child and adolescent population and by identifying and providing interventions to youth at-risk for mental health problems early in their lives, the number of children requiring intensive intervention is reduced, thereby allowing the resources to further strengthen universal and selected levels of intervention. This is particularly important in rural areas where such resources are even more limited. The Response to Intervention (RtI) model, used increasingly in education, incorporates similar premises in identifying children at risk of school failure through the use of a problem-solving approach (Gresham, 2006). The proposed problem-solving, mutitiered model discussed next integrates key concepts from the education and mental health literature as a framework for comprehensive delivery of home and school interventions in rural settings.

Tier 1: Universal

The initial tier incorporates services that are available to all students regardless of risk status. A team of key stakeholders including parents, school personnel, and community representatives determines a population-based method for identifying areas of risk or need specific to their local school and community and develops system-wide efforts to address these areas. By building social and emotional competence and addressing areas of need, typically 80–85% of students are successfully supported at this level. Information is collected regarding which students are at greater risk and a system is in place to refer these students for selected or targeted support at Tier 2.

Tier 2: Selected or Targeted Support

Once students have been identified through universal screening efforts as demonstrating continued behavioral or social emotional difficulties after Tier 1 efforts and determined to be at risk of more severe problems, targeted interventions are developed, implemented, and monitored for those individuals. Selected interventions should be highly efficient, produce rapid response, and be delivered in small groups or in the general setting with consultation from support personnel (Gresham, 2008). With the addition of effective Tier 2 supports, an additional 10–15% of students should have their needs met sufficiently to be successful in the school setting.

Tier 3: Targeted, Intensive

For students with whom Tier 1 and 2 efforts are not sufficient to remediate academic or social, emotional and behavioral difficulties, intensive intervention efforts with frequent progress monitoring are needed. Individual problem-solving that incorporates a functional behavioral assessment is typically required for the small percentage of children requiring this level of service delivery. Specialized personnel are often utilized at this level as children or adolescents may require multisystem interventions involving families and community agencies as well as individual therapy in order to make treatment gains.

INCORPORATING AN ECOLOGICAL PERSPECTIVE

When considering a service delivery model that allows for the provision of comprehensive home and school interventions, incorporating a social ecological perspective (Bronfenbrenner, 1979) has been shown to be a useful framework. Rones and Hoagwood (2000), in a review of research on school-based mental health services, demonstrated that the effectiveness of implemented programs was linked to the use of multicomponent interventions that addressed the child within an ecological framework and included various teachers, parents, and peers. Ecologically oriented prevention and intervention efforts involve using parents, educational stakeholders, and community resources, such as businesses and churches, as part of efforts to create environments that promote wellness and positive child and adolescent development. As previously discussed, capitalizing on the strengths of a rural community's social capital inherent in already existing relationships may offset some of the challenges of limited resources (Bauch, 2001). Meaningful involvement of the rural community is a reachable goal given (a) the generational roots which connect community members; (b) the sense of trust, belongingness, and cohesion; and (c) the likelihood that business owners have children who attend the local schools and/or have graduated from the local school. Mobilizing existing resources by recruiting, training, and supporting key individuals in the community to facilitate mental health efforts provides for expansion of such services and an ability to assist greater numbers of children and families (Power, 2003). Further, sustainability of a service delivery model such as the one proposed over time requires incorporation and coordination of all available resources across the various systems that impact on child development.

Family School Partnerships

Consideration of the interaction and support between home and school is a key factor in delivering comprehensive services for children and adolescents in rural areas. Family school partnerships require adopting a collaborative approach which involves relationship building and trust, as well as effective communication, to reduce barriers due to differences in culture, expectations, or history (Minke, 2006). Esler, Godber, and Christenson (2008) describe parents who are true partners as engaged rather than passive receivers of information. Specific activities used to engage families will differ based upon family and community characteristics and needs. For those families for whom general and universal strategies are not effective, more directed and targeted interactions may be necessary (Christenson, 2010). School staff members have a responsibility to provide an environment conducive to relationship building, to facilitate family involvement in the child's school experience, and to engage in an ongoing process of collaborating with family members in order to support students (NASP, 2005).

Family school partnerships are important at all levels within a multitiered model. At Tier 1, parents and educators work together in universal promotion of overall health and well-being (e.g., meeting physical health needs, promoting early literacy and social skill development and school readiness) and in creating population-based prevention programs that promote key initiatives relevant to the community. Fostering both individual and family resiliency at this level has been shown to be an important component in strengthening the mental health and social competence of children and adolescents (Harvey, 2007; Heflinger & Christens, 2006). At Tier 2, identified at-risk youngsters are taught specific needed skills in the school setting, and through collaboration between home and school, these skills can be reinforced in and generalized to the home and community setting. With regard to Tier 3, a careful consideration of all factors impacting on the child or adolescent's difficulties is required, and multiple change agents are needed in order to establish meaningful interventions. Thus, family and school personnel must work together in decision-making regarding intervention development and implementation (including the decision to involve outside agencies).

As schools implement a problem-solving process from universal through targeted and strategic interventions to address academic and behavioral needs of students, it is important to identify roles that parents can take within each level (Miller & Kraft, 2008). In addition to participating with their own child, representative family members should also be included in all aspects of planning, implementing, and evaluating a service delivery model for the community.

Interagency Collaboration

In cases where children or adolescents need intensive intervention, the access and use of available resources in the community and the coordination of these resources are key considerations. Position papers of several professional associations representing school support personnel (e.g., NASP and the American Counseling Association [ACA]) call for an integration of school mental health services with those of community service providers to provide a seamless continuum of interventions that meet the needs of children and adolescents in a more comprehensive manner. For example, the extent to which services are available and a coordinated effort is made for collaboration among agencies (such as primary health care providers, educators, children's services, juvenile justice, and mental health centers) will determine how effective and efficient needed services may be. In rural areas, where there are few agencies serving many individuals, agencies can work to maximize their impact by understanding the unique needs of the families they serve and the degree to which each agency may meet one or more elements of service. Open discussion between agency representatives often occurs informally in rural settings as their work is completed. However, formal information exchange and collaboration may be helpful to ensure comprehensive service delivery without duplication of efforts. Such formal exchanges may also include an educational component, where expertise of members of various agencies is exchanged through professional development. Further, given the diversity of population demographics in rural communities, agency members should exchange their knowledge of the unique culture as well as strategies that may be effective in addressing the diverse needs of the families they serve (Beebe-Frankenberger, 2008).

CASE EXAMPLE

The following case example illustrates the use of a multitiered problem-solving model proposed for the provision of comprehensive services for children and adolescents in rural communities. This case illustration outlines assessment and intervention processes for a young child demonstrating significant academic and behavioral needs who attends a rural public school. The use of the case is intended to illustrate levels of services provided, involvement of family and key educational stakeholders in the intervention process, and referral to and collaboration with needed community agencies. As discussed previously, needs are identified early in the child's academic career by school personnel, and the school is integral in problem-solving, assisting the family in obtaining needed services, and collaborating with outside agencies to coordinate interventions across the home and school setting. It should be noted that the information provided is from an actual case addressed by a school in a rural community, thus while the case illustrates many of the points discussed previously, some weaknesses and areas of suggested improvement are also identified.

History and Background

Jane, a 5-year-old African American female, was enrolled in a regular education kindergarten (K) classroom. This K classroom was considered an inclusion class in which children with special needs were integrated into the classroom through the implementation of their Individualized Education Programs (IEP). The classroom was staffed by a certified classroom teacher and a full-day paraprofessional. In addition, a certified special education teacher joined staff for part of the school day. This rural school (town population = 686, county population = 23,421) included 36.9% Caucasian students, 62.5% African American students, and <1% Hispanic or Asian. Seventy-nine percent of children attending this school qualified for free or reduced lunch.

Prior to enrollment in K, Jane was enrolled in full-day regular education state-funded pre-kindergarten (PK) class on the same school campus. This PK classroom was fully integrated into the school campus, using the same transportation (school bus services) and cafeteria as the rest of the school. PK children participated in similar activities across the school year as the K through 4th grade students who attended the school (e.g., holiday programs, field day activities). In addition, two of Jane's older siblings attended this local school.

During PK, difficulties were documented for Jane in all areas of school functioning. Specifically, Jane exhibited noncompliance with classroom and bus rules as well as routines across the school year. A Behavior Intervention Plan (BIP) was implemented for Jane, which provided access to preferred activities when compliance for specified periods of the day was achieved. Severe tantrums were addressed by alerting Jane to transitions in activities and providing a quiet place with adult supervision to calm down. In using the Developing Skills Checklist (CTB/McGraw-Hill, 1990) to assess academic readiness, needs for improvement were noted in many areas, including fine motor skills, following directions, participating in class activities, and recognizing letters, numbers, and shapes. While Jane clearly demonstrated continued need for school interventions, her behavior was managed throughout the PK school year with the use of the BIP. Upon entering K, Jane's difficulties were again evident and services were initiated in the new academic year.

Universal Interventions (Tier 1)

Partnering With Families

The identified school begins building relationships with families as children enter school each year, by inviting parents to work with staff toward each child's successful school experience. At the start of each school year, families were provided with two opportunities to meet the child's classroom teacher as follows: (a) a scheduled conference (PK and K) or Open House (first through fourth grade) or (b) a Parent–Teacher Organization meeting held during the first month of school, during which parents meet classroom staff, visit classrooms, and receive grade-level information. In addition, each child was provided with a "Home-School Communication Folder" in which parents and teachers exchange written notes. A Parent Resource Center was available on campus, which provided written materials regarding topics such as developmental stages and parenting techniques.

School-Wide Positive Behavioral Interventions and Supports

A school-wide Positive Behavioral Interventions and Supports (PBiS) plan was implemented beginning the first day of school in order to establish rules and routines, to connect with students, and to reinforce students for following the required procedures. This plan included verbal review of expectations, modeling and prompting of specific appropriate behaviors across school settings (e.g., classroom, bathroom, hallway, school bus, etc.), and review of behavioral expectations when needed (McKevitt & Braaksma, 2008). Children had daily opportunities to earn tokens that could be exchanged for tangible items or preferred activities. Monthly meetings of the PBiS committee were held to monitor behavioral performance of students, to plan activities, and to modify the PBiS plan as needed.

Monitoring of Behavioral and Academic Progress

PK and K children carried a daily report card home each day, which contained a teacher rating of behavior for the day, and was signed by the parent each night (Riley-Tillman, Chafouleas, & Briesch, 2007). For Jane's K classroom, the daily report card included a daily rating of child behavior across the school day with three possible levels indicated: good, fair, poor.

Child academic progress in reading and mathematics was screened three times annually using grade-level DIBELS® Next probes (Good & Kaminski,

2011). In the area of mathematics, AIMSweb® Kindergarten probes were used (Clarke & Shinn, 2004). The current published benchmark goals were used to identify children in need of closer progress monitoring and/or intervention. Monthly meetings of the Response to Intervention (RTI) team were held to review benchmark and progress monitoring data of children across all grades.

Tier 1 Results

Documentation of Jane's academic and behavioral progress during the first 4 weeks of school indicated performance below expectation in the areas of classroom and school behavior, early reading skills, and early numeracy skills. A rating of "poor" was obtained on greater than 50% of days on the Daily Report Card. Specific behavioral difficulties included verbal and physical noncompliance (stating "no" when a request was made of her, not walking with peers from one location to another, not remaining in designated area), aggression toward adults when redirected, and daytime wetting accidents. The intensity of these noncompliant behaviors was described as severe. During the fourth week of school, a parent/teacher conference was held to discuss observations of school behavior and behavioral difficulties evidenced in other settings and to receive information provided by parents that may be impacting on the child's behavior at school. At this time, Jane's parent reported consistent difficulty with compliance in the home setting as well.

The obtained score on the first benchmark period for DIBELS® Next (First Sounds Fluency) was below the cutoff. Jane's teacher began monthly progress monitoring and daily observation of participation and performance in early literacy activities in the classroom.

Strategic Interventions (Tier 2)

Problem-Solving Committee (PSC)

In cases where documentation of academic progress through benchmarking data or behavioral progress through daily rating of behaviors indicate a need for more intensive services, the classroom teacher completes a referral to the PSC. This committee comprises a committee manager, a school administrator, and a regular and special education teacher for the child's grade level. The parent is invited to this problem-solving meeting, and it is scheduled at a time convenient for the family. Data collected through implementation of the universal strategies are reviewed. Through one or more meetings, a plan of action is identified, with input from all participants, and progress is monitored as this plan is implemented.

Tier 2 Results

Jane was provided with a Behavioral Intervention Plan (BIP) that was developed in collaboration with her mother, who attended meetings of the PSC.

This committee also requested participation of the school counselor and a representative from the local pupil appraisal agency, the role of which is to provide the professionally trained specialists (e.g., school psychologists, school social workers, educational diagnosticians.) required by law to assess and determine the educational need of any child who may require specialized educational services because of various conditions. In this case, the representative from the pupil appraisal agency and the counselor were selected for their expertise in addressing behavioral concerns in young children. Jane's BIP targeted two behaviors to be exhibited throughout the school each day (hands to self and follows directions), and feedback was provided (good, fair, poor) for each behavioral goal following each scheduled activity. Percentage of time periods in which a rating of "good" was earned was calculated for each target behavior as an outcome measure. An 80% success rate across the two behaviors each day led to a reward. Across the first two weeks of implementation of the BIP, success on the two behavioral goals was inconsistent. Compliance with the first goal (hands to self) averaged 75% (range = 16–100%). Compliance with the second goal (follows directions) averaged 69% (range 16–100%). On five of the eight days that she attended school, Jane physically resisted following directions by crying and using aggression, requiring adult supervision in an alternate setting (administrator's office) until she was calm. On two of these days, Jane's mother was asked to come to school for a conference to inform her of Jane's severe noncompliance and to include her in continued problem solving. On the three remaining days, passive noncompliance was observed, that is, Jane did not follow instructions, but she did not disrupt others.

With regard to academic interventions and progress monitoring activities, participation was limited on several days due to disruptive behavior. According to her plan, Jane was scheduled to receive small-group or individual review and direct instruction within the classroom setting on a daily basis and weekly progress monitoring. Jane frequently missed the academic interventions outlined for her due to her noncompliance; thus, no progress was demonstrated in the areas of reading and math. Progress monitoring indicated no change in Jane's First Sounds Fluency score after 4 weeks. In early numeracy, progress monitoring indicated no change in Jane's performance on the four different probes.

Intensive Interventions (Tier 3)

Problem-Solving Committee
Where strategic (Tier 2) interventions are judged by the Problem Solving Committee (PSC) to be ineffective, the committee develops an alternate intervention plan that incorporates a more intensive evaluation of factors impacting on the problem behavior. Tier 2 data are considered, and additional assessment,

such as functional assessment or diagnostic academic screening, may aid in problem solving. This targeted (Tier 3) intervention includes more intensive supports for the student in terms of time, involvement of and individualized interaction with staff members, and frequency of contacts. Progress is monitored more frequently due to the severity of concerns. When a student is provided with a Tier 3 intervention, the staff considers a referral for the family to outside agencies (e.g., physician or mental health agency) as appropriate, because professional staff are not typically available in the school setting with sufficient expertise to address needs that extend to the home setting. Active family partnering is solicited at this time, and staff membership remains the same for this problem solving and intervention planning effort (including the school counselor and pupil appraisal representative engaged at the former PSC meetings).

Tier 3 Results

Owing to the severity of problem behavior (aggression toward others, physical noncompliance, severe tantrums), the family was referred to a local mental health agency for evaluation. This referral was made in order to provide the family with a resource to address continued noncompliance in the home setting.

In the school setting, for any child with whom data-based problem solving across a minimum of two individualized, evidence-based interventions does not result in improved performance, a referral for evaluation for special education eligibility should be completed. A referral for a special education evaluation was made for Jane. In addition, the BIP was reviewed, and an indirect functional behavior assessment was conducted through parent and teacher interview (Riley-Tillman et al., 2007). Counseling interventions at school were added which involved a daily "check-in" procedure, as well as meetings with the school counselor to review behavioral expectations and provide one-on-one attention.

Collaboration with referral agencies was accomplished through the sharing of documentation, primarily through Jane's mother. The child's physician provided documentation of a medical diagnosis (enuresis) and a recommendation for intervention within the school setting (e.g., regular schedule of bathroom visits). An evaluation report was provided by the mental health agency to the school staff which provided documentation of psychiatric diagnoses and prescribed medication. Recommendations for classroom accommodations were included in the agency's report.

The school provided documentation regarding Jane's behavioral and academic performance to the other agencies to assist in evaluation and intervention planning. Through the evaluation process completed at school, Jane was determined eligible for special education services under classifications of Speech/Language Impairment and Developmental Delay. On her IEP, goals were identified in the academic, behavioral, communication, and self-help areas. She was provided with small-group and/or individualized instruction daily for academic skills, interventions to improve expressive language, continued implementation of her BIP, and interactions with the school-based counselor. Throughout the evaluation process and thereafter, Jane's mother was provided with documentation of Jane's school behavior in order to inform the mental health agency staff of her progress.

Case Summary and Suggested Improvements

Jane's case provides an example of the manner in which comprehensive services can be provided in a rural setting by using the school as the central change agent, partnering with the parent in decision-making and intervention, and involving other agencies as needed. While many strengths were identified in the use of the multitiered problem-solving approach, there are several elements that could be strengthened to better illustrate a "best practice" approach.

Tier 1
Meaningful efforts in terms of universal interventions are related to the degree to which parents are truly active in the opportunities that are given. In this rural school, the Parent Resource Center is rarely accessed and does not contain current information. To strengthen efforts in this area, staff could disseminate resources when parents visit the school or when conferences are held. Information that is shared could be tailored to the individual family's needs (Christenson, 2004). Parent education topics could be tied to universal interventions, such as modeling and reinforcing behavioral expectations or using effective strategies to help children acquire early learning skills. In addition, schools can work to increase parental attendance at planning meetings where universal intervention planning takes place based on the needs of the school population.

Tier 2
While the PSC committee did monitor and move to the next level of intervention quickly (after 2 weeks of intervention), the documented needs exhibited by Jane in PK, coupled with the severity of the behavior resulting in missed instructional time, suggests a need to have accessed Tier 3 directly. Completion of functional analysis of behavior was needed to inform individualized intervention, and it would have been helpful to access the local psychologist or another professional with expertise in this area to assist with problem analysis and intervention planning. In Jane's case, earlier referral to available agencies was likely warranted as well.

Tier 3
In this case example, the family was referred to two different agencies. The family selected an agency that provided an evaluation, prescribed medication,

and scheduled monthly visits to monitor progress. Progress monitoring at these monthly appointments was based upon verbal report by the mother. True collaboration with the mental health agency might have involved more extensive communication between the school personnel, parent, and agency. Collaboration between schools and community agencies can be improved through establishing a formal system of communication, where representatives from each agency discuss and create documents that will include the most vital information needed for each agency serving the child (with documented permission from the child's parent for such disclosures to occur). For example, a progress report document prepared by school staff with specific data regarding behavioral and academic progress could have been helpful for agency staff in medication management assessment. Other forms of collaboration might include joint meetings, telephone calls, or video conferences between agency and school representatives to discuss the child, with the parent actively involved in this conversation (Shaw & Woo, 2008). Another identified shortcoming in the service delivery for this family is the fact that the family chose not to seek services from a more distant agency. This agency could have provided counseling services on a weekly basis, which may have helped to address behavioral issues in the home. However, the distance of approximately 15 miles away was a barrier to the family and this service was rejected. As such, within Tier 3 services, rural shortages in providers become more evident. Students requiring intervention at this level may not be able to locally receive the intensive care necessary for progress to be made. Future research should focus on novel ways to engage in Tier 3 intervention activities in rural settings (e.g., telehealth), particularly given the potential for establishing a telehealth center within school settings.

CONCLUSION

Shapiro (2006) comments that "we know that the strongest future for our children lies not in the remediation of problems that emerge, but in preventing problems from ever emerging" (p. 264). This is especially true in the provision of comprehensive mental health services to children and adolescents in rural communities where barriers such as transportation, stigma, and inadequate numbers of service providers are readily observed. While not unique to rural communities, the literature regarding comprehensive mental health programming has provided evidence of positive outcomes such as improvements in the social emotional functioning of children and adolescents, reduction of risky behaviors, and less restrictive placements for youth with mental health disorders (Nastasi & Varjas, 2008). Conceptualizing the provision of home and school interventions within a comprehensive model such as the one discussed in this chapter is supported by current thinking and research in mental health and education. By using the school as the central component of a multitiered problem-solving model that emphasizes prevention and early intervention (and utilizes the strengths inherent in rural communities such as informal networks of collaboration, family involvement.), effective service delivery of home and school interventions can be achieved. The proposed model should be viewed as a framework for service delivery that can be implemented within local communities based on careful consideration of the unique needs and resources of that community. Implementation and sustainability of such a model require consideration of the "fit" of various elements within the local ecology of the community. For example, the role of key mental health service providers may change depending on the availability and strengths of other individuals in the community to supplement those roles.

Commitment from local stakeholders, identification and coordination of internal resources, and training of school and community personnel in providing meaningful prevention activities and selected and targeted interventions are key elements in achieving comprehensive mental health services for children and adolescents. For rural schools, ensuring that strong efforts toward collaboration exist is one step in the right direction. Positive outcomes for children result when collaborative efforts are designed to fill gaps in the local service network for the unique rural setting.

REFERENCES

Adelman, H. S., & Taylor, L. (2010, July). Creating successful school systems requires addressing barriers to learning and teaching. *The F. M. Duffy Reports, 15*(3).

Bauch, P. A. (2001). School-community partnerships in rural schools: Leadership, renewal, and a sense of place. *Peabody Journal of Education, 76*(2), 204–221.

Beebe-Frankenberger, M. (2008). Best practices in providing school psychological services in rural setting. In A. Thomas, & J. Grimes (Eds.), *Best practices in school psychology* (pp. 1785–1807). Bethesda, MD: National Association of School Psychologists.

Bidwell, S. (2001). *Successful models of rural health service delivery and community involvement in rural health: International literature review.* Christchurch, New Zealand: Centre for Rural Health.

Bronfenbrenner, U. (1979). *The ecology of human development.* Cambridge, MA: Harvard University Press.

Brown, M. B., & Bolen, L. M. (2003). School-based health centers: Strategies for meeting the physical and mental health needs of children and families. *Psychology in the Schools, 40*(3), 279–287.

Child and Adolescent Health Measurement Initiative. (2007). *National survey of children's health, data resource center for child and Adolescent Health.* Retrieved from www.nschdata.org.

Christenson, S. L. (2004). The family–school partnership: An opportunity to promote learning competence of all students. *School Psychology Review, 33*(1), 83–104.

Christenson, S. L. (2010). Engaging with parents: The power of information, responsiveness to parental need, and ongoing support for the enhanced competence of all students. *Communique, 39*(1), 20-24.

Clarke, B., & Shinn, M. E. (2004). *Test of Early Numeracy (TEN): Administration and scoring of AIMSweb early numeracy measures for use with AIMSweb.* Eden Prairie, MN: Edformation.

Costello, E. J., Gordon, P., Keeler, M. S., & Angold, A. (2001). Poverty, race/ethnicity, and psychiatric disorder: A study of rural children. *American Journal of Public Health, 91*(9), 1494-1498.

CTB/McGraw-Hill. (1990). *Developing skills checklist.* Monterey, CA: Author.

Esler, A. N., Godber, Y., & Christenson, S. L. (2008). Best practices in collaborating with medical personnel. In A. Thomas, & J. Grimes (Eds.), *Best practices in school psychology V* (pp. 1707-1717). Bethesda, MD: National Association of School Psychologists.

Esveld, L. E., & Boody, R. M. (1997, October). *Interagency collaboration: A view from the rural principal's chair.* Revised version of a paper first presented at the 16th Annual Meeting ofthe Mid-Western Educational Research Association, Chicago, IL.

Foster, S., Rollefson, M., Doskum, T., Noonan, D., Robinson, G., & Teich, J. (2005). *School mental health services in the United States, 2002-2003.* Rockville, MD: U.S. Department of Health and Human Services.

Good, R. H., III, & Kaminski, R. A. (Eds.). (2011). *Dynamic Indicators of Basic Early Learning Skills: DIBELS® Next Assessment Manual.* Eugene, OR: Dynamic Measurement Group, Inc.

Gresham, F. M. (2006). Response to Intervention. In G. G. Bear, & K. M. Minke (Eds.), *Children's needs III: Development, prevention, and intervention* (pp. 525-540). Washington, DC: National Association of School Psychologists.

Gresham, F. M. (2008). Best practices in diagnosis in a multitier problem-solving approach. In A. Thomas, & J. Grimes (Eds.), *Best practices in school psychology V* (pp. 937-952). Bethesda, MD: National Association of School Psychologists.

Harvey, V. S. (2007). Schoolwide methods for fostering resiliency. Retrieved from National Association of School Psychologists website: http://www.nasponline. org/resources/principals/schoolresiliency.pdf

Heflinger, C. A., & Christens, B. (2006). Rural behavioral health services for children and adolescents: An ecological and community psychology analysis. *Journal of Community Psychology, 34,* 379-400.

Maag, J. W., & Katsiyannis, A. (2010). School-based mental health services: Funding options and issues. *Journal of Disability Policy Studies, 21*(2), 173-180.

Macgarvey, A. (2005). Rural youth education and support program: The Casterton Experience. *Rural Society, 15*(2), 133-147.

McKevitt, B. C., & Braaksma, A. D. (2008). Best practices in developing a positive behavior support system at the school level. In A. Thomas, & J. Grimes (Eds.), *Best practices in school psychology V* (pp. 735-747). Bethesda, MD: National Association of School Psychologists.

Merikangas, K. R., He, J. P., Brody, D., Fisher, P. W., Bourdon, K., & Koretz, D. S. (2010). Prevalence and treatment of mental disorders among US children in the 2001-2004. *Pediatrics, 125*(1), 75-81.

Miller, D. D., & Kraft, N. P. (2008). Best practices in providing school psychological services in rural settings. In A. Thomas, & J. Grimes (Eds.), *Best practices in school psychology V* (pp. 937-952). Bethesda, MD: National Association of School Psychologists.

Minke, K. M. (2006). Parent–teacher relationships. In G. G. Bear, & K. M. Minke (Eds.), *Children's needs III: Development, prevention, and intervention* (pp. 73-85). Washington, DC: National Association of School Psychologists.

Nastasi, B. (2004). Meeting the challenges of the future: Integrating public health and public education for mental health promotion. *Journal of Educational & Psychological Consultation, 15*(3/4), 295-312.

Nastasi, B. K., & Varjas, K. (2008). Best practices in developing exemplary mental health programs in schools. In A. Thomas, & J. Grimes (Eds.), *Best practices in school psychology V* (pp. 1349-1360). Bethesda, MD: National Association of School Psychologists.

National Association of School Psychologists. (2005). *Home-school collaboration* (Position Statement). Bethesda, MD: Author.

National Association of School Psychologists. (2008). *The importance of school mental health services* (Position Statement). Bethesda, MD: Author.

Power, T. J. (2003). Promoting children's mental health: Reform through interdisciplinary and community partnerships. *School Psychology Review, 32*(1), 3-16.

Riley-Tillman, T. C., Chafouleas, S. M., & Briesch, A. M. (2007). A school practitioner's guide to using daily behavior report cards to monitor student behavior. *Psychology in the Schools, 44*(1), 77-89.

Rones, M., & Hoagwood, K. (2000). School-based mental health services: A research review. *Clinical Child Family Psychological Review, 3*(4), 223-241.

Sawyer, D., Gale, J. A., & Lambert, D. (2006). *Rural and frontier mental and behavioral health care: Barriers, effective policy strategies, best practices*. Waite Park, MN: National Association of Rural Mental Health.

Shapiro, E. (2006). Are we solving the big problems? *School Psychology Review, 35*(2), 260-265.

Shaw, S. R., & Woo, A. H. (2008). Best practices in collaborating with medical personnel. In A. Thomas, & J. Grimes (Eds.), *Best practices in school psychology* (pp. 1707-1717). Bethesda, MD: National Association of School Psychologists.

Short, R. J. (2003). Commentary: School psychology, context, and population-based practice. *School Psychology Review, 32*(2), 181-184.

III

Working with Specific Populations and Issues

12

Substance Use and Abuse in Rural America

JENNIFER D. LENARDSON, DAVID HARTLEY, JOHN A. GALE, AND KAREN B. PEARSON

INTRODUCTION

*R*ural America may seem an unlikely setting for new trends in substance abuse. Over the last 10 years, however, the research community and mainstream media have described a remarkable rise and recognition of substance abuse far from urban centers. These rural areas, often characterized by limited economic opportunity and lengthy distances to the next town, continue to be plagued by the abuse of alcohol, marijuana, and inhalants, and have been infiltrated by methamphetamine and prescription drug abuse among vulnerable rural populations including adolescents, young adults, and Native Americans. Historically, rates of substance abuse between rural and urban areas are comparable; however, recent studies have found greater use of alcohol, OxyContin/oxycodone, and methamphetamine among rural youth than urban in the past year (Lambert, Gale, & Hartley, 2008). Rural areas have long been characterized by limited health care resources especially for specialty services such as substance abuse treatment (Schur & Franco, 1999), emphasizing the need for substance abuse prevention and providing an uncertain context for treatment and recovery.

The fragility of the rural health system (discussed in Chapter 1) generally has implications for substance abuse recognition, treatment, and recovery, and the barriers to overall rural health contribute to difficulties in implementing substance abuse prevention and treatment programs in rural areas (e.g., provider shortages, long travel distances, lack of public transportation). This chapter compares rural and urban areas and the rural continuum (where available) for prevalence of substance use and abuse, efforts to prevent substance abuse, treatment availability and accessibility, and continuing care and long-term support for abstinence. It also presents models of service delivery that address resource limitations common to rural areas.

PREVALENCE OF RURAL SUBSTANCE USE AND ABUSE

Understanding patterns of substance use prevalence as well as variations in those patterns across rural and urban areas is necessary to effectively target resources as well as prevention and treatment interventions to existing and emerging problems. While national studies reveal little difference in the prevalence of substance use across the broad categories of rural and urban (Compton, Thomas, Stinson, & Grant, 2007; Hasin, Stinson, Ogburn, & Grant, 2007; Thomas & Compton, 2007), these studies may obscure the patterns of substance use across smaller geographic areas and their subpopulations. Risk factors for substance use may be similar across the broad conceptualization of rural and urban, but vary by the demographic and socioeconomic characteristics of small towns (Donnermeyer, 1992; Oetting, Edwards, & Kelly, 1997; Van Gundy, 2006). In this discussion, examination of rural adjacency to urban areas, in addition to general rural status, allows for a continuum of rurality to be considered (urban, rural adjacent, rural nonadjacent). The distinction is important because rural residency near centralized and highly populated urban areas may improve rural residents' access to economic opportunities and health care services, thus minimizing the impact that rural living has upon substance abuse risk factors in these areas.

Patterns of Substance Use

N.b. For the following sections, the rural continuum was classified as follows by consolidating the 2003 Rural Urban Continuum Codes. We classified metropolitan counties as urban; non-metropolitan counties with any urban population of any size adjacent to a metropolitan area as rural-adjacent; non-metropolitan counties with an urban population of 20,000 or more that is not adjacent to a metropolitan area as rural large; and non-metropolitan counties with an urban population of 2,500 to 19,999 and nonmetropolitan counties that are completely rural or have an urban population less than 2,500 that are not adjacent to a metropolitan area as rural small-medium.

Regardless of location, alcohol is the most commonly used and abused substance. Looking specifically at problem use, data from the 2002–2004 National Survey on Drug Use and Health indicate that prevalence of binge drinking (i.e., 5 or more alcohol beverages on one occasion within the last 30 days) ranges from 14.2% in rural adjacent counties to a high of 16.6% in

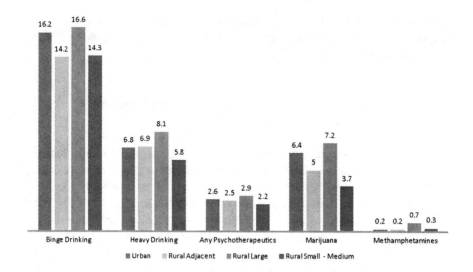

FIGURE 12.1

Past month substance use by location: Annual average percent, 2002–2004.
Source: Gale: Unpublished tabulations of the 2002–04 National Survey on Drug Use and Health

large rural counties, while rates for heavy drinking (i.e., binge drinking on five or more occasions within the last 30 days) range from 5.8% in medium/small rural counties to a high of 8.1% in large rural counties (Figure 12.1—see definitions of rurality above). The dangers of binge and heavy drinking include long-term physical risks (including dependency as well as metabolic, circulatory, digestive, and cardiovascular problems) and short-term risks due to impaired judgment (including driving under the influence and risky social behaviors).

Marijuana is the most commonly used illicit substance with past month rates-of-use that range from 3.7% in small or medium rural counties to 7.2% in large rural counties. The nonmedical use of any psychotherapeutic (i.e., pain reliever, tranquilizer, stimulant, and/or sedative) is the next highest category of illicit drug use with rates that range from 2.2% in small or medium rural counties to 2.9% in large rural counties. Use rates are much lower for the nonmedical use of individual psychotherapeutics (data not shown).

As mentioned earlier, national comparisons of substance abuse prevalence rates across all urban and rural areas tend to obscure patterns of use across smaller geographic areas and their subpopulations. A national study of the rates of substance use by youth and young adults confirms this observation. Although further study is needed to identify the specific reasons for these variations in the rates of substance use across the urban–rural continuum, earlier studies suggest that differences in racial and ethnic composition of these areas as well as differences in cultural, demographic, and economic factors known to influence substance use may help to explain these differences in prevalence rates (Conger, 1997).

Patterns of Substance Abuse by Demographic and Socioeconomic Characteristics

In her 2006 study of rural substance abuse, Van Gundy (2006) found that substance abuse in rural areas varies by social and economic characteristics. While educational attainment has not been shown to be related to alcohol use among rural young adults (aged 18–25) and older adults (aged 26+), fewer years of education is related to illicit drug use for young adults. According to Van Gundy (2006), youth (aged 12–17) from low-income rural families are more likely to abuse illicit drugs than youth from high-income families. Unemployment is also positively related to high rates of illicit drug use. While gender is not related to substance abuse among youth, substance abuse is higher among adult men than among adult women.

Van Gundy also found that substance abuse rates vary across racial and ethnic groups, though rates differ when socioeconomic status and other factors are considered. Among rural young adults, African Americans report the lowest rates of alcohol abuse (10%). Native Americans and Asian/Pacific Islanders report the highest rates (20%), followed by Whites (18%) and Hispanics (15%). For rural youth, 14% of Native Americans abuse alcohol compared to 11% for Asian/Pacific Islanders, 9% for Hispanics, 7% for Whites, and 2% for African Americans. Among adults 26 and older, alcohol abuse ranges from a high of 14% for Native Americans to a low of approximately 3% for African Americans. Illicit drug abuse also varies by race for youth, but not for young or older adults. Among youth, Native Americans have the highest rate of illicit drug use at 13%, followed by Whites and Hispanics at roughly 5% each, and African Americans and Asian/Pacific Islanders at 2% each (Van Gundy, 2006).

Specific Substance Use Issues in Rural Communities

Nonmedical use of prescription drugs is a growing national problem and one that heavily impacts on rural areas. While the rate of prescription drug use grew by 212% between 1992 and 2003 nationally, rural youth are 26% more likely than urban youth to have used prescription drugs nonmedically, adjusting for race, health, and other drug and alcohol use (Moon, 2010). Factors associated with prescription drug abuse among rural youth include poor health status, presence of a major depressive episode, and other drug (marijuana, cocaine, hallucinogens, and inhalants) and alcohol use (Havens, Young, & Havens, 2010).

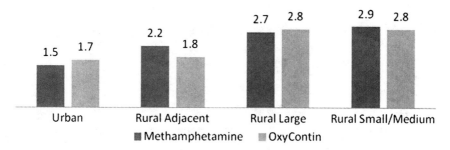

FIGURE 12.2

Percent of young adults (aged 18–25) using methamphetamine and OxyContin by location.

Source: Hartley, D. (2007). *Substance abuse among rural youth: A little meth and a lot of booze* (Research & Policy Brief No. 35A). Portland, ME: Maine Rural Health Research Center

Some, though not all, rural young adults have higher use rates of methamphetamine, prescription drugs, and alcohol compared to their urban peers. Young adults in small rural areas use methamphetamine (meth) and Oxy-Contin at rates nearly twice those of their peers in urban areas (Figure 12.2) (Hartley, 2007; Lambert et al., 2008). At least part of the greater use of meth in rural areas can be attributed to the fact that the drug is relatively easily manufactured using inexpensive chemicals readily available in rural agricultural industries as well as the fact that rural areas, with their lower population densities, greater isolation, and supply of little used barns and farmhouses on remote roads, provide the privacy necessary to produce the drug without detection.

In addition to the severe physiological (e.g., poor physical health and acute and long-term psychological and behavioral problems) and personal (e.g., family and child neglect, irregular work performance, and criminal behavior) effects suffered by meth addicts, meth abuse exerts a devastating toll on rural families and children, economies, law enforcement, social services, and the environment (Donnermeyer & Tunnel, 2007; Jefferson County Meth Action Team, 2008; Weisheit, 2004). The family effects of meth abuse include child abuse, neglect, endangerment, removal of children from the family, and exposure to toxic chemicals or contaminated foods from meth production (ibid.). Societal effects include the strain and economic costs absorbed by rural schools, hospitals, emergency rooms, treatment agencies, social service agencies, and the legal and criminal justice systems in coping with the consequences of meth abuse. Environmentally, meth production produces up to five pounds of toxic waste that contaminate local water systems, soil, property, and buildings as well as provide serious risk of fire, explosion, and exposure to hazardous chemicals (Donnermeyer & Tunnel 2007). Small rural communities frequently do not have the resources to address these problems (Johnson, 2004).

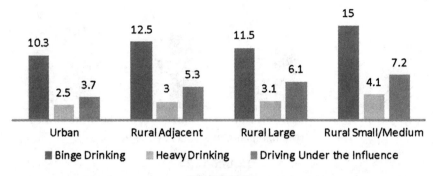

FIGURE 12.3
Percent of youth (aged 12–17) abusing alcohol by location.
Source: Hartley, D. (2007). *Substance abuse among rural youth: A little meth and a lot of booze*
(Research & Policy Brief No. 35A). Portland, ME: Maine Rural Health Research Center

Alcohol abuse is also substantially higher among youth and young adults in specific rural communities. Youth from the smallest rural areas are more likely than their urban peers to have used alcohol and to have engaged in binge drinking, heavy drinking, and driving under the influence (Figure 12.3) (Hartley, 2007; Lambert et al., 2008). In large rural areas, nearly half of young adults report binge drinking during the last month and 20% report heavy drinking, compared to 41% and 15% of urban young adults.

Driving under the influence of either alcohol or drugs is a significant risk behavior and is more common among young adults and within rural communities (Figures 12.3 and 12.4). In large rural communities, 33% of young adults have driven under the influence compared to 28% of young adults in rural adjacent and 29% in urban communities. Driving under the influence is

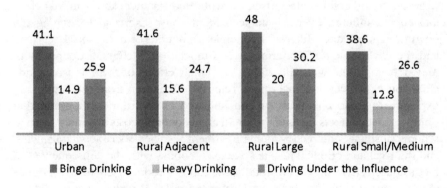

FIGURE 12.4

Percent of young adults (aged 18–25) abusing alcohol by location.
Source: Hartley, D. (2007). *Substance abuse among rural youth: A little meth and a lot of booze*
(Research & Policy Brief No. 35A). Portland, ME: Maine Rural Health Research Center

lower overall among youth; however, prevalence rates are higher in both small and large rural communities compared to urban communities. These patterns can be explained, in part, by the lack of public transportation in rural communities.

PREVENTION

At the national, state, and local levels, efforts to reduce the need for intervention and treatment of substance abuse have focused variously on early intervention, responsible use, and increasingly on primary prevention (Carnevale Associates, 2005). Since evidence suggests that those who become addicted to substances typically start using such substances in their adolescent years, primary prevention has focused largely on youth.

Review of Prevention Theory and Practice

As with all health promotion efforts, preference is given to promotion interventions that have been proven effective; that is, those that are "evidence-based." As a result, prevention of substance abuse has focused largely on youth, toward the goal of developing healthy behaviors early in life. For over 20 years, schools have attempted to address substance abuse in youth through programs such as Drug Abuse Resistance Education (*DARE*), an early effort that teaches students decision-making skills to avoid high-risk behavior. Prevention specialists have distinguished between programs that seek to help adolescents resist social influences to smoke, drink, or use drugs and programs that seek to develop an array of cognitive-behavioral personal and social skills (e.g., Botvin & Wills, 1985). Both types of prevention programs have the advantage of potentially addressing multiple risk behaviors. Substantial evidence demonstrates that adolescents who take risks by using alcohol are the same adolescents who smoke, experiment with drugs, have unprotected sex, and underperform in school. Correspondingly, a majority of interventions addressing youth substance abuse embrace the "gateway hypothesis," which assumes that substance abuse often begins with the illegal use of legal substances, that is, tobacco and alcohol (Pentz & Li, 2002). Discussions on prevention often feature smoking and drinking prevention as an attempt to break the gateway process. An extensive review of the inventory of prevention programs that target youth, either through social influence or personal skills approaches, found 70 such programs (Winters Fawkes, Fahnhorst, Botzet, & August, 2007). The evidence base for these programs varies, and unfortunately many do not focus upon the specific context of rural youth.

The probability that a young person will become involved with illegal substances is determined, in part, by both risk factors and protective factors.

The two approaches described above are loosely aligned with these two determinants. Attempts to help adolescents resist social influences are focused on risk factors, while those that build social skills are focused on protective factors. Prevention strategies often involve reducing risk factors and enhancing protective factors. This is sometimes accomplished at the community or state level rather than the individual level.

The *Life Skills Training* model is an example of a school-based program that teaches students the skills needed to resist social pressure to use substances, including tobacco, marijuana, and alcohol (Botvin & Griffin, 2002). Because it is implemented primarily in the school, it can be as effective with rural children as with urban children, as demonstrated in rigorous evaluations (Spoth, Randall, Trudeau, Shin, & Redmond, 2008). Because local culture affects social pressure in both positive and negative ways, some programs use the positive aspects of the community culture to build resistance to social pressure and to strengthen each child's confidence. One such program is *Project Venture*, a year-round program designed to develop skills, self-confidence, teamwork, cooperation, and trust among at-risk Native American youth. *Project Venture* includes a summer camp, 9-month school curriculum, and extensive community service (Hall, 2004).

While programs targeting individual risk behaviors have shown some success (Botvin & Griffin, 2002), community-level approaches suggest that environmental influences on youth often do not support the acquisition of good decision-making skills. Environmental or ecological models of prevention target whole communities, rather than individual children, and seek to change the standards of acceptable behavior in a neighborhood, town, or state. National surveys that gather data on substance use and abuse, such as the National Survey on Drug Use and Health, have begun to ask questions about perceptions of the acceptability of certain risky behaviors such as "To what extent do you agree with the following statement: 'My parents think it is not wrong or a little wrong for me to drink.'" Some other examples indicate the direction that environmental prevention has gone in recent years: "To what extent do you agree: 'A kid in my neighborhood who drinks won't be caught by police.' OR 'It would be easy to get alcohol if I wanted to.'" As these questions suggest, environmental prevention efforts target the home and community environment. As one prevention specialist stated: "Holding youth solely responsible for underage drinking is like blaming fish for dying in a polluted stream" (attributed to Laurie Leiber, Center on Alcohol Awareness, Berkeley, CA).

Applying Theory and Practice to Rural Populations

Interventions that derive from perceived acceptability of risky behaviors include parent education and zero-tolerance police enforcement policies regarding youth drinking and retail sales to minors. An example of such an evidence-based environmental program is *Community Trials Intervention to Reduce High-Risk Drinking*, which employs the following strategies:

1. Using zoning and municipal regulations to restrict alcohol access through alcohol outlet density control;
2. Enhancing responsible beverage service by training, testing, and assisting beverage servers and retailers in the development of policies and procedures to reduce intoxication and driving after drinking;
3. Increasing law enforcement and sobriety checkpoints to raise actual and perceived risk of arrest for driving after drinking;
4. Reducing youth access to alcohol by training alcohol retailers to avoid selling to minors and those who provide alcohol to minors; and
5. Forming coalitions to implement and support interventions that address each of these prevention components (Substance Abuse & Mental Health Services Administration [SAMHSA], 2008; Treno, Gruenewald, Lee, & Remer, 2007).

Environmental strategies are thought to be easier to implement because they do not target specific individuals and have potential to impact on whole populations. Such "campaigns" often involve multiple interventions, including various media (signs, radio and television spots, press conferences, etc.) as well as stepped up law enforcement, school-based health promotion, and the participation of community leaders (National Institute on Drug Abuse [NIDA], 2003). Rural communities may have an advantage in implementing such interventions, since they tend to be small, with relatively easily identified opinion leaders, fewer retail outlets for the sale of alcoholic beverages, and an enhanced potential to engage the whole community delivering a message to the population efficiently. Rural communities have some disadvantages as well. They often have few resources to invest in a campaign, and the effects of interventions may be harder to measure due to the small population and lack of statistical power for outcome studies. This unfortunately impacts on the ability of new programs to build an "evidence base," thus making it difficult for rural-tailored programs to be developed and tested. Also, many rural communities have their own culture, values, and standards of behavior, which may include tolerance of teen drinking and of excessive adult drinking, even to the point of inconsistent enforcement of state laws. Often, interventions that involve youth not only as the "target population" but also as the designers and communicators of a program can have an impact beyond their own generation.

The *Rural Murals* project in Mendocino County, California, is an example of a low-cost environmental intervention in which youth are the designers of the medium and the message. Teams of youth design and produce murals to be posted in the community with a message designed to change social norms by dispelling "everybody does it" myths, and by presenting a positive drug- and alcohol-free lifestyle. After 9 years of experience with this program, an evaluation has found some evidence of success, citing drops in tobacco and alcohol use for some age groups, and marginal evidence of changes in perceptions (Rural Murals Project, 2001).

Mural design has also been a component of one of the most successful rural prevention interventions, the *Montana Meth Project*. Since 2005, this multifaceted statewide campaign has combined professionally produced media spots on television and radio with posters, press releases, billboards, and roadside murals developed by youth. Two years after launching the *Montana Meth Project*, adult meth use declined by 72% and meth-related crime decreased 62% (McGrath, 2008). The most recent television spots were directed by Academy Award nominee Wally Pfister. The project has been funded largely by private donations, and was recently cited as one of the most effective philanthropic endeavors in the world by Barron's magazine. In one of the first years of this statewide intervention, students designed and painted public service messages on the sides of barns in rural Montana. In 2010, the project included a Paint-the-State campaign described below:

> . . . [Paint-the-State is] a statewide public art contest that leverages the creativity of Montana's youth to communicate the risks of methamphetamine use. To compete in the contest, teens throughout the state poured hundreds of hours into creating large-scale murals, massive sculptures, mixed media installations, and even live performances. Nearly half of the entries were created by grassroots organizations and community groups including Boy Scout troops, 4-H and Future Farmers of America chapters, and local Boys & Girls clubs, with groups ranging in size from 50 to 100 participants. Everything from bulldozers and jagged pieces of mirror to demolished cars and papier-mâché were used to create art that depicted lives shattered by meth. (For more information, see http://www.paint-thestatemontana.org/)

On the basis of a review of prevention programs in rural areas, including those mentioned above, the following are suggested as key elements of successful rural prevention initiatives:

- Target youth, both in the schools and in the community;
- Combine individual-focused strategies with environmental strategies;
- Involve youth in design and communication strategies;
- Engage communities, including retail outlets and law enforcement; and
- When possible, coordinate local interventions with statewide (or multi-tribal) campaigns.

SUBSTANCE ABUSE TREATMENT

Prevention alone cannot fully address the substance abuse challenges faced in rural areas. Treatment programs must also be available for those engaged in abuse or dependence. However, substance abuse treatment overall and intensive services in particular are limited in rural areas, especially among counties not adjacent to urban areas. Since the use of specialty and intensive substance abuse services has been shown to positively affect use of continuing treatment (Straussner, 2004) and posttreatment abstinence (Greenfield et al., 2004; Mojtabi, 2005), the limited availability of these services in rural areas negatively impacts on long-term success. Additionally, the small range of services available in rural areas frequently precludes the individualized treatment approach and long-term follow-up recommended by professional organizations and other experts (American Society of Addiction Medicine, 2001, 2005; Center for Substance Abuse Treatment [CSAT], 2000; Sowers & Rohland, 2004). Providing substance abuse services in rural areas is challenged by the distribution and characteristics of providers (e.g., limited availability of specialty services and programs and travel distances to treatment). This section concludes with examples of treatment models with relevance to rural areas.

Distribution and Characteristics of Rural Providers

Overall, treatment services are relatively scarce in rural areas, with the most isolated rural areas least likely to host services. In 2006, only 9% of all 13,600 treatment facilities in the United States were located in a rural county not adjacent to an urban county, with nearly 80% of facilities located in an urban county. Though few treatment facilities are located in rural nonadjacent areas, comparing facilities to population reveals a greater supply of treatment facilities in rural areas, with 5.8 inpatient and outpatient facilities per 100,000 population in rural and 4.6 facilities in urban areas. However, limited service availability remains apparent for rural residents. Fewer inpatient and residential beds are located in rural areas (29.7 beds per 100,000 population) compared to urban areas (45.8 beds per 100,000 population; Lenardson, 2008).

Detoxification ("detox") services, one of the most basic substance use treatment programs, are a gateway to longer term treatment and include interventions designed to manage acute intoxication and withdrawal while minimizing the medical complications and/or physical harm caused by withdrawals from substance abuse. Unfortunately, the vast majority (82%) of rural residents live in a county without a detox provider (Lenardson, Race, & Gale, 2009). Most rural detox providers are located in large rural towns ($n = 149$), with a lesser concentration in small rural towns ($n = 67$) and a few in isolated rural areas ($n = 19$). Most detox providers serve patients from at least 50 miles away and often greater than 100 miles away. In isolated rural areas, nearly all

(95%) providers serve patients that live 51 or more miles from the facility. For alcohol abuse treatment, less than half of adults with alcohol dependence in most rural counties have a choice between two or more facilities within 15 miles (Johnson, 2004). Lack of patient choice may exacerbate any disconnect between available services and local norms and beliefs, resulting in treatment avoidance (Drug and Alcohol Services Information System, 2002).

Isolated rural areas more heavily rely on less intensive community resources for treatment services following detox. Across all rural areas, patients discharged from detox programs are commonly referred to outpatient programs. However, facilities in isolated rural areas make most of their post-discharge referrals to counseling and self-help groups and less frequently to residential treatment programs and partial hospital/intensive outpatient programs (Lenardson et al., 2009).

Lack of Intensive Services and Special Programs

The continuum of substance abuse treatment services needed to effectively treat a range of patients at different stages of illness are limited in rural areas (including detoxification (detox), inpatient, partial hospital, intensive outpatient, outpatient, and residential care), and specialized, intensive services are often not available. Nearly all facilities across rural and urban areas provide intake, assessment, referral, and treatment (Lenardson, 2008). However, far fewer rural facilities provide detoxification, day treatment, and long-term residential treatment, especially among facilities located in rural, not adjacent, places. For example, nearly all opioid treatment programs (OTPs—programs that use methadone and other medications to treat heroin and other opiate addictions) were located in urban areas in 2006. The extremely limited supply of OTPs in rural areas could be related to the need for an adequate supply of patients to fund this type of program as well as perceived lack of privacy for specialty substance abuse treatment in rural areas (Fortney et al., 2004). Additionally, rural areas may have difficulty recruiting specialty providers to staff these programs. The urban location of OTPs may deter treatment for rural patients since opioid treatments are typically dispensed on a daily basis, requiring prohibitive travel (Mann, 2004).

Special substance abuse patient populations have been shown to need key services for successful treatment outcomes, such as family therapy for adolescents or co-occurring mental health treatment for those with dual diagnoses. Nationally, less than half of treatment facilities with special programs provide these key services (Olmstead & Sindelar, 2004), and the extent to which rural treatment providers offer these programs or services is unclear. Detox providers located in isolated rural areas are less likely than providers in small and large rural towns to offer programs or groups for adolescents, co-occurring disorders, pregnant women, and criminal justice clients (see Figure 12.5). In contrast,

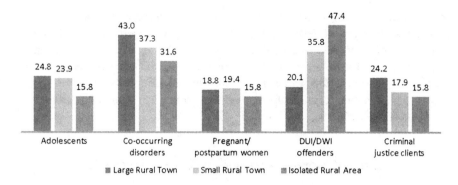

FIGURE 12.5

Percent of detox programs offering program for special populations by location.

Source: Lenardson, Race, & Gale (2009). *Availability, characteristics, and role of detoxification services in rural areas.* Portland, ME: Maine Rural Health Research Center

providers in isolated rural areas are more likely to offer special programs or groups for DUI/DWI offenders (Lenardson et al., 2009). The Office of National Drug Control Policy has revamped its National Youth Anti-Drug Media Campaign to concentrate on substances most often abused by adolescents and is focusing the anti-meth portion of its activities on rural and small suburban communities as well as American Indian and Native Alaskan communities (Office of National Drug Control Policy [ONDCP], 2010a). The President's FY 2011 budget requests a $25 million increase for training and delivery of brief interventions and addiction treatment within community health centers, and an additional $4 million in new funding to add behavioral health counselors and other addiction specialist to IHS facilities (Humphreys & McLellan, 2010).

Challenges to Treatment Accessibility

In addition to the geographic barriers created by long travel distances to services, access to substance abuse treatment services in rural areas may be challenged by detox treatment capacity and confidentiality concerns. Approximately one-third of rural detox providers have a formal waiting list for patients wishing to access services and one-third are unable to admit one or more patients within 2 months. When providers are unable to admit, patients are referred to the hospital emergency department or a provider outside their community, indicating inadequate local capacity (Lenardson et al., 2009). The desire for anonymity in small, close-knit communities during substance abuse treatment may also compromise willingness to seek treatment in local settings (Calloway, Fried, Johnson, & Morrissey, 1999). Patients receiving behavioral health through tribal sources or the Indian Health Service were concerned with issues of confidentiality and having to receive care at facilities where friends and relatives work (Duran et al., 2005). In an examination of barriers to receipt of substance abuse treatment, rural outpatients identified confidentiality as a primary reason why they felt uncomfortable receiving treatment (e.g., negative reactions from family, employers) in contrast to urban outpatients (Davis, 2009).

Treatment Models With Relevance for Rural Providers

Treatment models with relevance for rural providers address the shortcomings of existing services. In the case of primary care, delivering treatment during a physician office visit builds on existing service providers and may address confidentiality because of the generalized nature of a primary care practice. Telehealth (defined below and discussed in Chapter 10) and residential services may help address travel distances and confidentiality concerns; telehealth additionally expands treatment options.

Role of Primary Care in Identifying and Treating Substance Abuse

Primary care may play an important role in rural substance abuse treatment given the lack of specialty providers in rural areas, the likelihood of providers' regular and long-term patient contact, and the ability of the primary care setting to remove stigma associated with specialized treatment facilities. In fact, substance abuse services were one of the first mental health programs put forth as being highly needed in integrated care models (see Chapter 9). A federal consensus panel recommends that primary care clinicians include routine substance abuse screenings during office visits, brief interventions for less severe problems, assessment and treatment, referrals to specialists, and procedures to assure confidentiality (CSAT, 1997). Brief interventions within primary care and hospital settings have been shown effective in reducing substance abuse and across a variety of substances including cigarettes, alcohol, marijuana, opiates, and tranquilizers (ONDCP, 2010b; Smith, Eisenberg, & Bukstein, 2008).

Buprenorphine is an alternative to methadone for treating withdrawal from heroin, prescription pain medicine, and other opioids and was approved for office-based treatment of opioid dependence in 2002. This allows physicians with appropriate training and certification to provide detox or long-term maintenance for as many as 100 patients at a time. Since 2002, the number of physicians qualified to prescribe buprenorphine has increased continuously, primarily among addiction specialists or psychiatrists, but also among family and internal medicine specialists, which greatly expands treatment capacity. The mean number of patients treated has also increased (Arfken, Johanson, di Menza, & Schuster, 2010). Barriers to further expansion include medication cost, difficulty obtaining reimbursement for physician services, and lack of adequate patient counseling (Arfken et al., 2010). No studies to date have examined the use of buprenorphine in rural practices, but the prescribing authority of primary care physicians and the potential flexibility in service site present possibilities for rural providers. In-home use of buprenorphine has been shown successful in urban settings and may have potential for rural areas, as at-home use greatly minimizes travel burden (Lee, Grossman, DiRocco, & Gourevitch, 2008; Sohler et al., 2010).

As an example of a successful training and collaboration program specific to rural health, McCarty, Rieckmann, Green, Gallon, and Knudsen (2004) describe the Opiate Medication Initiative for Rural Oregon Residents. The initiative trained primary care physicians, nurse practitioners, drug abuse counselors, and pharmacists from seven rural counties in the use of buprenorphine and supported the development of community-based service models. Training was provided over a day and a half regarding buprenorphine for treatment of opiate dependence. County-based teams were formed among participants and each team drafted clinical protocols that included assessment, referral, and treatment. The training facilitated new relationships among different providers and improved physician confidence in working with treatment facilities and caring for patients undergoing withdrawal. Following the training, 10 of 17 physicians sought federal authorization to write buprenorphine prescriptions (McCarty et al., 2004).

Telehealth

While empirical evidence is needed to assess telehealth effectiveness for substance abuse, small studies have reported high levels of patient satisfaction with mental health services (Simpson, Doze, Urness, Hailey, & Jacobs, 2001; Skinner & Latchford, 2006) as well as diagnosis and treatment for specific mental health conditions (Hilty, Luo, Morache, Marcelo, & Nesbitt, 2002). In a study of partial and poor responders for opioid dependency, the addition of Internet-based video conferencing for group therapy to other types of in-person treatment was satisfactory to patients and therapists; patients were also able to achieve abstinence and return to less intensive services within several weeks (King et al., 2009). Potential issues to overcome include practitioner reluctance to incorporate telehealth into existing service delivery, patient lack of required technology, data security concerns, and uncertain reimbursement (CSAT, 2009). Additionally, other limitations include lack of direct eye contact and the potential for poor quality connectivity affecting sound and image (McGinty, Saeed, Simmons, & Yildirim, 2006). Additional strengths and challenges of telehealth are addressed in Chapter 10. Overall, the ability of telehealth services to decrease travel burden and increase access to all health services, including substance abuse treatment, indicate it is a crucial line of investigation for ongoing research into treatment modalities in rural populations.

Residential Service Options

Residential programs have the advantage of minimizing transportation barriers since patients live at the facility during treatment. The *Rural Women's Recovery Program* is located in a residential addiction and mental health treatment facility located in southeastern Ohio. The program follows a gender-specific treatment model and uses individualized treatment plans. Patients receive group and individual counseling and educational programming on the biological, psychological, social, and spiritual factors of addiction. The program has been certified by the Ohio Department of Drug Addiction Services and the Commission on Accreditation of Rehabilitation Services (Health Recovery Services, 2010). Rural in-home service options have been used in the past to address transportation and confidentiality barriers in rural areas (e.g., Adams & Ward, 1995); however, few are currently in operation and provider shortages may put this out of reach for many communities. In addition, the lower absolute numbers of individuals needing treatment in rural communities tends to push such residential facilities into more populated and urbanized areas.

CONTINUING CARE AND LONG-TERM SUPPORT

Posttreatment efforts to sustain recovery are important in maintaining continued substance use abstinence (McKay, Lynch, Shepard, & Pettinati, 2005; McKay, Merikle, Mulvaney, Weiss, & Koppenhaver, 2001) and discharge planning that transitions patients from treatment to continuing care supports continued abstinence (McKay et al., 2005; Schaefer, Harris, Cronkite, & Turrubiartes, 2008). Forms of long-term support include self-help groups, individual therapy, brief check-ups, peer and group counseling, and telephone-based counseling. The research literature has little to say about the availability and role of continuing care and long-term support in rural communities. Numerous studies refer informally to the limited number of 12-step meetings per week in rural areas compared to availability in urban areas. Transportation difficulties remain a factor posttreatment and patients undergoing continuing care without access to transportation are less likely to maintain abstinence than patients with access (Schaefer et al., 2008). Long-term support may be compromised if the client feels group therapy attendance may unintentionally reveal substance use to community members. Continuing care interventions that bring care to the patient, through aggressive outreach or the use of low burden delivery systems (e.g., telephone), have an advantage over traditional clinic-based approaches (McKay, 2009). These approaches may be particularly useful in rural areas.

Various approaches and models from the literature may be useful for promoting long-term support in rural areas. As described by SAMHSA's *Recovery Month Toolkit*, community coalitions can be built to promote education about addiction, treatment, and recovery (CSAT, 2010). Coalitions can include a diverse group of organizations such as substance abuse treatment providers as well as law enforcement, social and educational agencies, religious organizations, veterans or military groups, child welfare organizations, and mental health organizations. This model may be useful to rural communities in customizing a coalition and activities to home town needs. Through the Drug Free Communities program, federal grant money is available to community coalitions for youth drug prevention efforts. In FY 2010, 62% of awards went to rural communities (ONDCP, 2010c). Faith-based organizations may also be useful in recovery and support efforts for rural communities (Hartman, Arndt, Barbaer, & Wassink, 2006). Faith communities provide a consistent source of social support free from associations with past substance abuse behavior and often already provide some services such as lunch programs, spiritual counseling, and space for self-help group meetings.

At the federal level, substance abuse treatment funding is targeting providers and patients in rural communities. Begun in 2004, Access to Recovery (ATR) is a grant program awarded to competing states and tribes that provides vouchers for the provision of substance abuse treatment and recovery support services (http://www.atr.samhsa.gov). Vouchers are given to patients in the early stages of recovery and are to be used for support services such as facilitating return to employment, transportation to self-help meetings or follow-up medical appointments, or peer-to-peer counseling. The President's FY 2011 budget included a 10% requested increase to the Access to Recovery grant program (Humphreys & McLellan, 2010). Although ATR may positively impact on *financial* access to services, the program does not specifically target rural areas and may not be useful in rural areas with limited service availability or lengthy travel distances.

CONCLUSION

The prevalence of substance abuse among rural youth and young adults emphasizes the importance of developing intervention programs that target rural communities, particularly communities in small and remote areas. Substance abuse prevention generally targets alcohol and tobacco as initiation substances and is attentive to youth in order to stop substance use early or ideally before it begins. Prevention efforts are intended to address social influences that put youth at risk and provide social skills to resist pressure to use substances, and target individuals as well as their environment. However, a culture of drinking tolerance in many rural communities has made community-based prevention a challenge.

Few substance abuse treatment facilities operate in rural areas, particularly among the most remote rural counties. Where facilities exist, access to intensive services and the full range of professionally recommended services is limited. Travel distances for detox services are lengthy and access to specialty programs for patients for specific needs is incomplete. Treatment models should build on existing primary care and safety net providers and community resources and consider incorporating new technology approaches that could address distance and confidentiality issues. Despite the importance of continuing care and long-term support in abstinence following treatment, little research has examined the availability and role of these services in rural communities. Like other forms of substance abuse treatment, continued recovery services are likely in short supply and, where they exist, group arrangements in small communities may exacerbate confidentiality concerns. Continued financial support and additional research on the prevention and treatment needs of rural areas is essential to decreasing substance abuse in these areas.

REFERENCES

Adams, K. M., & Ward, C. C. (1995). A case management model utilizing in-home treatment services for rural AODA clients: The Family and Children's Center Model. In *Treating alcohol and other drug abusers in rural and frontier areas: TAP 17.* (DHHS Publication No. SMA 95-3054). Rockville, MD: U.S. Department of Health and Human Services, Substance Abuse and Mental Health Services Administration.

American Society of Addiction Medicine. (2001). Preface. In D. Mee-Lee (Ed.), *ASAM patient placement criteria for the treatment of substance-related disorders* (2nd Rev. ed.). Chevy Chase, MD: Author.

American Society of Addiction Medicine. (2005). *Public policy statement on treatment for alcoholism and other drug dependencies.* Chevy Chase, MD: Author.

Arfken, C. L., Johanson, C.-E., di Menza, S., & Schuster, C. R. (2010). Expanding treatment capacity for opioid dependence with office-based treatment with buprenorphine: National surveys of physicians. *Journal of Substance Abuse Treatment, 39*(2), 96–104.

Botvin, G. J., & Griffin, K. W. (2002). Life skills training as a primary prevention approach for adolescent drug abuse and other problem behaviors. *International Journal of Emergency Mental Health, 4*(1), 41–47.

Botvin, G. J., & Wills, T. A. (1985). Personal and social skills training: Cognitive-behavioral approaches to substance abuse prevention. *National Institute of Drug Abuse Research Monograph, 63,* 8–49.

Calloway, M., Fried, B., Johnson, M., & Morrissey, J. (1999). Characterization of rural mental health service systems. *Journal of Rural Health, 15*(3), 296–307.

Carnevale Associates. (2005). *SAMHSA's Strategic Prevention Framework.* (Information Brief). Darnestown, MD: Carnevale Associates, LLC.

Center for Substance Abuse Treatment. (1997). Guide to substance abuse services for primary care clinicians (SMA 97-3139). In K. Allen, R. L. Brown, D. Czechowicz, L. S. Foley, W. A. Glover, P. J. Greer, G. Hill, S. W. Long, E. A. Renz, R. K. Ries, S. H. School (Eds.), *Treatment Improvement Protocol (TIP) Series* (24 ed.). Rockville, MD: U.S. Department of Health and Human Services, Substance Abuse and Mental Health Services Administration.

Center for Substance Abuse Treatment. (2000). *Changing the conversation: Improving substance abuse treatment* (SMA 00-3480). Rockville, MD: U.S. Department of Health and Human Services, The National Treatment Plan Initiative.

Center for Substance Abuse Treatment. (2009). *Considerations for the provision of e-therapy.* (SMA 09-4450). Rockville, MD: U.S. Department of Health and Human Services, Substance Abuse and Mental Health Services Administration.

Center for Substance Abuse Treatment. (2010). Join the voices for recovery: Now more than ever! In *National alcohol and drug abuse recovery month toolkit.* Rockville, MD: U.S. Department of Health and Human Services, Substance Abuse and Mental Health Services Administration.

Compton, W. M., Thomas, Y. F., Stinson, F. S., & Grant, B. F. (2007). Prevalence, correlates, disability, and comorbidity of DSM-IV drug abuse and dependence in the United States: Results from the national epidemiologic survey on alcohol and related conditions. *Archives of General Psychiatry, 64*(5), 566–576.

Conger, R. (1997). The special nature of rural America. In E. Robertson, Z. Sloboda, G. Boyd, L. Beatty, & N. Kozel (Eds.), *Rural substance abuse: State of knowledge and issues.* (pp. 1–5). Rockville, MD: U.S. Department of Health and Human Services, National Institutes of Health, National Institute on Drug Use.

Davis, W. M. Jr. (2009). *Barriers to substance abuse treatment utilization in rural versus urban Pennsylvania* (Unpublished doctoral dissertation). Indiana University of Pennsylvania, Indiana, PA.

Donnermeyer, J. F. (1992). The use of alcohol, marijuana, and hard drugs by rural adolescents: A review of recent research. In R. Edwards (Ed.), *Drug use in rural American communities* (pp. 31–75). New York: Haworth Press.

Donnermeyer, J. F., & Tunnell, K. (2007). In our own backyard: Methamphetamine manufacturing, trafficking and abuse in rural America. *Rural Realities, 2*(2), 1–11.

Drug and Alcohol Services Information System. (2002). *Distance to substance abuse treatment facilities among those with alcohol dependence or abuse.* (DASIS Report). Arlington, VA: Office of Applied Studies, Substance Abuse and Mental Health Services Administration.

Duran, B., Oetzel, J., Lucero, J., Jiang, Y., Novins, D. K., Manson, S., . . . Beals, J. (2005). Obstacles for rural American Indians seeking alcohol, drug, or mental health treatment. *Journal of Consulting and Clinical Psychology, 73*(5), 819–829.

Fortney, J., Mukherjee, S., Curran, G., Fortney, S., Han, X., & Booth, B. (2004). Factors associated with perceived stigma for alcohol use and treatment among at-risk drinkers. *Journal of Behavioral Health Services and Research, 31*(4), 418–429.

Greenfield, L., Burgdorf, K., Chen, X., Porowski, A., Roberts, T., & Herrell, J. (2004). Effectiveness of long-term residential substance abuse treatment for women: Findings from three national studies. *American Journal of Drug and Alcohol Abuse, 30*(3), 537–350.

Hall, M. (2004). *Project venture: SAMHSA model program.* Rockville, MD: U.S. Department of Health and Human Services, Substance Abuse and Mental Health Administration.

Hartley, D. (2007). *Substance abuse among rural youth: A little meth and a lot of booze.* (Research & Policy Brief No. 35A). Portland, ME: University of Southern Maine, Muskie School of Public Service, Maine Rural Health Research Center.

Hartman, J. C., Arndt, S., Barbaer, K., & Wassink, T. (2006). An environmental scan of faith-based and community reentry services in Johnson County, Iowa. In *The National Rural Alcohol and Drug Abuse Network Awards for Excellence*, 2004 (pp. 49–58). Rockville, MD: U.S. Department of Health and Human Services, Substance Abuse and Mental Health Services Administration.

Hasin, D. S., Stinson, F. S., Ogburn, E., & Grant, B. F. (2007). Prevalence, correlates, disability, and comorbidity of DSM-IV alcohol abuse and dependence in the United States: Results from the National Epidemiologic Survey on Alcohol and Related Conditions. *Archives of General Psychiatry, 64*(7), 830–842.

Havens, J. R., Young, A. M., & Havens, C. E. (2010). Nonmedical prescription drug use in a nationally representative sample of adolescents: Evidence of greater use among rural adolescents. *Archives of Pediatric and Adolescent Medicine, 165*(3), 250–255. doi: 10.1001/archpediatrics.2010.217

Health Recovery Services. (2010). *Rural Women's Recovery Program*. Retrieved from http://www.hrs.org/residential.html

Hilty, D. M., Luo, J. S., Morache, C., Marcelo, D. A., & Nesbitt, T. S. (2002). Telepsychiatry: An overview for psychiatrists. *CNS Drugs, 16*(8), 527–548.

Humphreys, K., & McLellan, A. T. (2010). Brief intervention, treatment, and recovery support services for Americans who have substance use disorders: An overview of policy in the Obama administration. *Psychological Services, 7*(4), 275–284.

Jefferson County Meth Action Team. (2008). *Methamphetamine in Jefferson County: Understanding the impact of methamphetamine abuse: Issue paper & recommendations*. Port Townsend, WA: Jefferson County Meth Action Team.

Johnson, D. (2004, March). *Policing a rural plague: Meth is ravaging the Midwest–Why it's so hard to stop*. Retrieved from http://www.msnbc.msn.com/id/4409266/site/newsweek

King, V. L., Stoller, K. B., Kidorf, M., Kindbom, K., Hursh, S., Brady, T., . . . Brooner, R. (2009). Assessing the effectiveness of an Internet-based videoconferencing platform for delivering intensified substance abuse counseling. *Journal of Substance Abuse Treatment, 36*(3), 331–338.

Lambert, D., Gale, J. A., & Hartley, D. (2008). Substance abuse by youth and young adults in rural America. *Journal of Rural Health, 24*(3), 221–228.

Lee, J. D., Grossman, E., DiRocco, D., & Gourevitch, M. N. (2008). Home buprenorphine/naloxone induction in primary care. *Journal of General Internal Medicine, 24*(2), 226–232.

Lenardson, J. D. (2008). *Unpublished tabulations of the 2006 National Survey of Substance Abuse Treatment Services*. Portland, ME: University of Southern Maine, Muskie School of Public Service, Maine Rural Health Research Center.

Lenardson, J., Race, M., & Gale, J. A. (2009). *Availability, characteristics, and role of detoxification services in rural areas*. (Working Paper No. 41). Portland, ME: University of Southern Maine, Muskie School of Public Service, Maine Rural Health Research Center.

Mann, B. (2004). Profile: Methadone treatments for heroin addicts. [Radio transcript]. Bob Edwards. Host. *NPR Morning Edition*. Online Ed. Retrieved from http://www.npr.org

McCarty, D., Rieckmann, T., Green, C., Gallon, S., & Knudsen, J. (2004). Training rural practitioners to use buprenorphine: Using the Change Book to facilitate technology transfer. *Journal of Substance Abuse Treatment, 26*(3), 203–208.

McGinty, K., Saeed, S., Simmons, S., & Yildirim, Y. (2006). Telepsychiatry and e-mental health services: Potential for improving access to mental health care. *Psychiatric Quarterly, 77(4)*, 335–342.

McGrath, M. (2008). *Methamphetamine in Montana: A follow-up report on trends and progress.* Helena, MT: Montana Department of Justice.

McKay, J. R. (2009). Continuing care research: What we have learned and where we are going. *Journal of Substance Abuse Treatment, 36*(2), 131–145.

McKay, J. R., Lynch, K. G., Shepard, D. S., & Pettinati, H. M. (2005). The effectiveness of telephone-based continuing care for alcohol and cocaine dependence: 24-month outcomes. *Archives of General Psychiatry, 62*(2), 199–207.

McKay, J. R., Merikle, E., Mulvaney, F. D., Weiss, R. V., & Koppenhaver, J. M. (2001). Factors accounting for cocaine use two years following initiation of continuing care. *Addiction, 96*(2), 213–225.

Mojtabi, R. (2005). Use of specialty substance abuse and mental health services in adults with substance use disorders in the community. *Drug and Alcohol Dependence, 78*(3), 345–354.

Moon, M. A. (2010). Rural adolescents more likely than urban ones to abuse prescription drugs. *Internal Medicine News Digital Network.* Retrieved from http://www.inter nalmedicinenews.com/news/adolescent-medicine/single-article/rural-adolescents-more-likely-than-urban-ones-to-abuse-prescription-drugs/64587a7088.html

National Institute on Drug Abuse. (2003). *Preventing drug abuse among children and adolescents: A research-based guide for parents, educators and community leaders.* Bethesda, MD: Author.

Oetting, E. R., Edwards, R. W., & Kelly, K. B. F. (1997). Risk and protective factors for drug use among rural American youth. In E. B. Robertson, Z. Slobda, G. M. Boyd, L. Beatty, & N. J. Kozel (Eds.), *Rural substance abuse: State of knowledge and issues. NIDA Research Monograph 168* (pp. 90–130). Rockville, MD: U.S. Department of Health and Human Services, National Institutes of Health, National Institute on Drug Abuse.

Office of National Drug Control Policy. (2010a). *National youth anti-drug media campaign [fact sheet].* Retrieved from http://www.whitehouse.gov/sites/default/files/ondcp/Fact_Sheets/national_youth_anti_drug_page_media_campaign_fact_sheet_7-16-10.pdf

Office of National Drug Control Policy. (2010b). *Screening, brief intervention, referral & treatment.* Retrieved from http://www.whitehousedrugpolicy.gov/treat/screen_brief_intv.html

Office of National Drug Control Policy. (2010c). *White house drug policy director awards $85.6 million to local communities to prevent youth drug use [press release].* Retrieved from http://www.whitehousedrugpolicy.gov/pda/083110.html

Olmstead, T., & Sindelar, J. (2004). To what extent are key services offered in treatment programs for special populations. *Journal of Substance Abuse Treatment, 27*, 9–15.

Pentz, M. A., & Li, C. (2002). The gateway theory applied to prevention. In D. B. Kandel (Ed.), *Stages and pathways of drug involvement: Examining the gateway hypothesis* (pp. 139–157). New York, NY: Cambridge University Press.

Rural Murals Project. (2001). *Environmental prevention.* Retrieved from http://www. ruralmurals.org/prevention.shtml

Schaefer, J. A., Harris, A. H., Cronkite, R. C., & Turrubiartes, P. (2008). Treatment staff's continuity of care practices, patients' engagement in continuing care, and abstinence following outpatient substance-use disorder treatment. *Journal of Studies on Alcohol and Drugs, 69*(5), 747–756.

Schur, C. L., & Franco, S. J. (1999). Access to health care. In T. C. Ricketts (Ed.), *Rural health in the United States* (pp. 25–37). New York, NY: Oxford University Press.

Simpson, J., Doze, S., Urness, D., Hailey, D., & Jacobs, P. (2001). Evaluation of a routine telepsychiatry service. *Journal of Telemedicine and Telecare, 7*(2), 90–98.

Skinner, A. G., & Latchford, G. (2006). Attitudes to counseling via the Internet: A comparison between in-person counseling clients and Internet support group users. *Counseling and Psychotherapy Research, 6*(3), 158–163.

Smith, J. G., Eisenberg, S. G., & Bukstein, O. G. (2008, June). *Managing substance abuse disorders in primary care settings.* Presented at the Blending Science and Treatment NIDA Conference, Cincinnati, OH.

Sohler, N. L., Li, X., Kunins, H. V., Sacajiu, G., Giovanniello, A., Whitley, S. et al. (2010). Home- versus office-based buprenorphine inductions for opioid-dependent patients. *Journal of Substance Abuse Treatment, 38*(2), 153–159.

Sowers, W. E., & Rohland, B. (2004). American Association of Community Psychiatrists' principles for managing transitions in behavioral health services. *Psychiatric Services, 55*(11), 1271–1275.

Spoth, R. L., Randall, G. K., Trudeau, L., Shin, C., & Redmond, C. (2008). Substance use outcomes $5\frac{1}{2}$ years past baseline for partnership-based, family–school preventive interventions. *Drug and Alcohol Dependence, 96*(1–2), 57–68.

Straussner, S. L. A. (2004). Assessment and treatment of clients with alcohol and other drug abuse problems: An overview. In S. L. A. Straussner (Ed.), *Clinical work with substance-abusing clients.* (2nd ed., pp. 3–36). New York, NY: The Guilford Press.

Substance Abuse & Mental Health Services Administration, Center for Substance Abuse Prevention, NREPP database. (2008). *Community trials intervention to reduce high-risk drinking.* Retrieved from http://www.nrepp.samhsa.gov/ViewIntervention.aspx?id=9

Thomas, Y. F., & Compton, W. M. (2007). Rural populations are not protected from drug use and abuse. *Journal of Rural Health, 23*(Suppl.), 1–3.

Treno, A. J., Gruenewald, P. J., Lee, J. P., & Remer, L. G. (2007). The Sacramento Neighborhood Alcohol Prevention Project: Outcomes from a community prevention trial. *Journal of Studies on Alcohol and Drugs, 68*(2), 197–207.

Van Gundy, K. (2006). *Reports on rural America: Substance abuse in rural and small town America.* Durham, NH: University of New Hampshire, Carsey Institute.

Weisheit, R. A. (2004). *The impact of methamphetamine on Illinois communities: An ethnography.* Normal, IL: Illinois State University, Department of Criminal Justice Sciences.

Winters, K. C., Fawkes, T., Fahnhorst, T., Botzet, A., & August, G. (2007). A synthesis review of exemplary drug abuse prevention programs in the United States. *Journal of Substance Abuse Treatment, 32*(4), 371–380.

13

Suicide in Rural Areas: Risk Factors and Prevention

COURTNEY CANTRELL, SARAH VALLEY-GRAY, AND
RALPH E. CASH

INTRODUCTION

Suicide is the third leading cause of death among adolescents and is predicted to become the second in all age groups in the world by 2020 (United States [U.S.] Department of Health and Human Services, n.d.). Suicide rates increase with age, are higher among men, and are lower in African Americans. While the suicide rate for Caucasian men increases with age, the rate is either constant or decreases after age 65 for all other ethnic groups (Gibbons, Hur, Bhaumik, & Mann, 2005). Women attempt suicide approximately three to four times as often as men, but men complete suicide about four times as often as their female counterparts (six times as often in the 20–24 age group) because they are more likely to use firearms (Dresang, 2001).

Suicide deaths occur more frequently in nonmetropolitan, rural, less densely populated regions (Goldsmith, Pellmar, Kleinman, & Bunney, 2002), and the rate of suicide completions is higher in rural areas (Centers for Disease Control and Prevention [CDC], 2007; Institute of Medicine, 2002; New Freedom Commission Subcommittee on Rural Issues [NFC-SRI], 2004). In fact, suicide rates, particularly in the rural west, are three times the rate found in urban areas (Mulder et al., 2001). U.S. suicide statistics vary by region, potentially reflecting the population-level impact of rural suicide disparities: in 2005 the suicide rates were 12.1 per 100,000 in the West; 11.8 per 100,000 in the South; 11.1 per 100,000 in the Midwest; and 8.1 per 100,000 in the Northeast. Adjusted suicide rates are particularly high in rural areas of the western U.S. and Alaska (Goldsmith et al., 2002). According to Forrest (1988), 30 out of 1000 rural adolescents in the study attempted suicide in a 1-month period, while the national average is 2 out of 1000.

Despite this pronounced disparity among rural populations, the majority of studies investigating the incidence of and interventions for individuals who are suicidal utilize urban samples. This chapter summarizes the literature on suicide in rural settings within the United States, recognizing the considerable diversity that exists from one rural region of the country to another (Letvak, 2002).

RISK FACTORS FOR SUICIDE IN RURAL AREAS

Individuals in rural areas tend to have more suicide completions than their urban counterparts (Dresang, 2001). The most significant variable may not be location, but instead, other characteristics shared more often by rural residents (Rost, Owen, Smith, & Smith, 1998). Suicide completions are associated with a variety of risk factors, including geographic and interpersonal isolation; stressful cultural variables within the community; low socioeconomic status; lack of career opportunities; limited access to health care, especially mental health resources; a culture of pride and secrecy; and access to lethal means (Hirsch, 2006), all of which can disproportionately impact on those who live in rural areas. The combined effects of these variables can be exponential. In fact, individuals who live in rural areas frequently experience the "triple jeopardy" of being rural, poor, and uninsured (Rowland & Lyons, 1989). Pfeffer (2002) concluded that the most efficacious way to reduce risk and to prevent suicide within rural areas is to recognize and to respond to the specific risk factors within the community. The most important of these risk factors includes access to lethal means, geographic and social isolation, cultural values which limit help-seeking behaviors, and the stigma associated with mental illness.

Access to Lethal Means

Compared to their urban counterparts, suicide attempts among individuals from rural areas more frequently result in lethality because their methods are more likely to involve firearms and pesticides (Branas, Nance, Elliott, Richmond, & Schwab, 2004; Dembling & Merkel, 2003; Dresang, 2001; Pasewark & Fleer, 1993; Sadowski & Munoz, 1996; Svenson, Spurlock, & Nypaver, 1996; World Health Organization [WHO] in collaboration with UNEP, 1990). Suicide is a major cause of gun deaths in rural areas (Dresang, 2001), and there is an associated increased risk of suicide when a gun is owned (Kellermann et al., 1992; Miller, Azrael, & Hemenway, 2002). Firearm ownership is particularly high in rural areas for sport and hunting. Consequently, suicides in rural areas are more likely to be completed by rifles or shotguns than by handguns, as is typically seen in urban areas (Dodge, Cogbill, Miller, Landercasper, & Strutt, 1994; Hargarten, Karlson, O'Brien, Hancock, & Quebbeman,

1996). Self-poisoning is largely a rural phenomenon and is the most common method of suicide completion worldwide (WHO in collaboration with UNEP, 1990). Approximately two-thirds of all pesticide poisonings are suicidal acts (Jeyaratnam, 1990), resulting in 220,000 deaths annually around the globe (WHO, 2003).

Geographic and Social Isolation

Rural areas tend to encompass wide geographic regions, resulting in expanses of land that are sparsely populated and potentially quite isolating (United Stated Department of Agriculture [USDA], 2003). As a result of this geographic isolation, residents tend to become self-reliant for survival. Individuals from rural areas who complete suicide are more likely to have lacked a close, intimate relationship than their urban counterparts (Isometsa et al., 1997; Turvey, Stromquist, Kelly, Zwerling, & Merchant, 2002). This isolation, coupled with the stigma attached to seeking out mental health treatment, may help to explain the delay in rural areas of seeking help for problems in general, particularly among men (Wainer & Chesters, 2000). Overall, there is decreased dependency upon seeking outside resources such as mental health care (Lawrence & Ndiaye, 1997), which only serves to exacerbate existing mental health conditions.

Urbanization and lack of vocational opportunity have resulted in many individuals leaving their rural communities, creating a loss of relationships, a decreased sense of togetherness, and feeling of loneliness among rural residents (Gerrard, 2003). These variables of interpersonal and social isolation are routinely associated with suicide in general and are particularly challenging given the environmentally imposed limitations for social connections within rural communities (Dorling & Gunnell, 2003; Renwick, Olsen, & Tyrrell, 1982; Shajahan & Cavanagh, 1998).

Culture of the Community

Rural communities are considered "high context cultures" where people rely on one another for support in a variety of social organizations (Wenger, 1992). When distressed, individuals frequently try to help themselves alone or to seek informal support from family, spouses, neighbors, friends, and religious organizations rather than mental health professionals (Blank, Mahmood, Fox, & Guterbock, 2002; Fox, Merwin, & Blank, 1995). Strong allegiances are held to family, church, country, and community, which create a higher tolerance for other individual differences among members of the community (Buckwalter, Smith, & Castor, 1994; Eckersley, 2002; Heffernan, 1999; Scott, Ciarrochi, & Deane, 2003; Wodarski, 1983). Mental health services are often stigmatized; consequently, individuals look to physicians or religious leaders for assistance with problems which might, in other settings, be considered as mental health issues (Holzer & Ciarlo, 2000; Meystadt, 1984).

The lifestyles within rural communities promote rugged independence. As a result, suicidal thoughts and behaviors may be neglected because of the independence mandate (Crawford & Brown, 2002). Challenges, particularly those associated with mental illness, are often kept within the family. This creates a sense of shame about mental illness, resulting in less knowledge and understanding of risk factors for and prevention of suicide. This stigma of shame makes for a greater suicide risk, since mental illness can run in families, and shame about previous family suicides can preclude getting help for others who are at risk.

Stigma

As discussed in more detail in Chapter 4, the stigma associated with mental illness tends to be magnified in rural settings (Hoyt, Conger, Valde, & Weihs, 1997). For example, in research conducted by Komiti, Judd, and Jackson (2006), the majority of rural residents sampled reported concern that members of their community would gossip about a person diagnosed with a mental illness and would be suspect of someone who was hospitalized for emotional difficulties. Stigma and lack of privacy associated with mental health problems are additional stressors for individuals who may be suicidal, as well as for their families. Rural residents frequently fail to recognize the need for mental health treatment, even following a positive screening for a mental disorder, the diagnosis of a psychiatric disorder, or a psychoeducational evaluation. In fact, in an investigation of rural southerners, 90% had not sought treatment 1 month after receiving a psychiatric diagnosis, while 81% did not feel the need for treatment despite the fact that they were referred to nearby agencies for services (Fox, Blank, Berman, & Rovnyak, 1999). Of those who screened positive and discussed their diagnosis with family and friends, a mere 13% were encouraged to seek out services (Fox et al., 1999). Refusal or avoidance of services appears to be based largely upon the culture of the community and likely has a dramatic impact on the increased prevalence of suicides in rural areas.

SUICIDE IN RURAL AREAS: PREVENTION, INTERVENTION, AND SYSTEMS OF CARE

The field of rural mental health has been neglected by both researchers and policy-makers (Blank, Fox, Hargrove, & Turner, 1995). The few studies that have been conducted in rural regions have included samples from single geographic areas, so generalizability is questionable (Jameson & Blank, 2007).

Nonetheless, there has been a recent push by federal agencies to respond to the needs in rural areas, which have been deemed special populations for increased focus in the areas of health, mental health, drug and alcohol abuse, and prevention and intervention (U.S. Department of Health and Human Services, 2005). Similarly, organized public policy advocacy movements have typically not been implemented in rural regions (Bjorklund & Pippard, 1999). Public policy issues which should be addressed in rural communities include deinstitutionalization, disparity in health insurance for mental health care, and the importance of the integration of mental health care with general health care (Letvak, 2002).

Creating an effective, systematic suicide prevention, intervention, and postvention plan in rural areas involves responding to the multiple issues unique to this population. Bushy (2000) described social resources within the context of a three-tier system. The first tier consists of family and friends. The second tier includes local emergency services, community members, and religious organizations, as well as schools and churches, which are often the centers of community activities in rural areas (Bushy, 1998). The third tier is composed of formal supports that require a fee for service. Historically, rural residents tend to prefer the first and second tiers (Lee, 1998). This is understandable, given the perceived lack of confidentiality and stigma in the context of receiving formalized services (Howland, 1995). It is important to note, however, that while support from family members and friends is highly valued in rural communities, it does not necessarily equate to successful outcomes when more intense intervention is required.

Prevention

There tends to be a lack of knowledge and a culture of avoidance surrounding the incidence of suicide, particularly in rural areas. The severity of the problem is frequently ignored, and minimal education is provided (Hirsch, 2006). To combat this significant public health problem, effective, evidence-based prevention strategies must be implemented. In particular, a systematic plan of action should be devised with a focus on preventive mental health care. Factors that demonstrably work to prevent suicide include school-based suicide prevention curricula (Aseltine & DeMartino, 2004; Kalafat, 2003), gatekeeper training (King & Smith, 2000), crisis centers (Lester, 1997), patient education (Mann et al., 2005), means restriction (Hawton, 2002; Kruesi et al., 1999), and bridging prevention and treatment (Shaffer et al., 2004).

Spoth (1997) recommends strategies to target involvement in prevention efforts, such as recruitment, retention, and compliance and indicates that interventions should be sensitive to local culture and customs with incentives for participation. Providing education to community members and professionals about the warning signs associated with suicide is an essential aspect of suicide prevention. In particular, individuals should take note of the following symptoms: changes in eating or sleeping patterns; neglect of personal appearance; the onset of depressed, sad, angry, or aggressive moods; setbacks or losses academically or vocationally; alcohol or substance abuse; self-mutilation; withdrawal from connections with family or friends; a loss of interest in pleasurable activities; and perfectionism or harsh self-criticism (Cash, 2011). Suicidality should be described as a disease, similar to other biological disorders, to assist in bringing an end to the stigma associated with it. Protective factors should be strengthened, and school and community resources linked. Education targeting knowledge of the warning signs of suicide should be employed within schools as well as other public and private agencies.

Community members should not only be educated regarding the urgent danger signs of suicide, but should also be taught how to respond, such as removing firearms from the house or carefully securing them. Individuals who are at risk should routinely be asked about suicidal ideation, intent, and plans. All individuals who express thoughts or feelings of suicide should be taken seriously and should be provided with an opportunity to express their feelings in a nonjudgmental manner. An actively suicidal person should never be left alone. While one may become angry, the individual's anger must not prevent others from taking control of the situation. Interdisciplinary collaboration is critical, and discharge plans from inpatient psychiatric services must provide meaningful treatment, supports, and case management (Bushy, 2000).

The National Strategy for Suicide Prevention (U.S. Department of Health and Human Services, 2001) acknowledged the need for evidence-based practices for the prevention of suicide and suicidal behavior. To address this need, the Evidence-Based Practices Project (EBPP) to prevent suicide was created in 2002. The EBPP fosters collaboration between the Suicide Prevention Resource Center (SPRC) and the American Foundation for Suicide Prevention (AFSP) funded by the Substance Abuse and Mental Health Services Administration (SAMHSA). The initial goals were to evaluate the effectiveness of suicide prevention efforts and to create an online registry of evidence-based prevention programs. The resulting registry can be accessed at the SPRC website (www.sprc.org). Given the limited availability of specialized health care services, particularly in the area of mental health, rural residents receive most, if not all, of their health care from primary care physicians, nurse practitioners, and physicians' assistants (American Psychological Association Office of Rural Health, 1995; Guralnick, Kemele, Stamm, & Sister-Grieving, 2003; National Rural Health Association, 1999; Yuen, Gerdes, & Gonzales, 1996). Moreover, rural primary care practitioners treat more cases of depression without consultation or referral to a specialty provider than urban primary care physicians (Hartley, Korsen, Bird, & Agger, 1998; Lambert & Agger, 1995). These practitioners are in a unique position to detect self-destructive behavior and to assist with suicide prevention efforts

(Hawton, 1993). However, they may not be aware of the specific questions to ask to determine the potential for suicidality (Jencks, 1985; Kessler, Cleary, Burke, 1985). Questions surrounding suicidality and previous suicide attempts tend not to be part of a standard medical interview. In fact, 60% of physicians were unaware of previous suicidal behavior among their patients who ultimately died by suicide (Ashkenassy, Clark, Zinn, & Richtsmeiser, 1992; Pirkis & Burgess, 1998). This is of particular relevance, as the majority of individuals who either attempt or complete suicide consult with a helping agency or professional during the month prior to an attempt, and up to half do so within a week of their attempt (Davis, 1992). Because of the lack of additional suicide prevention resources in rural areas, primary care providers are an essential component of any suicide prevention/intervention program to be implemented in those communities.

The provision and increased availability of formalized continuing education programs, either live or in a web-based format, will allow practitioners to develop knowledge and to increase competence in providing mental health support in rural areas where specialty services are limited (Jameson & Blank, 2007). However, knowledge alone is insufficient. Mental health practitioners must gain the trust of the community, as they are frequently perceived as outsiders (Long, 1993). Moreover, they should seek opportunities to understand and to appreciate deeply the unique culture of the rural community. Furthermore, behaving in a manner that facilitates community acceptance, such as dressing in a way that is consistent with community expectations, needs to be considered (Jameson & Blank, 2007). It is critical to identify and to take into account a multitude of factors to gain acceptance within the rural community, including cultural, economic, health, religious, and political variables (Nelson, Pomerantz, Schwartz, 2007).

Particularly in rural areas, suicide prevention practices should include general gun safety measures. Few patients bring up the topic of gun safety with their physicians, and only 30% of physicians surveyed reported discussing firearm safety with their patients (Camosy, 1996). Moreover, Barkin, Duan, Fink, Brook, and Gelberg (1998) reported that while 80% of physicians felt that they should counsel their patients regarding firearm safety and the risks of gun ownership, only 38% actually did so. These findings suggest that physicians have a unique, but underutilized, opportunity to educate patients regarding the possible dangers in owning a firearm and potentially addressing suicide prevention, particularly in rural communities (Dresang, 2001). Intra-individual protective factors against suicide that should be nurtured include positive self-esteem, sobriety and avoidance of drugs and alcohol as a means to cope, a sense of hope and plans for the future, good mental and physical health, a relationship with a counselor or therapist, pets, medication compliance, a sense of duty to others, school and job success, limited access to lethal means, cultural and religious beliefs that discourage suicide, the development of resiliency factors, and enhancement of coping skills.

Intervention

As discussed throughout this text, accessibility, availability, and acceptability are the three primary variables that limit the provision of mental health services in rural areas in general, and are particularly problematic when considering the challenges associated with individuals who are at risk of suicide (U.S. Department of Health and Human Services, 2005). Poverty, low levels of education, and a failure to understand the nature of psychiatric problems are barriers to seeking treatment (President's Commission on Mental Health, 1978), and may result in a minimization of the symptoms associated with suicide. Traditional psychotherapy, consisting of once-a-week sessions within the context of the therapist–patient relationship, is not the most effective treatment modality for rural mental health conditions (Falcone & Rosenthal, 1982). Instead, expectations within rural culture require brief, time-limited interventions which emphasize symptom reduction (Edgerton, 1983).

Given these significant challenges in providing mental health services in rural settings, technology is a promising and important tool for suicide prevention. Advances in technology have permanently changed communication patterns and altered the traditional association of rural areas with extreme isolation. Telehealth generally refers to the use of technology to provide information, while telemedicine refers to the use of telehealth services for the provision of patient care (Stamm & Peredina, 2000). Telemedicine has the potential for linking people in rural and remote areas to psychologists in urban areas (Bischoff, Hollist, Smith, & Flack, 2004) and is discussed in detail in Chapter 10. Innovative uses of technology, including broadband Internet and videoconferencing, can provide services to isolated rural areas which lack mental health providers and serve as important strategies for prevention of and intervention in factors associated with suicide.

Telemedicine has also proven effective in the treatment of anxiety and depression, disorders often associated with suicide (Proudfoot et al., 2003). In particular, one program, Beating the Blues, has demonstrated efficacy in urban areas of the United Kingdom in reducing depression, anxiety, and suicidal ideation (Van Den Berg, Shapiro, Bickerstaffe, & Cavanagh, 2004). However, the use of manualized, evidenced-based treatments using telemedicine technology in rural areas has received little research attention. At this point, such technology is a promising field for future research with great potential for increasing access to and acceptability of care, a critical element preventing suicide and intervening with suicidal individuals.

Systems of Care

As discussed in Chapter 9, integrating general health care and mental health service systems is particularly advisable in rural areas (Kane & Ennis, 1996).

A comprehensive system of care allows for the integration of mental health and primary health services in one location and may provide a unique setting to address pre-suicidal behaviors in rural areas. Such a model improves early identification of suicidality, facilitates timely interventions, and provides enhanced monitoring (Kane & Ennis, 1996). The collaboration of mental health professionals and physicians provides a powerful team to make available the psychoeducation, assessment, consultation, crisis intervention, and treatment necessary to respond effectively to potentially suicidal patients and their families (Morris, 1997).

Any formal health care system needs to fit in with the informal helping system in rural areas (Lee, 1998). The emphasis of any plan should be on the communal nature of rural areas and should target this for successful prevention and intervention, emphasizing protective factors (Gerrard, 2003) and using clergy and physicians as gatekeepers (Lipschitz, 1995; Marshfield Clinic, 2003; Mulder & Chang, 1997). Establishing traditional and nontraditional suicide prevention/intervention mechanisms, including telephone follow-up services, telemental health, crisis lines, computer-based telecommunications, traveling counselors, and social clubs and self-help groups can be effective (Agee, Blank, Fox, Burkett, & Pezzoli, 1997; Jong, 2004; LaMendola, 1997; Mishara & Daigle, 1997; Oyama et al., 2005; Ratnayeke, 1998; Strawn, Hester, & Brown, 1998).

Natural supports, a given within most rural communities, can serve as protective factors that can be encouraged and developed in mental health treatment. However, the utilization of such social networks and supports has not been formally integrated into traditional care (Kane & Ennis, 1996). Social relationships that serve to support mental health interventions, especially when individuals are at risk for suicide, should include family, friends, aides, confidants, medicine men, and shamans (D'Augelli, 1982; Hill, 1985). Family members are particularly important, as they can provide 24-hour case management and residential support to their mentally ill family members who may be suicidal (Kane & Ennis, 1996). Clergy frequently serve as counselors and provide in-residence help for individuals diagnosed with psychiatric disorders. Moreover, systems and agencies such as places of worship, schools, and clinics can serve as support. These supports serve as adjuncts to traditional suicide prevention/intervention services and provide a means of communication between the client and mental health professionals (Bachrach, 1983; Hargrove, 1982; Kelley & Kelley, 1985). Given the lack of mental health services in rural areas, law enforcement personnel are frequently responsible for those with mental health emergencies (Larson, Beeson, & Mohatt, 1993); unfortunately, appropriate training in handling mental health emergencies may not be readily available for rural law enforcement and should be included in any plan to ensure appropriate response to those with mental illness (especially those who are suicidal).

Nurturing strong partnerships between primary care physicians and mental health care providers encourages the coordination of services and the continuity of care (Starfield, 1992).

Psychologists and other mental health specialists who serve in rural settings should be advocates for mental health services through the provision of psychoeducation within the community and collaboration with primary care physicians. Mental health practitioners should provide education to primary care physicians to ensure that they have access to evidence-based interventions for the treatment of depression and other mental disorders as well as to suicide prevention and intervention protocols (Kelly, Howard, & Smith, 2007).

REFERENCES

Agee, E., Blank, M. B., Fox, J. C., Burkett, B. M., & Pezzoli, J. (1997). The introduction of computer-assisted telephone support in a community mental health center. *Journal of Rural Community Psychology, E1*(1). Retrieved from http://www.marshall.edu/jrcp/vole1/vol_e1_1/vole1no1.html

American Psychological Association Office of Rural Health. (1995). *Caring for the rural community: An interdisciplinary curriculum.* Washington, DC: American Psychological Association.

Aseltine, R. H. Jr., & DeMartino, R. (2004). An outcome evaluation of the SOS suicide prevention program. *American Journal of Public Health, 94*(3), 446-451. doi: 10.2105/AJPH.94.3.446

Ashkenassy, J. R., Clark, D. C., Zinn, L. D., & Richtsmeiser, A. J. (1992). The nonpsychiatric physician's responsibilities for the suicidal adolescent. *New York State Journal of Medicine, 92,* 97-103.

Bachrach, L. (1983). Psychiatric services in rural areas: A sociological overview. *Hospital and Community Psychiatry, 34*(3), 215-226.

Barkin, S., Duan, N., Fink, A., Brook, R., & Gelberg, L. (1998). The smoking gun: Do clinicians follow guidelines on firearm safety counseling? *Archives of Pediatric Adolescent Medicine, 275,* 1762-1764.

Bischoff, R., Hollist, C., Smith, C., & Flack, P. (2004). Addressing the mental health needs of the rural underserved: Findings from a multiple case study of a behavioral telehealth project. *Contemporary Family Therapy: An International Journal, 26*(2), 179-198.

Bjorklund, R., & Pippard, J. (1999). The mental health consumer movement: Implications for rural practice. *Community Mental Health Journal, 35*(4), 347-359.

Blank, M., Fox, J., Hargrove, D., & Turner, J. (1995). Critical issues in reforming rural mental health service delivery. *Community Mental Health Journal, 31*(6), 511-524.

Blank, M., Mahmood, M., Fox, J., & Guterbock, T. (2002). Alternative mental health services: The role of the black church in the South. *American Journal of Public Health, 92*(10), 1668-1672.

Branas, C. C., Nance, M. L., Elliott, M. R., Richmond, T. S., & Schwab, C. W. (2004). Urban–rural shifts in intentional firearm death: Different causes, same results. *American Journal of Public Health, 94,* 1750-1755.

Buckwalter, K., Smith, M., & Castor, C. (1994). Mental and social health of the rural elderly. In R. Coward, C. N. Bull, G. Kubulka, & J. Gallchu (Eds.), *Health services for rural elders* (pp. 203-232). New York: Apresquer. doi: 10.3109/01612849409009384

Bushy, A. (1998). Health issues of a woman in rural environments. An overview. *Journal of the American Woman's Medical Association, 53*, 53-56.

Bushy, A. (2000). *Orientation to nursing in the rural community.* Thousand Oaks, CA: Sage.

Camosy, P. (1996). Incorporating gun safety into clinical practice. *American Family Physician, 54*, 971-980.

Cash, R. (October, 2011). Suicide: Preventable tragedy. Invited continuing education presentation at Nova Southeastern University Center for Psychological Studies, Davie, FL.

Centers for Disease Control and Prevention (CDC). (2007). *Preventing suicide: Program activities guide.* Retrieved from http://www.cdc.gov/violenceprevention/pdf/Preventing Suicide-a.pdf

Crawford, P., & Brown, B. (2002). Like a friend going round: Reducing the stigma of mental health care in rural communities. *Health and Social Care in the Community, 10*, 229-238.

D'Augelli, A. R. (1982). Future directions for paraprofessionals in rural mental health, or how to avoid giving indigenous helpers civil service ratings. In P. Kellerand Murray (Eds.), *Handbook of rural community mental health* (pp. 210-223). New York: Human Sciences Press.

Davis, A. (1992). Suicidal behavior among adolescents: It's nature and prevention. In R. Kosky, H. S. Eshkevari, & G. Kneebone (Eds.), *Breaking out: Challenges in adolescent mental health in Australia* (pp. 89-101). Canberra: Australian Government Publishing Service.

Dembling, B., & Merkel, L. (2003). *Suicide in Virginia, 1979-1996: Working paper.* Southeastern Rural Mental Health Research Center, University of Virginia.

Dodge, G., Cogbill, T., Miller, G., Landercasper, J., & Strutt, P. (1994). Gunshot wounds: 10-year experience of a rural, referral trauma center. *American Journal of Surgery, 60*, 410-404.

Dorling, D., & Gunnell, D. (2003). Suicide: The spatial and social components of despair in Britain, 1980-2000. *Transactions of the Institute of British Geographers, 28*, 442-460.

Dresang, L. (2001). Gun deaths in rural and urban settings: Recommendations for prevention. *Guns and Violence Prevention, 14*(2), 107-115. Retrieved from www.jabfm.org/cgi/reprint/14/2/107.pdf

Eckersley, R. (2002). Taking the prize or paying the price? Young people and progress. In L. Rowling, G. Martin, & L. Walker (Eds.), *Mental health promotion and young people: Concepts and practice* (pp. 70-81). Sydney, Australia: McGraw-Hill Australia.

Edgerton, J. W. (1983). Models of service delivery. In A. W. Childs, & G. B. Melton (Eds.), *Rural psychology.* New York: Plenum Press.

Falcone, A. M., & Rosenthal, T. L. (1982). *Delivery of rural mental health services.* Cleveland, OH: Synapse Inc.

Forrest, S. (1988). Suicide and the rural adolescent. *Adolescence, 23*(90), 341-346.

Fox, J. C., Blank, M., Berman, J., & Rovnyak, V. (1999). Mental disorders and help seeking in a rural impoverished population. *International Journal of Psychiatry in Medicine, 29*(2), 181-195.

Fox, J., Merwin, E., & Blank, M. (1995). De facto mental health services in the rural south. *Journal of Health Care for the Poor and Underserved, 6*, 434-469.

Gerrard, N. (2003). *Farm stress: Resiliency in rural people.* Regina, Saskatchewan, Canada: Saskatchewan Agriculture and Food.

Gibbons, R., Hur, K., Bhaumik, D., & Mann, J. (2005). The relationship between antidepressant medication use and rate of suicide. *The American Journal of Psychiatry, 163*(11), 163-172. doi:10.1176/appi.ajp.163.11.1898

Goldsmith, S., Pellmar, T., Kleinman, A., & Bunney, W. (Eds.). (2002). *Reducing suicide: A national imperative.* Washington, DC: The National Academies Press.

Guralnick, S., Kemele, K., Stamm, B. H., & Sister-Grieving, A. M. (2003). Rural geriatrics and gerontology. In B. H. Stamm (Ed.), *Rural behavioral health care: An interdisciplinary guide 1* (pp. 193-2002). Washington, DC: American Psychological Association.

Hargarten, S., Karlson, T., O'Brien, M., Hancock, J., & Quebbeman, E. (1996). Characteristics of firearms involved in fatalities. *Journal of American Medical Association, 275*, 42-45.

Hargrove, D. S. (1982). An overview of professional considerations in the rural community. In P. Keller, & J. Murray (Eds.), *Handbook of rural community mental health* (pp. 169-182). New York: Human Sciences Press.

Hartley, D., Korsen, N., Bird, D., & Agger, M. (1998). Management of patients with depression by rural primary care practitioners. *Archives of Family Medicine, 7*, 139-145.

Hawton, K. (1993). Suicide prevention by general practitioners. *British Journal of Psychiatry, 162*(3), 422.

Hawton, K. (2002). United Kingdom legislation on pack sizes of analgesics: Background, rationale, and effects on suicide and deliberate self-harm. *Suicide and Life-Threatening Behavior, 32*(3), 223-229. doi: 10.1521/suli.32.3.223.22169

Heffernan, J. B. (1999). *Mental health and ministry: The vital connection* (Report No. 7). Kansas City, MO: National Association for Rural Mental Health.

Hill, C. E. (1985). Folk beliefs and practices. In L. Jones, & R. Parlour (Eds.), *Psychiatric services for underserved rural populations* (pp. 27-37). New York: Brunner and Mazel.

Hirsch, J. (2006) A review of the literature on rural suicide: risk and protective factors, incidence, and prevention. *The Journal of Crisis Intervention and Suicide Prevention, 27*(4), 189-199. doi:10.1027/0227-5910.27.4.189

Holzer, C. E. III, & Ciarlo, J. (2000). *Mental health service utilization in rural and nonrural areas.* Denver, CO: Frontier Mental Health Services Resource Network, University of Denver.

Hoyt, D., Conger, R., Valde, J., & Weihs, K. (1997). Psychological distress and help seeking in rural America. *American Journal of Community Psychology, 25*(4), 449-470.

Howland, R. (1995). The treatment of persons with dual diagnoses in a rural community. *Psychiatric Quarterly, 66*(1), 33-49. doi: 10.1007/BF02238714

Institute of Medicine. (2002). Reducing suicide: A national imperative. *National Academy of Science.* Retrieved from National Institute of Mental Health website: http://www.nimh.nih.gov/health/topics/suicide-prevention/reducing-suicide-a national-imperative.shtml

Isometsa, E., Heikkinen, M., Henriksson, M., Marttunen, M., Aro, H., & Lonnqvist, J. (1997). Differences between urban and rural suicides. *Acta Psychiatrica Scandinavica, 95*, 297-305. doi:10.1111/j.1600-0447.1997.tb09635.x

Jameson, J., & Blank, M. (2007). The role of clinical psychology in rural mental health services: Defining problems and developing solutions. *Clinical Psychology: Science and Practice, 14*(3), 283-298. doi: 10.1111/j.1468-2850.2007.00089.x

Jencks, S. (1985). Recognition of mental distress and diagnosis of mental disorders in primary care. *Journal of American Medical Association, 253*(13), 1903-1907.

Jeyaratnam, J. (1990). Acute pesticide poisoning: A major global health problem. *World Health Statistics Quarterly, 43*, 139-144.

Jong, M. (2004). Managing suicides via videoconferencing in a remote northern community in Canada. *International Journal of Circumpolar Health, 63*(4), 422-428.

Kalafat, J. (2003). School approaches to youth suicide prevention. *The American Behavioral Scientist, 46*(9), 1211-1223. doi: 10.1177/0002764202250665

Kane, C., & Ennis, J. (1996). Health care reform and rural mental health: Severe mental illness. *Community Mental Health Journal 32*(5), 445-462. doi: 10.1007/BF02251045

Kellermann, A. L., Rivara, F. P., Somes, G., Reay, D. T., Francisco, J., Banton, J. G. et al. (1992). Suicide in the home in relation to gun ownership. *New England Journal of Medicine, 327*(7), 467-472.

Kelley, P., & Kelley, V. R. (1985). Supporting natural helpers: A cross-cultural study. *Social Casework: The Journal of Contemporary Social Work, 66*, 358-366.

Kelly, M., Howard, A., & Smith, J. (2007). Early intervention in psychosis: a rural perspective. *Journal of Psychiatric and Mental Health Nursing, 14*, 203-208. doi: 10.1111/j.1365-2850.2007.01064.x

Kessler, L., Cleary, I'D., & Burke, J. (1985). Psychiatric disorders in primary care. *Archives of General Psychiatry, 42*(6), 583-586.

King, K. A., & Smith, J. (2000). Project SOAR: A training program to increase school counselors' knowledge and confidence regarding suicide prevention and intervention. *Journal of School Health, 10*, 402-407.

Komiti, A., Judd, F., & Jackson, H. (2006). The influence of stigma and attitudes on seeking help from a GP for mental health problems. *Social Psychiatry and Psychiatric Epidemiology, 41*(9), 738-745. doi: 10.1007/s00127-006-0089-4

Kruesi, M. J. P., Grossman, J., Pennington, J. M., Woodward, P. J., Duda, D., & Hirsch, J. G. (1999). Suicide and violence prevention: Parent education in the emergency department. *Journal of the American Academy of Child and Adolescent Psychiatry, 38*(3), 250-255.

Lambert, D., & Agger, M. S. (1995). Access of rural AFDC Medicaid beneficiaries to mental health services. *Health Care Financing Review, 17*(1), 133-145.

LaMendola, W. (1997). *Telemental health services in frontier areas: Provider and consumer perspectives* (Report No. 19). Denver, CO: Frontier Mental Health Services Network.

Larson, M. L., Beeson, P. G., & Mohatt, D. F. (1993). *Taking rural into account: A report of the National Public Hearing on Rural Mental Health*. St. Cloud, MN: National Association for Rural Mental Health and the Federal Center for Mental Health Services.

Lawrence, J., & Ndiaye, S. (1997). Prevention research in rural communities: Overview and concluding comments. *Prevention Research of Community Psychology, 25*(4), 545–562.

Lee, H. (1998). *Conceptual basis for rural nursing.* New York: Springer Publishing Co.

Lester, D. (1997). The effectiveness of suicide prevention centers: A review. *Suicide and Life-Threatening Behavior, 21*(3), 304–310.

Letvak, S. (2002). The importance of social support for rural mental health. *Issues of Mental Health, 23,* 249–261. doi: 10.1080/016128402753542992.

Lipschitz, A. (1995). Suicide prevention in young adults (age 18–30). *Suicide and Life Threatening Behavior, 25*(1), 155–170.

Long, K. (1993). The concept of health. *The Nursing Clinics of North America, 28*(1), 123–130.

Mann, J., Apter, A., Bertolote, J., Beautrais, A., Currier, D., Haas, A. et al. (2005). Suicide prevention strategies: A systematic review. *Journal of the American Medical Association. 294*(16), 2064–2074.

Marshfield Clinic. (2003). *Rural suicide prevention: Seeds of safety.* Marshfield, WI: National Children's Center for Rural and Agricultural Health and Safety.

Meystadt, D. (1984). Religion and the rural population: Implications for social work. *Social Casework, 65,* 219–226.

Miller, M., Azrael, D., & Hemenway, D. (2002). Household firearm ownership and suicide rates in the United States. *Epidemiology, 13,* 517–524.

Mishara, B. L., & Daigle, M. S. (1997). Effects of different telephone intervention styles with suicidal callers at two suicide prevention centers: An empirical investigation. *American Journal of Community Psychology, 25*(6), 861–885. doi: 10.1023/ A:1022269314076

Morris, J. A. (1997). The rural psychologist in the hospital emergency room. In J. A. Morris (Ed.), *Practicing psychology in rural settings: Hospital privileges and collaborative care* (pp. 81–96). Washington, DC: American Psychological Association.

Mulder, P., & Chang, A. (1997). Domestic violence in rural communities: A literature review and discussion. *Journal of Rural Community Psychology, E1*(1). Retrieved from http://www.marshall.edu/jrcp/vole1/vol_e1_1/vole1no1.html

Mulder, P. L., Kenken, M. B., Shellenberger, S., Constantine, M. G., Streigel, R., Sears, S. F., & ... Hager, A. (2001). *The behavioral health care needs of rural women.* Retrieved from http://www.apa.org/rural/ruralwomen.pdf

National Rural Health Association. (1999). *Rural policy positions.* Retrieved from http://www.ruralhealthweb.org/go/left/policy-and-advocacy/policy-documents-and-statements/official-policypositions/archived-policy-positions

Nelson, W., Pomerantz, A., & Schwartz, J. (2007). Putting "rural" into psychiatry residency training programs. *Academic Psychiatry, 31*(6), 423–429. doi: 10.1176/ appi.ap.31.6.423

New Freedom Commission on Mental Health. (2004). *Subcommittee on rural issues: Background paper.* Retrieved from http://govinfo.library.unt.edu/mentalhealth commission/subcommittee/Sub_Chairs.htm

Oyama, H., Watanabe, N., Ono, Y., Sakashita, T., Takenoshita, Y., & Taguchi, M. (2005). Community-based suicide prevention through group activity for the elderly successfully reduced the high suicide rate for females. *Psychiatry & Clinical Neurosciences*, *59*(3), 337-344.

Pasewark, R., & Fleer, J. (1993). Suicide in Wyoming, 1960-1975. *Journal of Rural Community Psychology*, *12*, 39-41.

Pfeffer, C. (2002). Suicide in mood disordered children and adolescents. *Child & Adolescent Psychiatric Clinics of North America*, *11*(3), 639-647. doi: 10.1016/S1056-4993(02)00012-3.

Pirkis, J., & Burgess, P. (1998). Suicide and recency of health care contacts: A systematic review. *British Journal of Psychiatry*, *173*, 462-474.

The President's Commission on Mental Health. (1978). *Report to the President*. Washington, DC: U.S. Government Printing Office.

Proudfoot, J., Goldberg, D., Mann, A., Everitt, B., Marks, I., & Gray, J. A. (2003). Computerized, interactive, multimedia cognitive-behavioural program for anxiety and depression in general practice. *Psychological Medicine*, *33*(2), 217-227.

Ratnayeke, L. (1998). Reaching the suicidal in rural communities. In R. J. Kosky, H. S. Eshkevari, R. D. Goldney, & R. Hassan (Eds.), *Suicide prevention: The global context* (pp. 269-271). New York: Plenum.

Renwick, M. Y., Olsen, G. G., & Tyrrell, M. S. (1982). Suicide in rural New South Wales: Comparison with metropolitan experience. *Medical Journal of Australia*, *1*(9), 377-380.

Rost, K. M., Owen, R. R., Smith, J., & Smith, G. R., Jr. (1998). Rural-urban differences in service use and course of illness in bipolar disorder. *Journal of Rural Health*, *14*(1), 3643.

Rowland, D., & Lyons, B. (1989). Triple jeopardy: Rural, poor, and uninsured. *Health Services Research*, *23*(6), 975-1004.

Sadowski, L., & Munoz, S. (1996). Nonfatal and fatal firearm injuries in rural county. *Journal of American Medical Association*, *275*(22), 1762-1764.

Scott, G., Ciarrochi, J., & Deane, F. (2003). The increasing incidence of suicide: Economic development, individualism, and social integration. In P. Hunout (Ed.), *The erosion of the social link in the economically advanced countries*, part 1, (pp. 1-40). *The International Scope Review*, *5*(9).

Shaffer, D., Scott, M., Wilcox, H., Maslow, C., Hicks, R., Lucas, C. P. et al. (2004). The Columbia Suicide Screen: Validity and reliability of a screen for youth suicide and depression. *Journal of the American Academy of Child and Adolescent Psychiatry*, *43*(1), 1-9.

Shajahan, P. M., & Cavanagh, J. T. (1998). Admission for depression among men in Scotland, 1980-1995: retrospective study. *British Medical Journal*, *316*, 1496-1497.

Spoth, R. (1997). Challenges in defining and developing the field of rural mental disorder preventive intervention research. *American Journal of Community Psychology*, *25*(4), 425-448. doi:10:1023/A:1024603504781

Stamm, B. H., & Peredina, D. A. (2000). Evaluating psychosocial aspects of telemedicine and telehealth systems. *Professional Psychology: Research and Practice*, *31*, 184-189.

Starfield, B. (1992). *Primary care: Concept evaluation and policy*. New York: Oxford University Press.

Strawn, B. D., Hester, S., & Brown, W. S. (1998). Telecare: A social support intervention for family caregivers of dementia victims. *Clinical Gerontologist*, *18*(3), 66-69.

Svenson, J. E., Spurlock, C., & Nypaver, M. (1996). Pediatric firearm-related fatalities. Not just an urban problem. *Archives of Pediatrics Adolescent Medicine, 150*(6), 583–587.

Turvey, C., Stromquist, A., Kelly, K., Zwerling, C., & Merchant, J. (2002). Financial loss and suicidal ideation in a rural community sample. *Acta Psychiatrica Scandinavica, 106*(5), 373–380. doi:10.1034/j.1600-0447.2002.02340.x

U.S. Department of Agriculture Economic Research Service. (2003). Measuring rurality: Rural–urban continuum codes. Retrieved from http://www.ers.usda.gov/briefing/rurality/RuralUrbCon/

U.S. Department of Health and Human Services. (n.d.). *Healthy People 2000. Midcourse Review and 1995 Revisions.* Washington, DC: Author.

U.S. Department of Health and Human Services. (2005). *Mental Health and Rural America*: 1994–2005. Retrieved May, 23, 2011, from Health Resources and Service Administration website: ftp://ftp.hrsa.gov/ruralhealth/RuralMentalHealth.pdf

U.S. Department of Health and Human Services. (2001). *National strategy for suicide prevention: Goals and objectives for action.* Retrieved from http://www.ncbi.nlm.nih.gov/books/NBK44281/pdf/TOC.pdf

Van Den Berg, S., Shapiro, D. A., Bickerstaffe, D., & Cavanagh, K. (2004). Computerized cognitive-behaviour therapy for anxiety and depression: A practical solution to the shortage of trained therapists. *Journal of Psychiatric and Mental Health Nursing, 11*(5), 508–513. doi:10.1111/j.1365-2850.2004.00745.x

Wainer, J., & Chesters, J. (2000). Rural mental health: Neither romanticism nor despair. *Australian Journal of Rural Health, 8*(3), 141–147.

Wenger, A. (1992). Transnational nursing and health care issues in urban and rural contexts. *Journal of Transcultural Nursing, 4*(2), 4–10.

Wodarski, J. S. (1983). Rural community mental health practice. Baltimore: University Park Press.

World Health Organization. (2003). The world health report: Shaping the future. Retrieved from http://www.who.int/whr/2003/en/

World Health Organization in collaboration with UNEP. (1990). *Public health impact of pesticides used in agriculture.* Geneva: World Health Organization.

Yuen, E., Gerdes, J., & Gonzales, J. (1996). Patterns of rural mental health care: An exploratory study. *General Hospital Psychiatry, 18*(1), 14–21.

14

Providing Mental Health Services for Racial, Ethnic, and Sexual Orientation Minority Groups in Rural Areas

ISHAN WILLIAMS, DERICK WILLIAMS, AMANDA PELLEGRINO, AND JACOB C. WARREN

INTRODUCTION

*R*eports have consistently demonstrated that stark disparities exist in the receipt of overall health care, and specifically in mental health care, for minority groups (Freiman & Zuvekas, 2000; Kirby, Taliaferro, & Zuvekas, 2006; Lasser, Himmelstein, & Woolhander, McCormick, & Bor, 2002; Smedley, Stith, & Nelson, 2003; Zuvekas, Taliaferro, 2003). A number of factors have surfaced that partially explain some of the disparities, such as health insurance coverage and socioeconomic differences (Kirby et al., 2006). However, Kirby and colleagues (2006) suggest that other factors may also play a part, such as attitudes toward risk, perceptions of discrimination or bias in the health care system, and other social and cultural beliefs that affect seeking care. All these factors potentially have a stronger effect in rural areas, where overall economic and social conditions influence a number of health outcomes (particular for minorities). A better understanding is needed of the underlying causes of mental health care disparities among rural minorities (including minorities from racial/ethnic groups and sexual orientation groups) if overall treatment and access to treatment for mental health is to be improved.

RACIAL AND ETHNIC DISPARITIES IN RURAL AREAS

Research into the underlying processes surrounding racial and ethnic disparities in receiving mental health care services has shown that African Americans and Hispanic populations receive less mental health treatment even when age,

229

gender, and insurance status are controlled for in the analysis (Goodwin, Koenen, Hellman, Guardino, & Struening, 2002; Han & Liu, 2005; Padgett, Patrick, Burns, & Schlesinger, 1994; Zito, Safer, Zuckerman, Gardner, & Soeken, 2005). While effective treatments exist for many mental health disorders, it is well documented that many receive no treatment or are undertreated. This problem is particularly acute for African Americans and Hispanics (Freiman & Zuvekas, 2000; Han & Liu, 2005; Hines-Martin, Malone, Kim, & Brown-Piper, 2003; Lasser et al., 2002; Mueller, Patil, & Boilesen, 1998; Padgett et al., 1994; Phillips, Mayer, & Aday, 2000). For example, the Mexican American Prevalence and Services Survey (MAPSS) showed that 71% of Mexican Americans with diagnosed disorders received no mental health services in a calendar year (Vega et al., 1998). Harman, Edlund, and Fortney (2004), using the Medical Expenditure Panel Survey (MEPS; Hauenstein et al., 2006), also found that African Americans and Latinos were about half as likely as non-Hispanic Whites to fill a prescription for an antidepressant. Also using MEPS data, Han and Liu (2005) found that African Americans were 8.3% less likely than non-Hispanic Whites to fill a prescription for psychotropic medications used to treat mental illness.

According to Davis (2005), 25% of the African American population has been diagnosed with a mental health disorder. In 2003, the California Black Women's Project found that 60% of African American women experience symptoms of depression. This number may be higher for those who experience chronic disease, as chronic disease has been linked to depression and other mental health issues in this population (Artinian, Washington, Flack, Hockman, & Jen, 2006; Centers for Disease Control and Prevention, 2004). One way in which African American women cope with mental health issues is by utilizing mental health services; yet many researchers have reported lower utilization rates of using mental health services by African American women when compared to their White counterparts, and even African American men (e.g., Breslau, Kendler, Su, Gaxiola-Aguilar, & Kessler, 2005). Thus, it is important to recognize other ways in which African American women manage their mental health issues. It is known throughout the literature that many African American populations use informal sources of support to cope with mental health issues. Spirituality and religiosity (Gill, Barrio Minton, & Myers, 2010; Yick, 2008), other resources such as church, family, and friends (Abrams, Dornig, & Curran, 2009; Matthews & Hughes, 2001), and informal helping relationships with neighbors and coworkers (Matthews & Hughes, 2001) have been cited as resources for coping and may be even more beneficial in rural areas where access to traditional mental health services is limited. However, research has not confirmed whether these resources are sufficient to meet the needs created by chronic mental health issues such as depression.

While fully controlled outcome studies have not been conducted, help-seeking behaviors increase when African American women are referred for treatment by informal resources (Jackson, Neighbors, Gurin, 1986). Ward,

Clark, and Heidrich (2009) found that African American women reported individual and group counseling to be beneficial in controlling mental health issues. Women reported many different coping resources such as physical activities (e.g., exercise), spiritual behaviors (e.g., reading the Bible, praying, and counseling with pastors), social activities (e.g., using family and friends as support and visiting community support activities), seeking professional help, and other coping activities (e.g., journaling) for mental health concerns. Knowing this, it appears that a strength-based holistic approach to mental health treatment would be beneficial in meeting the needs of rural African American communities, and for women in particular.

Differences in mental health care among minorities have been documented extensively for urban populations; however, there is limited information on mental health treatment in rural areas. Rural populations have higher rates of comorbidities and adverse outcomes, including greater rates of hospitalization and suicide (Breslau et al., 2005; Kroenke, Spitzer, & Williams, 2001; Rost et al., 1998a; Rost, Zhang, Fortney, Smith, & Smith, 1998b; World Health Organization, 2007). Minority populations, who frequently experience disparities in the incidence, prevalence, seriousness of disease, and in access to care, may bear a disproportionate burden from mental illness and the associated reduction of quality-of-life in rural areas (U.S. Department of Health and Human Services, 2001; Williams, 2005). Additional barriers include discrimination and stigma, which often contribute to minorities not receiving mental health treatment (Lau & Gallagher-Thompson, 2002).

Much remains to be learned about factors that contribute to racial/ethnic disparities in rural mental health treatment services that affect the provision of rural mental health care. For example, poverty is common among rural residents, even more so among rural minority populations. Research indicates that African Americans and other minorities are less likely to be insured, more likely to live in poverty, and more likely to use emergency services or seek mental health treatment from a primary care provider than from a mental health specialist (Chow, Jaffee, & Snowden, 2003; Pingatore, Snowden, Sansone, & Klinkman, 2001). More than one-third of nonmetropolitan African Americans, Hispanics, and Native Americans have poverty-level incomes, almost three times the poverty rate for nonmetropolitan Whites. Correspondingly, nonmetropolitan poverty rates are highest in the South, where rural African Americans are concentrated, and in the West, where most rural Hispanics are located (Dalaker & Naifeh, 1997). In 2004, the poverty rates of rural residents, Latinos, African Americans, and Native Americans ranged from 21.8% to 26.8%; however, the poverty rate for similar ethnic groups living in metropolitan statistical areas (MSAs) was only 14.5% during the same time frame. Similarly, the unemployment rates in rural populations are almost three times the national average (Rural Healthy People, 2010). This likely contributes to the continued higher poverty rates among rural ethnic minority populations versus metropolitan populations, greatly impacting on their ability to afford mental health services (even if they are available). The high rate of poverty among rural minorities likely contributes to nontreatment rates as much as race and ethnicity, cost of treatment, and place of residence.

Another study conducted by Petterson, Williams, Hauenstein, Rovnyak, and Merwin (2009) examined not only MSAs, but also different levels of rurality. Results indicated smaller differences in treatment rates for ethnic minorities compared to non-Hispanic Whites. The authors suggest this result may be a consequence of the scarcity of mental health providers in rural areas, which may lead people to rely more heavily on primary care. Further, the authors suggest that there may be smaller differences across race because mental health treatment is more likely to be administered in conjunction with non-mental health treatment.

Other studies have shown that urban non-Hispanic Whites are more likely to receive mental health treatment than rural residents of any race/ethnicity. For example, Alegría et al. (2002) found that urban non-Hispanic Whites are more likely to receive specialty mental health treatment than Latinos or African Americans regardless of socioeconomic status. Interestingly, race was not a significant factor in predicting who receives treatment in rural areas among those classified as nonpoor. This finding illustrates the problem of limited access to mental health treatment for all people in rural areas. Yet, when combining race and ethnicity with low socioeconomic status, the ability to receive mental health treatment may be less accessible.

Barriers to Provision of Mental Health Services for Rural Minorities

Economic conditions and insufficient mental health services create barriers in rural populations, and especially among persons from ethnic minority groups (Gamm, Stone, & Pittman, 2003). As indicated above, poverty rates are higher in rural areas than metropolitan areas. Approximately 59% of African Americans in the South are poorer than their urban counterparts. Poverty has been found to interact with rural status, further impacting on health outcomes for ethnic minorities (Markstrom, Stamm, Stamm, Berthold, & Running Wolf, 2003). Research has indicated, however, that ethnic minorities from a disadvantaged socioeconomic status have increased utilization of mental health *emergency* services (Snowden, Masland, Libby, Wallace, & Fawley, 2008). Further investigation in the provision of mental health services among rural minorities could further elucidate this phenomenon; however, it is possible that treatment is delayed until crisis situations arise, at which point the emergency room becomes the only place available to receive services (especially for the rural uninsured).

Even for rural minorities who can afford mental health care, it is frequently inaccessible or personally unacceptable for a variety of reasons. As discussed throughout this text, there is resounding evidence showing an insufficient number of mental health and generalist providers in rural areas (Merwin, Hinton, Dembling, & Stern, 2003; Merwin, Snyder, & Katz, 2006; National Rural Health Association, 1999). This insufficient number of providers often results in rural families having to travel long distances to obtain care, which continues to limit access (Arcury, Preisser, Gesler, & Powers, 2005; Fortney, Rost, Zhang, & Warren, 1999). Further, general distrust of professionals among minorities (Corbie-Smith, Thomas, & St. George, 2002; Fox, Blank, Rovnyak, & Barnett, 2001; Fox, Merwin, & Blank, 1995) and stigmatization of mental health problems (Menke & Flynn, 2009; Ward et al., 2009) have been associated with African Americans' lack of seeking mental health services when available (Murry, Heflinger, Suiter, & Brody, 2011; Sirey et al., 2001). Given the stigma associated with obtaining mental health care services and the limited number of facilities providing mental health services in rural areas, rural residents may opt out of receiving care due to the lack of anonymity. Moreover, higher rates of poverty and stigma regarding mental health among rural minorities make the likelihood of seeking care low (Lau & Gallagher-Thompson, 2002; Murry et al., 2011). Thus, the answer to the lack of mental health utilization among rural minorities is multifold, focusing on affordability, accessibility, and acceptability.

Many reasons for the existing disparities, and strategies to remedy these disparities, remain unexplained (Zuvekas & Taliaferro, 2003). Compared to Caucasians, ethnic minorities may underestimate their need for mental health services. Kimerling and Baumrind (2005) suggest that overall African American, Hispanic, and Asian women are less likely to seek specialty mental health treatment compared to White women. Additionally, these researchers suggest that even after controlling for perceived need for mental health treatment, insurance status, poverty, and mental distress, variations in access based on race and ethnicity persist. Similar disparities have been reported in rural areas; however, there have been attempts in reducing these disparities in access and use of mental health treatment. In particular, Diaz-Perez, Farley, and Cabanis (2004) utilized a mobile unit to help identify mental health needs among immigrant Mexicans in rural Colorado. This strategy was found to be effective in getting the rural immigrants to a health care home for follow-up. Once minorities have communicated their unique needs and these issues have been examined, future research can focus on how best to address the inequalities among rural and urban populations, in particularly among minorities, as well as reducing the stigma associated with mental health.

THE IMPACT OF SEXUAL ORIENTATION ON MENTAL HEALTH IN RURAL AREAS

Much of the research involving sexual minorities including lesbians, gay, bisexual, and questioning (LGBQ) individuals residing in rural areas is either qualitative in nature or restricted in geographic area (Boulden, 2001; Cody & Welch,

1997; Eldridge, Mack, & Swank, 2006; Kennedy, 2010; Leedy & Connolly, 2007; McCarthy, 2000; Oswald & Culton, 2003; Willging, Salvador, & Kano 2006a). While this may limit the generalizations that can be made from the results, these studies have yielded information that is consistent, valuable, and rich in detail about this under-researched population. Although research involving gender minorities (e.g., transgendered persons) residing in rural areas would inform the understanding of this population, there are very few studies that include transgendered individuals, and these have been almost exclusively conducted in urban areas. In addition, the literature on rural lesbians is very limited; therefore, the majority of the discussion below focuses on rural gay men.

Studies involving LGBQ individuals who reside in rural areas indicate they may be more vulnerable than their nonrural counterparts to psychological risk factors related to exposure to victimization and discrimination, higher levels of internalized heterosexism due to increased levels of religiosity, isolationism and lack of social opportunities with other LGBQ individuals, lack of familial and social support, and decreased comfort level of disclosing sexual identity to others (Kennedy, 2010; Leedy & Connolly, 2007; McCarthy, 2000; Preston, D'Augelli, Kassab, & Starks, 2007; Willging et al., 2006a). Additionally, research has suggested that many practitioners in rural areas may not be aware of the best practices for LGBQ individuals (Willging, Salvador, & Kano 2006b). While there are many challenges, there are also many proposed solutions for improving rural life for LGBQ individuals.

Heterosexism

Rural living is associated with conservatism, religiosity, uniformity, gossip, social conformity, and heterosexual culture (Bell & Valentine, 1995; Oswald, 2002). Residing in a rural area has been shown to be correlated with being more likely to harbor attitudes of heterosexism, or discriminatory attitudes or actions directed toward sexual minorities (Snively, Kreuger, Stretch, Watt, & Chadha, 2004). Some factors found to predict increased likelihood of heterosexism among rural residents are fear of HIV/AIDS, male gender, religiosity or fundamentalism, conservative political orientation, and less contact with LGBQ individuals (Eldridge et al., 2006; Hopwood & Connors, 2002; Snively et al., 2004). Social institutions are also involved with perceptions of heterosexism; schools in particular were identified by LGBQ individuals in rural Wyoming as institutions fraught with high levels of heterosexism (Leedy & Connolly, 2007). With heterosexism more likely in rural than urban areas, rural areas may be more dangerous environments for LGBQ individuals to navigate (which can have a direct impact on their mental health).

Furthermore, exposure to heterosexism and stigma from others can create internalized heterosexism within LGBQ individuals, which is when an LGBQ individual harbors negative or prejudiced thoughts and feelings about homosexuality, as well as possibly acting in discriminatory ways toward other LGBQ individuals. Kennedy (2010) found that gay men in rural Ontario, Canada, continued to harbor negative feelings, guilt, and low self-esteem as adults stemming from their childhood experience of religion in their family of origin. As a result, many of these men had since rejected organized religion (a frequent source of social interaction and support in rural areas; Kennedy, 2010). Internalized heterosexism was a common theme found in interviews with 85% of a sample of gay men living in rural areas of New England (Cody & Welch, 1997). The men had experienced and internalized negative oppressive messages from parents, teachers, members of the clergy, and peers, which had caused the men to feel ashamed and guilty about their sexual orientation. Some had even sought mental health assistance to change their sexual orientation (so-called "conversion therapies"). Many reported experiencing continuing heterosexist treatment from others (Cody & Welch, 1997). Similarly, gay men living in rural Wyoming minimized the frequent experience of verbal and physical violence against themselves and others for being gay, which Boulden (2001) asserts is evidence of internalized heterosexism. Additionally, Boulden (2001) suggests that the fact the gay men accepted that they had to hide their sexual orientation publicly to be accepted within their rural communities was also indicative of internalized heterosexism, since the gay men did not challenge the oppression. Other studies have also suggested that a number of LGBQ individuals in rural areas conceal their sexual identity in public to be accepted within their communities (Bell & Valentine, 1995; Leedy & Connolly, 2007; McCarthy, 2000; Oswald & Culton, 2003). These researchers suggest that such an admission of feelings of shame and guilt or lack of indignation about experienced oppression by LGBQ individuals residing in rural areas may be evidence of internalized heterosexism. However, other explanations for these behaviors may involve self-preservation strategies and cultural norms specific to rural communities.

Invisibility and "Don't Ask, Don't Tell"

As discussed above, some LGBQ individuals attempt to conceal their sexual identity within the rural environment. LBGQ individuals have consistently reported to researchers that they fear coming out to their rural neighbors because they may be victimized, discriminated against, or ostracized (Bell & Valentine, 1995; Cody & Welch, 1997; McCarthy, 2000; Oswald & Culton, 2003). In one study, LGBQ individuals who lacked confidence and a sense of belongingness in their rural New Mexico communities reported experiencing fear of disclosure as a major stressor (Willging et al., 2006a). Those same LGBQ individuals reported being fearful of disclosing their sexual or gender identity to mental health providers for fear of bias, discrimination, and negative response (Willging et al., 2006a).

Boulden (2001) discovered an unspoken "don't ask, don't tell" mentality between gay men and their rural neighbors. A hyperawareness of surroundings and others was a common theme in the interviews Boulden (2001) conducted, and men reported guarding against purposefully revealing their homosexuality in front of their neighbors in order to be accepted in the community. Participants described how they were careful to be on guard in public and not engage in behaviors such as holding hands with their partners, referring to their partners by pet names, or acting in ways that could be perceived as effeminate (Boulden, 2001). Oswald and Culton (2003) found that LGBQ individuals living in nonmetropolitan Illinois also felt the need to forgo drawing attention to their sexuality in public in their rural surroundings to ensure safety. Similarly, LGBQ individuals surveyed by Leedy and Connolly (2007) in Wyoming also indicated that they refrained from exhibiting behavior in public that would indicate their sexual orientation. The gay men in rural Wyoming described developing public personas to improve their quality of life and ease of existence in rural culture, especially in community and work settings (Boulden, 2001). The hyperawareness and fear of discovery prompt LGBQ individuals in rural areas to attempt to remain invisible in their surroundings for safety and social motivations.

Leedy and Connolly (2007) posited that their respondents may have been selective about coming out to coworkers, friends, and neighbors based on the nature of anticipated response, because the respondents rated the reactions of their coworkers, friends, and neighbors as neutral or generally positive. This anticipatory planning regarding whom to reveal their sexual identity to seems consistent with the caution reported by LGBQ individuals residing in rural areas concerning how to navigate the heterosexist landscape of rural community life.

However, many of the gay men interviewed by Boulden (2001) believed that many of their neighbors knew of or suspected their sexual orientation. Participants reported that other men in the community would avoid socializing with them or would not come to the gay men's homes for fear that association with them would imply homosexuality. Thus, despite the gay men's efforts to hide their sexual identity in public, they felt many in the community were silently aware (hence the "don't ask, don't tell" label Boulden (2001) utilized to describe the interaction between the gay men and the heterosexual rural community).

Victimization and Discrimination

Despite attempts to remain invisible, LGBQ individuals residing in rural areas experience harassment, discrimination, and violence. Waldo, Hesson-McInnis, and D'Augelli (1998) found that heterosexist victimization, a term encompassing a range of victimization from verbal harassment to physical assault motivated by heterosexism, has similar correlates for young adults in urban and rural settings. Those individuals that do not conform to traditional gender stereotypes are more likely to be assumed to be LGBQ, and thus are more frequently targeted for victimization. Those individuals who are more open about their LGBQ sexual orientation are more likely to be victimized as well. The victimization leads to lowered self-esteem, which in turn exacerbates psychological distress. While suicidality is not a direct consequence of stressful life events, suicidality is frequently caused by a period of psychological turbulence initiated by stressful experiences. Thus, since victimization leads to lowered self-esteem which in turn leads to increased psychological distress, these experiences and the resulting stress are jointly predictive of suicidality. However, reducing life stressors and problems can improve self-concept and self-esteem while also reducing psychological distress, and should be explored with LGBQ clients (Waldo et al., 1998).

A very high proportion (71.2%) of LGBQ survey respondents from rural Wyoming reported they had suffered harassment and victimization (Leedy & Connolly, 2007). Some had experienced discrimination in regard to credit and banking decisions, tax benefits, entry into community groups, employment benefits, employment opportunities, and termination of employment. LGBQ individuals residing in the least densely populated counties in Wyoming indicated experiencing the highest levels of discrimination at institutional and personal or community levels (Leedy & Connolly, 2007). While only 10% of the gay men interviewed by Cody and Welch (1997) had been harassed in childhood or adolescence for being gay, 35% had been harassed for being gay as adults in rural northern New England. Boulden (2001) indicated the gay men he interviewed reported they could not even walk down the street with women without being verbally harassed. The same gay men had objects and trash thrown onto their lawns, and they received threatening phone calls as well (Boulden, 2001). This victimization was perpetrated despite attempts by the gay men to keep their sexuality as invisible as possible in public, as discussed in the previous section.

Unfortunately, LGBQ individuals may engage in maladaptive coping mechanisms to reduce the stressors and problems associated with rural life. When gay men experience intolerance from families, health care providers, and communities in rural areas they sometimes engage in risky sexual behavior to relieve the stress caused by intolerance, regardless of self-esteem and internalized heterosexism (Preston, et al., 2007). LGBQ individuals also have high rates of tobacco and alcohol consumption (Greenwood & Gruskin, 2007). Sadly, these maladaptive coping mechanisms often lead to serious negative health consequences including cancer, heart disease, pulmonary disease, stroke, renal disease, vascular disease, ulcers, liver disease, obesity, blood pressure, diabetes, and injury (Fagerström, 2002; Foster & Marriott, 2006).

Isolation

LGBQ individuals living in rural areas may be more susceptible to negative effects from victimization and discrimination because they feel isolated and have fewer opportunities to socialize with other LGBQ individuals through LGBQ-affirming organizations. LGBQ community support relieves psychological distress (Waldo et al., 1998); however, a lack of community-based LGBQ resources heightens feelings of social isolation among rural individuals (McCarthy, 2000; Willging et al., 2006b). Rural LGBQ residents are even more prone to isolation given the smaller populations and often conservative environment of rural living. Oswald and Culton (2003) found that LGBQ respondents in nonmetropolitan Illinois rated the lack of a community as the "worst thing" about living in a rural area, and they indicated the LGBQ community was too small, hidden, fragmented, and/or lacking in resources. Particularly, resources were lacking for individuals looking for committed relationships, same-sex couples, and parents with children, as the gay bars that were available seemed to cater to young and single LGBQ individuals (Oswald & Culton, 2003).

While LGBQ individuals residing in rural Wyoming reported being active in their geographic community and having social ties with other LGBQ individuals locally, they reported a lack of LGBQ-affirming services, especially in the less densely populated counties (Leedy & Connolly, 2007). Additionally, it is important to note that there are frequently no gay bars or bookstores, and there are no regular places for LGBQ individuals to congregate (Leedy & Connolly, 2007). Negative aspects of rural living found by Cody and Welch (1997) were lack of visible gay community, difficulty meeting similar people for establishing relationships or friendships, magnified sense of aloneness/difference/isolation, and too much introspection with little distraction. The gay men interviewed coped with these drawbacks by living near colleges/universities or visiting nearby cities (Cody & Welch, 1997).

Some gays and lesbians find a small group of gay or lesbian friends to socialize with in the rural areas, which functions as a small LGBQ community (Boulden, 2001; McCarthy, 2000). The groups go to dinner, socialize at each other's houses, go to the theater together, and other small group social activities. Yet, even these small groups are kept secret and underground to minimize the risk of being exposed to their heterosexist rural neighbors, and the small groups do not socialize with one another for the most part. To find and become an invited member of such a group can be quite challenging (Boulden, 2001; McCarthy, 2000). Despite these small informal LGBQ groups, there remains a paucity of LGBQ-affirming services and organizations in rural communities, which in itself raises the risk for LGBQ individuals feeling isolated, vulnerable, and psychologically distressed.

Lack of Support

LGBQ individuals can also lack support, understanding, and acceptance from family and friends. Half of the gay men interviewed by Cody and Welch (1997) who were living in rural New England indicated they experienced some sort of censorship by their families regarding their sexual orientation. Their families responded to the men's coming out declaration with silence, disinterest, ambivalence, or a lack of support. Some of the men had not verbally come out to their families, and instead had developed an unspoken understanding about their sexual orientation (Cody & Welch, 1997). While the gay men Boulden (2001) interviewed spoke about close relationships with their families in rural Wyoming, there was no indication about whether they were out to their families. Waldo et al. (1998) found that unsupportive family and friends were more likely to victimize or enable victimization of an LGBQ individual. On the other hand, supportive family and friends were found to be more likely to protect an LGBQ individual from victimization and offer resources to help an LGBQ individual avoid victimization (Waldo et al., 1998). Cody and Welch (1997) found that interviewees dealt with family censorship and lack of support by developing a family of choice from a group of close gay and nongay friends within their communities.

Mental Health Providers and Services
Unfortunately, despite being at risk for psychological distress due to heterosexism, victimization, discrimination, invisibility, isolation, and lack of familial and social support, LGBQ-affirming mental health services may not be readily available in many rural areas. Willging et al. (2006b) found that rural mental health providers lacked appropriate training to treat LGBQ individuals, reported individual and institutional forms of bias against LGBQ individuals in institutions proving mental health services in rural areas, assumed clients were heterosexual, isolated LGBQ individuals in treatment facilities, discouraged expression of sexual or gender identity disclosures in group therapy, and indicated many observed examples of fellow colleagues mistreating LGBQ individuals. Some mental health providers compensated for their biases by attempting to treat LGBQ individuals as no different from other clients (Willging et al., 2006b). This attempt at therapeutic neutrality is problematic because the mental health providers neglect confronting their own heterosexism and lack of training in LGBQ issues, as well as fail to consider the impact sexual and gender identity issues may have on the clients' mental health problems (Willging et al., 2006b). Additionally, even mental health providers knowledgeable about LGBQ issues struggled with whether to encourage LGBQ individuals to live more openly or continue to hide their identity in their rural communities, when both options could have detrimental effects (Willging et al., 2006b).

However, this lack of knowledge of and sensitivity to LGBQ issues may not be unique to practitioners in rural areas. Eliason and Hughes (2004) found that mental health practitioners and substance abuse counselors in urban areas of Chicago and rural areas of Iowa had little formal training in LGBQ issues, did not differ in knowledge of specific LGBQ issues that might influence alcohol and drug treatment, and lacked knowledge about legal issues such as domestic partnership and power of attorney, concepts of domestic partnership and internalized heterosexism, and issues related to family of origin and current family. Additionally, nearly half of the counselors both in the urban and rural areas reported negative or ambivalent attitudes about LGBQ individuals (Eliason & Hughes, 2004).

A lack of LGBQ social networks, fear of discrimination based on sexual or gender identity, misconceptions of mental illness and substance abuse, and financial concerns were some factors preventing LGBQ individuals from seeking mental health services in rural New Mexico (Willging et al., 2006a). Respondents indicated that they had experienced discrimination, inappropriate care, or premature discontinuation of care due to their sexual or gender identity when they sought mental health services in their communities. Several LGBQ individuals in the Willging et al. (2006a) study turned to religious institutions for treatment of emotional distress and substance abuse issues due to financial concerns, yet many of those individuals kept their sexual or gender identities secret while seeking religious assistance. Participants from Latino and Native American families reported that their family influenced their decision to utilize religious treatment options (Willging et al., 2006a).

LGBQ individuals sometimes report significantly *harmful* treatment from mental health professionals based on their sexual and gender identities, such as humiliation, laughter, and disparaging remarks (Willging et al., 2006a). Misconception about mental illness and substance abuse that prevent LGBQ individuals in rural areas from seeking mental health treatment include believing that mental illness is a sign of personal weakness that can be overcome by perseverance and hard work (Willging et al., 2006a). Access to LGBQ-affirming mental health services is limited in rural areas, and financial concerns as well as lack of referrals to such services due to limited LGBQ social networks prevent many LGBQ individuals from traveling to LGBQ-affirming providers in urban areas (Willging et al., 2006a). LGBQ individuals in nonmetropolitian areas in Illinois also assumed that seeking mental health services would require either a suppression of the topic of their sexuality or that their sexuality would be treated with therapeutic neutrality (Oswald & Culton, 2003). These research findings expose a critical area in which mental health practitioners need further specialized training, continuing education, and mandated practice standards to improve the care provided to LGBQ individuals, especially those residing in rural areas. Additionally, the relationship of mental health professionals and the LGBQ community may require repair due to the aforementioned experiences and any other unethical treatment of LGBQ individuals have suffered from mental health service providers.

A HOLISTIC APPROACH TO MENTAL HEALTH FOR RURAL MINORITIES

Many of the issues faced by minorities (even beyond mental health) are neglected or underserved (Crockett, Zlotnick, Davis, Payne, & Washington, 2008), and there is a lack of a strong evidence base for provision of mental health care focused on the cultural realities of rural minorities. Finding culturally sensitive solutions to positively provide mental health resources to rural minority populations is essential. One promising approach for the provision of mental health care to rural minorities is taking a holistic, wellness-based approach. Wellness provides a perspective for understanding human functioning and how individuals choose a way of life in order to live life more fully (Myers, Sweeney, & Witmer, 2000). A Wellness model is focused on the holistic treatment of individuals. Wellness has been theoretically conceptualized by several researchers (e.g., Ardell, 1988; Hettler, 1984; Myers & Sweeney, 2005a; Myers et al., 2000). One specific model that has been useful across cultures and across many different adult mental health populations is the Indivisible Self model of wellness (IS-Wel; Myers & Sweeney, 2005a).

The Indivisible Self-Wellness Model

The IS Wel is an evidence-based model created from analyzing data from over 5,000 persons over a 7-year period (Myers & Sweeney, 2008). It is a strength-based model that focuses on the interconnectedness of each aspect of a person's life (Myers & Sweeney, 2005a). The model features five second-order factors, termed as *Creative Self, Coping Self, Social Self, Essential Self*, and *Physical Self*, and one higher order factor, titled *Wellness*. These five factors emerged from 17 scales (i.e., five life tasks and 12 individual subtasks of self-direction) of a previous model (see Hattie, Myers, & Sweeney, 2004). The various aspects of this model are depicted in Figure 14.1. According to Myers and Sweeney (2005a), each dimension of the model is connected to the others, thus an individual's strength in one dimension can be used to enhance functioning and overcome deficits in other dimensions. This model has been examined across populations with respect to age, ethnic group, sexual orientation, and geographic location (e.g., rural location).

In addition to the higher-order factor and the second-order factors, the Indivisible Self model of wellness presents contextual variables or environments in which individuals function. These contexts are *local, institutional, global*, and *chronometrical* (Myers & Sweeney, 2005a). Local contexts include families, neighborhoods, and communities; institutional contexts are education, religion, government, business, and industry; global contexts are politics, culture, global events, environment, media, and community; and, finally, chronometrical contexts represent the perpetual, positive, and purposeful ways in which people change over time (Myers & Sweeney, 2005a).

THE INDIVISIBLE SELF:
An Evidence-Based Model Of Wellness

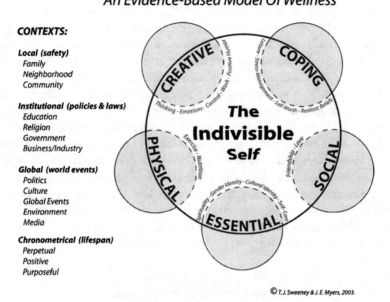

CONTEXTS:

Local (safety)
Family
Neighborhood
Community

Institutional (policies & laws)
Education
Religion
Government
Business/Industry

Global (world events)
Politics
Culture
Global Events
Environment
Media

Chronometrical (lifespan)
Perpetual
Positive
Purposeful

© T. J. Sweeney & J. E. Myers, 2003.

FIGURE 14.1
Indivisible self model of wellness

These contexts represent safety, policies and laws, world events, and lifestyle choices over the lifespan, respectively. Each context helps to understand individual behavior in relation to wellness and how the individual interacts with their environment, in this case specifically in the rural environment.

Wellness has been examined in relation to several mental health issues. Based on the IS-Wel and previous iterations of this model (e.g., Wheel of Wellness (Myers et al., 2000), the Five-Factor Wellness Inventory (5F-Wel; Myers & Sweeney, 2005b) was created to assess total wellness and the five factors. Using the 5F-Wel, mental health issues have been linked with wellness. Hermon and Hazler (1999) found a significant relationship between psychological well-being and wellness. They concluded that one's ability to self-regulate work, recreation, and leisure were significant contributors to undergraduate students' affective experience of psychological well-being ($R^2 = .35$). Gill et al. (2010) also found that wellness was significantly correlated with spirituality and religiosity.

More importantly, several empirical studies have been conducted that provide evidence of the effectiveness of using counseling wellness interventions. Myers and Sweeney (2008) summarize several studies that report positive effects of wellness interventions using pretest and posttest assessments of wellness across young adult and school-aged populations. Though it is not indicative that these studies included rural populations, Myers and Gill (2004) suggest that wellness strategies should be used to address mental health issues and the barriers to services for low-income rural women. Because of the complexities of rural living, and the systemic influence that rural life has upon all aspects of an individual's functioning, taking a holistic approach (specifically one guided by the 5F-Wel model) holds much promise in promoting mental health among rural minorities. By not focusing exclusively on mental health, the approach is able to impact the entire wellness of the individual—this may lead to not only improved outcomes, but also to rural minorities being more likely to accept treatment.

IMPLICATIONS FOR BEST PRACTICES AND RECOMMENDATIONS FOR THE FUTURE

Medically underserved populations and minorities who live in rural areas constitute a heterogeneous group. Understanding their challenges and potential solutions requires a variety of methods. While no one rural community looks exactly like another, there are consistent themes throughout communities that researchers and policy makers can pay attention to regarding the provision of quality mental health care services. Findings have consistently shown that rural residents are at a disadvantage relative to others for mental health treatment. Petterson et al. (2009) acknowledge that this disadvantage in rural areas is independent of minority status. This finding underscores the necessity of the pursuit of, examination, and provision of evidence-based practices and culturally competent mental health care to these diverse groups.

Racial and Ethnic Minorities

Evidence continues to suggest that there are variations in the provision of mental health services among diverse populations living in rural areas. Vega et al. (1998) found that the provision of service use was different for Mexican Americans living in rural areas when compared with those of urban users. Specifically, rural Mexican Americans were more likely to use general practitioners or informal service providers for their mental health problems. Using data from the National Comorbidity Survey, another study showed that rural residence was associated with less mental health treatment for African Americans and Latinos (Alegría et al., 2002). It is therefore imperative that future research builds on the current body of knowledge and continues to investigate the complexities and overlapping factors that contribute to mental health care service use among rural minorities. Important considerations include investigating how poor rates of mental health treatment and service use among minorities in rural areas could be a combination of the consequence of stigma, differences between consumers and professionals, and other traditional rural values that decrease the use of formal service use (Petterson et al., 2009; Philo, Parr, & Burns, 2003). In order to reduce disparities and improve access and resources for rural residents needing mental health care services, it seems essential to provide services that are tailored to the specific needs of the community.

Reduction of health care disparities in the rural community is a defined goal of best practice. To improve the quality of health care and the mental health care of a diverse population, there must be improved access to services (i.e., greater numbers of mental health providers, transportation to services). It is likely that access to a provider or a usual source of care will over time improve health outcomes (Beal, Doty, Hernandez, Shea, Davis, 2007). Further, the availability of quality services, supported by consumer advocacy programs is another way to improve the mental health care of rural residents. Many rural residents need advocacy help for access to care which gives voice to the need for personal, social, and community services. Advocacy can take various forms in practice, including self, peer, and specialty mental health advocacy. However, advocacy developed for African Americans and other minority communities must emphasize the interdependence with families and communities in the act of achieving an advocacy group (Rai-Atkins et al., 2002). Advocacy work will also be influenced by the concept of understanding racism and inequalities (McLean, Campbell, & Cornish, 2003; Newbigging & McKeown, 2007). These factors may not be solely associated with mental illness, but also influenced by being a member of a minority group.

Policies should be developed that involve consumers in the planning process of obtaining mental health services. Doty and Holmgren (2006) suggest that improving the continuity among the patients' relationship with their providers may reduce disparities in access, and this can be facilitated by including the patients' family in that process. Families frequently become the voice of patients in receiving mental health services and often reflect the patients' preferences. A universal best practice for those needing mental health care services is the provision of psychoeducation. For example, Coon, Thompson, Steffen, Sorocco, and Gallagher-Thompson (2003) found that women caregivers of older adults with dementia benefited from education about dementia that resulted in a reduction in caregiver depression. Other studies have shown that simply providing factual information to minority groups about mental illness may not be sufficient to reduce the myths associated with the disease or improve treatment or access to treatment (Alvidrez, Snowden, Rao, & Boccellari, 2009; Han, Chen, Hwang, & Wei, 2006; Jorm et al., 2003). As a result, psychoeducational interventions culturally tailored for African American populations may be more successful. Unfortunately, this strategy has rarely been used among rural African American populations. Alvidrez, Area'n, and Stewart (2005) sought the African American consumers' perspective regarding their concerns or challenges with mental health in order to develop a culturally tailored psychoeducational intervention. In this study, the psychoeducation was helpful in getting consumers to discuss mental health issues, but not necessarily change their treatment patterns.

It is necessary to ensure that rural minority families and consumers understand how to best navigate the mental health service system and know how to dispel the myths associated with mental illness in order to reduce associated disparities. It is not to say that "one size fits all," but strategies offered that can cover several mental illnesses or use a wellness approach, tailored by issues relevant to African Americans and/or Hispanics, is essential. Clearly, more work is needed to understand how rural people, in particular minority consumers, differ in their responsiveness to mental health information and to develop mental health interventions that are tailored to be culturally sensitive.

Sexual Orientation

Researchers have suggested many ways to improve the quality of life for LGBQ individuals living in rural areas. Leedy and Connelly (2007) recommend persuading human service providers and administrators to recognize and address their own heterosexism, as well as advocate for culturally competent services and programming for LGBQ individuals. State governments can require mandates, similar to racial and ethnic minority mandates, to require mental health providers to obtain training about LGBQ issues and recognize how their own attitudes and behaviors affect services provided to LGBQ individuals (Willging et al., 2006b). Preston, D'Augelli, Cain, and Schulze (2002) suggest utilizing peer gatekeepers and leaders to help address LGBQ health and mental health care issues in rural areas.

Oswald and Culton (2003) proposed many ways practitioners could help improve life for LGBQ individuals living in rural areas, including:

- Strengthen LGBQ-affirmative resources;
- Improve public support for LGBQ residents and pursue legal advocacy;
- Make contacts within the LGBQ community and distribute business cards among members or advertise within a LGBQ publication;
- Collaborate with the LGBQ community to develop programs to meet needs such as parenting classes, relationship enhancement groups, drug- and alcohol-free social events, retirement workshops, and legal rights classes;
- Offer community workshops to school, law enforcement, health care workers, and other community service providers on LGBQ issues; and
- Become an ally and advocate for LGBQ at local, state, and national level.

Snively (2004) proposes creating nonclinical-based gay/straight community-based groups for adolescents and young adults in rural areas, as young people need a nonschool, nonclinical acceptance-based group alternative that is not bound by bureaucracy. LGBQ adults can serve as mentors, volunteers, and board members for these groups, which may also be a way to strengthen LGBQ-affirming communities in rural areas for adults. Practitioners are cautioned to treat sexual orientation not as a problem, but rather collaborate with the rural LGBQ community to be an ally in order to advocate for an end to the oppression, discrimination, and victimization of LGBQ individuals (Boulden, 2001; Cody & Welch, 1997). By implementing any of these suggestions, mental health practitioners could actively improve rural life for LGBQ individuals.

CONCLUSION

As identified in this chapter, there are several barriers to mental health treatment in rural areas, and even more so among minority populations. These barriers impact on groups from minority racial, ethnic, and sexual orientation groups and can make them less likely to seek care in the midst of an environment of increased psychological stress. Reducing these barriers to mental health care in rural areas may both improve the overall health of Americans and reduce the disparities that still exist (Johnson, 2008). Murry et al. (2011) suggest a need for greater attention to public policy and the development of community advocacy groups in efforts to reduce and eliminate barriers among rural minorities seeking mental health treatment. Myers and Gill (2004) suggest a wellness approach to meet the mental health needs of individuals who live in rural areas. Understanding and encouraging minorities to voice their mental health needs will likely ignite rural families to seek appropriate mental health care and overcome the existing barriers to obtain care.

REFERENCES

Abrams, L. S., Dornig, K., & Curran, L. (2009). Barriers to service use for postpartum depression symptoms among low-income ethnic minority mothers in the United States. *Qualitative Health Research, 19*, 535–551.

Alegría, M., Canino, G., Rios, R., Vera, M., Calderon, J., Rusch, D. et al. (2002). Inequalities in use of specialty mental health services among Latinos, African Americans, and non-Latino whites. *Psychiatric Services, 53*(12):1547–1555.

Alvidrez, J., Areán, P. A., & Stewart, A. L. (2005). Psychoeducation to increase psychotherapy entry for older African Americans. *The American Journal of Geriatric Psychiatry, 13*, 554–561.

Alvidrez, J., Snowden, L. R., Rao, S. M., & Boccellari, A. (2009). Psychoeducation to address stigma in black adults referred for mental health treatment: A randomized pilot study. *Community Mental Health Journal, 45*, 127–136.

Arcury, T. A., Preisser, J. S., Gesler, W. M., & Powers, J. M. (2005). Access to transportation and health care utilization in a rural region. *Journal of Rural Health, 21*(1), 31–38.

Ardell, D. B. (1988). The history and future of the wellness movement. In J. P. Opatz (Ed.), *Wellness promotion strategies: Selected proceeding of the eighth annual National Wellness Conference*. Dubuque, IA: Kendall/Hunt.

Artinian, N. T., Washington, O. G. M., Flack, J. M., Hockman, E., & Jen, K. L. (2006). Depression, stress and blood pressure in urban African American women. *Progress in Cardiovascular Nursing, 21*, 68-75.

Bell, D. D., & Valentine, G. G. (1995). Queer country: Rural lesbian and gay lives. *Journal of Rural Studies, 11*(2), 113-122.

Beal, A. C., Doty, M. M., Hernandez, S. E., Shea, K. K., & Davis, K. (2007). *Closing the divide: How medical homes promote equity in health care: Results from the Commonwealth Fund 2006 Health Care Quality Survey*. The Commonwealth Fund: New York.

Breslau, J., Kendler, K. S., Su, M., Gaxiola-Aguilar, S., & Kessler, R. C. (2005). Lifetime risk and persistence of psychiatric disorders across ethnic groups in the United States. *Psychological Medicine, 35*, 317-327.

Boulden, W. T. (2001). Gay men living in a rural environment. *Journal of Gay & Lesbian Social Services: Issues in Practice, Policy & Research, 12*(3-4), 63-75. doi: 10.1300/J041v13n01_06

Centers for Disease Control and Prevention. (2004). *The burden of chronic diseases and their risk factors: National and state*. Retrieved from http://www.cdc.gov/nccdphp/burdenbook2004/pdf/burden_book2004.pdf

Chow, J. C., Jaffee, K., & Snowden, L. (2003). Racial/ethnic disparities in the use of mental health services in poverty areas. *American Journal of Public Health, 93*, 792-797.

Cody, P. J., & Welch, P. L. (1997). Rural gay men in northern New England: Life experiences and coping styles. *Journal of Homosexuality, 33*(1), 51-67. doi: 10.1300/J082v33n01_04

Corbie-Smith, G., Thomas, S. B., & St. George, M. (2002). Distrust, race, and research. *Archives of Internal Medicine, 162*(21), 2458-2463.

Coon, D. W., Thompson, L., Steffen, A., Sorocco, K., & Gallagher-Thompson, D. (2003). Anger and depression management: Psychoeducational skill training interventions for women caregivers of a relative with dementia. *Gerontologist, 43*(5), 678-689.

Crockett, K., Zlotnick, C., Davis, M., Payne, N., & Washington, R. (2008). A depression prevention intervention for rural low-income African American women at risk for postpartum depression. *Women's Mental Health, 11*, 319-325. doi: 10.1007/s00737-008-0036-3

Davis, K. (2005). *Decreasing discrimination and stigma associated with mental illness in the African American community*. Retrieved from http://promoteacceptance.samhsa.gov/update/archive/march2005.aspx

Dalaker, J., & Naifeh, M. (1997). *U.S. Bureau of the Census Current Population Reports Series P60-201, Poverty in the United States: 1997*. Washington, DC: U.S. Government Printing Office.

Diaz-Perez, Mde. J., Farley, T., & Cabanis, C. M. (2004). A program to improve access to health care among Mexican immigrants in rural Colorado. *Journal of Rural Health, 20*(3), Retrieved from http://www.ncbi.nlm.nih.gov/pubmed/15298101

Doty, M. M., & Holmgren, A. L. (2006). Health care disconnect: Gaps in coverage and care for minority adults. Findings from the Commonwealth Fund Biennial Health Insurance Survey (2005). *Issue Brief: Commonwealth Fund, 21*, 1-12.

Eldridge, V., Mack, L., & Swank, E. (2006). Explaining comfort with homosexuality in rural America. *Journal of Homosexuality*, *51*(2), 39-56. doi: 10.1300/J082v51n02_03

Eliason, M. J., & Hughes, T. (2004). Treatment counselor's attitudes about lesbian, gay, bisexual, and transgendered clients: Urban vs. rural settings. *Substance Use & Misuse*, *39*(4), 625-644. doi: 10.1081/JA-120030063

Fagerström, K. (2002). The epidemiology of smoking: Health consequences and benefits of cessation. *Drugs*, *62*, 21-29.

Freiman, M. P., & Zuvekas, S. H. (2000). Determinants of ambulatory treatment mode for mental illness. *Health Economics*, *9*, 423-434.

Fortney, J., Rost, K., Zhang, M., & Warren, J. (1999). The impact of geographic accessibility on the intensity and quality of depression treatment. *Medical Care*, *37*, 884-893.

Foster, R. K., & Marriott, H. E. (2006). Alcohol consumption in the new millennium—Weighing up the risks and benefits for our health. *Nutrition Bulletin*, *31*(4), 286-331. doi: 10.1111/j.1467-3010.2006.00588.x

Fox, J. C., Blank, M., Rovnyak, V. G., & Barnett, R. Y. (2001). Barriers to help seeking for mental disorders in a rural impoverished population. *Community Mental Health Journal*, *37*, 421-436.

Fox, J., Merwin, E., & Blank, M. (1995) De facto mental health services in the rural south. *Journal of Health Care for the Poor and Underserved*, *6*(4), 434-468.

Gamm, L. G., Stone, S., & Pittman, S. (2003). Mental health and mental disorders—A rural challenge. *Rural healthy people 2010: A companion document to healthy people 2010: Vol 1*. College Station, TX: Texas A&M University System Health Science Center, School of Rural Public Health, Southwest Rural Health Research Center.

Gill, C. S., Barrio Minton, C. A., & Myers, J. E. (2010). Spirituality and religiosity: Factors affecting wellness among low-income, rural women. *Journal of Counseling & Development*, *88*, 293-302.

Goodwin, R., Koenen, K. C., Hellman, F., Guardino, M., & Struening, E. (2002). Helpseeking and access to mental health treatment for obsessive-compulsive disorder. *Acta Psychiatrica Scandinavica*, *106*(2), 143-149.

Greenwood, G. L., & Gruskin, E. P. (2007). LGBT tobacco and alcohol disparities. In I. H. Meyer, & M. E. Northridge (Eds.), *The health of sexual minorities: Public health perspectives on lesbian, gay, bisexual, and transgender populations* (pp. 566-583). New York, NY: Springer Science + Business Media.

Han, D. Y., Chen, S. H., Hwang, K. K., & Wei, H. L. (2006). Effects of psychoeducation for depression on help-seeking willingness: Biological attribution versus destigmatization. *Psychiatry and Clinical Neurosciences*, *60*, 662-668.

Han, E., & Liu, G. G. (2005). Racial disparities in prescription drug use for mental illness among population in U.S. *Journal of Mental Health Policy Economics*, *8*(3), 131-143.

Harman, J. S., Edlund, M. J., & Fortney, J. C. (2004). Disparities in the adequacy of depression treatment in the United States. *Psychiatric Services*, *55*(12), 1379-1385.

Hattie, J. A., Myers, J. E., & Sweeney, T. J. (2004). A factor structure of Wellness: Theory, assessment, analysis, and practice. *Journal of Counseling & Development*, *2*, 354-364.

Hauenstein, E. J., Petterson, S., Merwin, E., Rovnyak, V., Heise, B., & Wagner, D. (2006). Rurality, gender, and mental health treatment. *Family & Community Health, 29*(3), 169-185.

Hermon, D. A., & Hazler, R. J. (1999). Adherence to a wellness model and perceptions of psychological well-being. *Journal of Counseling & Development, 77,* 339-343.

Hettler, B. (1984). Wellness: Encouraging a lifetime pursuit of excellence. *Health Values, 8,* 13-17.

Hines-Martin, V., Malone, M., Kim, S., & Brown-Piper, A. (2003). Barriers to mental health care access in an African American population. *Issues in Mental Health Nursing, 24*(3), 237-256.

Hopwood, M., & Connors, J. (2002). Heterosexual attitudes to homosexuality: Homophobia at a rural Australian university. *Journal of Gay & Lesbian Social Services: Issues in Practice, Policy & Research, 14*(2), 79-94. doi: 10.1300/J041v14n02_07

Jackson, J. S., Neighbors, H. W., & Gurin, G. (1986). Findings from a national survey of Black mental health: Implications for practice and training. In M. M. Miranda, & H. H. L. Kitano (Eds.), *Mental health research and practice* (pp. 91-116). Washington, DC: Department of Human Services National Institute of Mental Health.

Johnson, R. W. J. (2008). *Overcoming the obstacles of health.* New York: Robert Wood Johnson Foundation.

Jorm, A. F., Griffiths, K. M., Christensen, H., Korten, A. E., Parslow, R. A., & Rodgers, B. (2003). Providing information about the effectiveness of treatment options to depressed people in the community: A randomized controlled trial of effects on mental health literacy, help-seeking and symptoms. *Psychological Medicine, 33,* 1071-1079.

Kennedy, M. (2010). Rural men, sexual identity and community. *Journal of Homosexuality, 57*(8), 1051-1091. doi: 10.1080/00918369.2010.507421

Kimerling, R., & Baumrind, N. (2005). Access to specialty mental health services among women in California. *Psychiatric Services, 56*(6), 729-734. Retrieved from http://www.ncbi.nlm.nih.gov/pubmed/15939951

Kirby, J. B., Taliaferro, G., & Zuvekas, S. H. (2006). Explaining racial and ethnic disparities in health care. *Medical Care, 44*(5), 64-72.

Kroenke, K., Spitzer, R. L., & Williams, J. B. W. (2001). The PHQ9: Validity of a brief depression severity measure. *Journal of General Internal Medicine, 16*(9), 606-613.

Lasser, K. E., Himmelstein, D. U., Woolhander, S. J., McCormick, D., & Bor, D. (2002). Do minorities in the United States receive fewer mental health services than whites? *International Journal of Health Services, 3,* 567-78.

Lau, A. W., & Gallagher-Thompson, D. (2002). Ethnic minority older adults in clinical research programs: Issues and recommendations. *The Behavioral Therapist, 25*(1), 10-11.

Leedy, G., & Connolly, C. (2007). Out of the cowboy state: A look at lesbian and gay lives in Wyoming. *Journal of Gay & Lesbian Social Services: Issues in Practice, Policy & Research, 19*(1), 17-34. doi: 10.1300/J041v19n01_02

Markstrom, C. A., Stamm, B. H., Stamm, H. E., Berthold, S. M., & Running Wolf, P. (2003). Ethnicity and rural status in behavioral health care. In B. H. Stamm (Ed.), *Rural behavioral health care: An interdisciplinary guide* (pp. 231–243). Washington, DC: American Psychological Association.

Matthews, A. K., & Hughes, T. L. (2001). Mental health service use by African American women: Exploration of subpopulation differences. *Cultural Diversity and Ethnic Minority Psychology, 7*, 75–87.

McCarthy, L. (2000). Poppies in a wheat field: Exploring the lives of rural lesbians. *Journal of Homosexuality, 39*(1), 75–94. doi: 10.1300/J082v39n01

Mclean, C., Campbell, C., & Cornish, F. (2003). African-Caribbean interactions with mental health services in the UK: Experiences and expectations of exclusion as (re)productive of health inequalities. *Social Science & Medicine, 56*, 657–669.

Menke, R., & Flynn, H. (2009). Relationships between stigma, depression, and treatment in white and African American primary care patients. *Journal of Nervous and Mental Disease, 197*(6), 407–411. Retrieved from http://www.ncbi.nlm.nih.gov/pubmed/19525740

Merwin, E., Hinton, I., Dembling, B., & Stern, S. (2003). Shortages of rural mental health professionals. *Archives of Psychiatric Nursing, 17*, 42–51.

Merwin, E., Snyder, A., & Katz, E. (2006). Differential access to quality rural health care: Professional and policy challenges. *Family & Community Health, 29*, 186–194.

Mueller, K. J., Patil, K., & Boilesen, E. (1998). The role of uninsurance and race in health care utilization by rural minorities. *Health Services Research, 33*(3), 597–610.

Murry, V. M., Heflinger, C. A., Suiter, S. V., & Brody, G. H. (2011). Examining perceptions about mental health care and help-seeking among rural African American families of adolescents. *Journal of Youth and Adolescence, 40*(9), Retrieved from http://www.ncbi.nlm.nih.gov/pubmed/21259067

Myers, J. E., & Gill, C. S. (2004). Poor, rural and female: Under-studied, under-counseled, more at-risk. *Journal of Mental Health Counseling, 26*(3), 225–242.

Myers, J. E., & Sweeney, T. J. (2005a). The indivisible self: An evidence-based model of wellness. *Journal of Individual Psychology, 61*, 234–245.

Myers, J. E., & Sweeney, T. J. (2005b). *The five factor wellness inventory.* Palo Alto, CA: Mindgarden, Inc.

Myers, J. E., & Sweeney, T. J. (2008). Wellness counseling: The evidence base for practice. *Journal of Counseling & Development, 86*, 482–493.

Myers, J. E., Sweeney, T. J., & Witmer, J. M. (2000). The Wheel of Wellness counseling for wellness: A holistic model for treatment planning. *Journal of Counseling & Development, 78*, 251–266.

National Advisory Committee on Rural Health and Human Services. (2009). *The 2009 Report to the Secretary: Rural health and human services issues.* Retrieved from http://www.hrsa.gov/advisorycommittees/rural/2009secreport.pdf

National Rural Health Association. (1999). *Mental health in rural America.* Washington, DC: National Rural Health Association.

Newbigging, K., & McKeown, M. (2007). Mental health advocacy with black and minority ethnic communities: Conceptual and ethical implications. *Current Opinion in Psychiatry, 20*, 588–593.

Oswald, R. (2002). Who am I in relation to them? Gay, lesbian, and queer people leave the city to attend rural family weddings. *Journal of Family Issues, 23*(3), 323–348. doi: 10.1177/0192513X02023003001

Oswald, R., & Culton, L. S. (2003). Under the rainbow: Rural gay life and its relevance for family providers. *Family Relations, 52*(1), 72–81. doi: 10.1111/j.1741-3729.2003.00072.x

Padgett, D. K., Patrick, C., Burns, B. J., & Schlesinger, H. J. (1994). Ethnicity and use of outpatient mental health services in a national insured population. *American Journal of Public Health, 84*(2), 222–226.

Petterson, S., Williams, I. C., Hauenstein, E., Rovnyak, V., & Merwin, E. (2009). Race and ethnicity and rural mental health treatment. *Journal of Health Care for the Poor and Underserved, 20,* 678–694.

Phillips, K. A., Mayer, M. L., & Aday, L. A. (2000). Barriers to care among racial/ethnic groups undermanaged care. *Health Affairs, 19*(4), 65–75.

Philo, C., Parr, H., & Burns, N. (2003). Rural madness: A geographical reading and critique of the rural mental health literature. *Journal of Rural Studies, 19,* 259–281.

Pingatore, D., Snowden, L., Sansone, R. A., & Klinkman, M. (2001). Persons with depression symptoms and the treatments they receive: A comparison of primary care physicians and psychiatrists. *International Journal of Psychiatry and Medicine, 31,* 41–60.

President's New Freedom Commission on Mental Health. (2003). *Achieving the promise: Transforming mental health care in America. Final Report.* (DHHS Pub. No. SMA-03-3832). Rockville, MD. Retrieved from Mental Health Commission website: http://www.mentalhealthcommission.gov/reports/FinalReport/toc.html

Preston, D., D'Augelli, A. R., Cain, R. E., & Schulze, F. W. (2002). Issues in the development of HIV—Preventive interventions for men who have sex with men (MSM) in rural areas. *The Journal of Primary Prevention, 23*(2), 199–214. doi: 10.1023/A:1019968315959.

Preston, D., D'Augelli, A. R., Kassab, C. D., & Starks, M. T. (2007). The relationship of stigma to the sexual risk behavior of rural men who have sex with men. *AIDS Education and Prevention, 19*(3), 218–230. doi: 10.1521/aeap.2007.19.3.218

Rai-Atkins, A., Jama, A. A., Wright, N., Scott, S., Perring, C., Craig, G. et al. (2002). *Best practice in mental health: Advocacy for African, Caribbean and South Asian Communities.* York, UK: Joseph Rowntree Foundation.

Rost, K., Zhang, M., Fortney, J., Smith, J., Coyne, J., & Smith, Jr. G. R. (1998a). Persistently poor outcomes of undetected major depression in primary care. *General Hospital Psychiatry, 20*(1), 12–20.

Rost, K., Zhang, M., Fortney, J., Smith, J., & Smith, Jr. G. R. (1998b). Rural–urban differences in depression treatment and suicidality. *Medical Care, 36*(7), 1098–1107.

Rural Healthy People. (2010). *A companion document for rural areas.* Retrieved from http://www.srph.tamushsc.edu/rhp2010/

Sirey, J. A., Bruce, M. L., Alexopoulos, G. S., Perlick, D. A., Friedman, S. J., & Meyers, B. S. (2001). Stigma as a barrier to recovery: Perceived stigma and patient-rated severity of illness as predictors of antidepressant drug adherence. *Psychiatric Services, 52,* 1615–1620.

Smedley, B. D., Stith, A. Y., & Nelson, A. R. (eds). (2003). *Unequal treatment: Confronting racial and ethnic disparities in health.* Washington, DC: National Academies Press.

Snively, C. A. (2004). Building community-based alliances between GLBTQQA youth and adults in rural settings. *Journal of Gay & Lesbian Social Services: Issues in Practice, Policy & Research, 16*(3–4), 99–112. doi: 10.1300/J041v16n03_07

Snively, C. A., Kreuger, L., Stretch, J. J., Watt, J., & Chadha, J. (2004). Understanding homophobia: Preparing for practice realities in urban and rural settings. *Journal of Gay & Lesbian Social Services: Issues in Practice, Policy & Research, 17*(1), 59–81. doi:10.1300/J041v17n01_05

Snowden, L. R., Masland, M. C., Libby, A. M., Wallace, N., & Fawley, K. (2008). Racial/ethnic minority children's use of psychiatric emergency care in California's public mental health system. *American Journal of Public Health, 98*(1), 118–124.

U.S. Department of Health and Human Services. (2001). *Mental health: Culture, race, and ethnicity (Supplement to Mental Health: A Report of the Surgeon General).* Rockville, MD: Author.

Vega, W. A., Kolody, B., Aguilar-Gaxiola, S., Alderete, E., Catalano, R., & Caraveo-Anduaga, J. (1998). Lifetime prevalence of DSM-III-R psychiatric disorders among urban and rural Mexican Americans in California. *Archives of General Psychiatry, 55*(9), 771–778.

Waldo, C. R., Hesson-McInnis, M. S., & D'Augelli, A. R. (1998). Antecedents and consequences of victimization of lesbian, gay, and bisexual young people: A structural model comparing rural university and urban samples. *American Journal of Community Psychology, 26*(2), 307–334. doi: 10.1023/A:1022184704174

Ward, E. C., Clark, L. O., & Heidrich, S. (2009). African American women's beliefs, coping behaviors, and barriers to seeking mental health services. *Qualitative Health Research, 19*(11), 1589–1601. Retrieved from http://www.ncbi.nlm.nih.gov/pubmed/19843967

Willging, C. E., Salvador, M., & Kano, M. (2006a). Pragmatic help seeking: How sexual and gender minority groups access mental health care in a rural state. *Psychiatric Services, 57*(6), 871–874. doi: 10.1176/appi.ps.57.6.871

Willging, C. E., Salvador, M., & Kano, M. (2006b). Unequal treatment: Mental health care for sexual and gender minority groups in a rural state. *Psychiatric Services, 57*(6), 867–870. doi: 10.1176/appi.ps.57.6.867

Williams, I. C. (2005). Differences in emotional health between African American and Caucasian dementia caregivers: A contextual approach. *The Journal of Gerontology: Psychological Sciences, 60B*(6), 287–295.

World Health Organization. (2007). *Health statistics and health information systems.* Retrieved from http://www.who.int/healthinfo/statistics/en/

Yick, A. G. (2008). A metasynthesis of qualitative findings on the role of spirituality and religiosity among culturally diverse domestic violence survivors. *Qualitative Health Research, 18*(9), 1289–1306.

Zito, J. M., Safer, D. J., Zuckerman, I. H., Gardner, J. F., & Soeken, K. (2005). Effect of Medicaid eligibility category on racial disparities in the use of psychotropic medications among youths. *Psychiatric Services, 56*(2):157–163.

Zuvekas, S. H., & Taliaferro, G. S. (2003). Pathways to access: Health insurance, the health care delivery system, and racial/ethnic disparities, 1996–1999. *Health Affairs, 22*(2), 139–153.

15

Providing Mental Health Services for Women in Rural Areas

FRIEDA FARFOUR BROWN, SHANNON P. WARDEN,
AND AMANDA BROWN KOTIS

INTRODUCTION

*O*ne out of five women in the United States lives in a rural area. Yet, less than 10% of the patients served in mental health settings are located in rural areas. Rates of depression are equal to or higher than those in urban areas, and depressed patients are nine times more likely to be hospitalized in rural areas as in urban settings (Badger, Robinson, & Farley, 1999). Badger et al. (2009) also discuss in their journal article how issues of transportation, stigma, low socioeconomic level, and lack of access to services define the nature of the service delivery model as it exists today. These issues are particularly challenging for women in rural America who have more mental health issues than men, are often responsible when other family members suffer mental illnesses, make many of the health-related decisions in the family, and play a critical role in perpetuating or breaking intergenerational effects of mental illness (U.S. Department of Health and Human Services, 2002). Just as for other target rural groups, the challenges of accessibility, availability, and acceptability umbrella the nature of the service delivery models possible and practical for women in rural America (Health Resources and Service Administration, 2005). These problems are uniquely true for women who lack assistance from adult children, have diminished financial resources, and suffer the strain of stigma if they access mental health services.

In 1999, the Surgeon General issued a report on the state of mental health services in the United States. In response, the U.S. Department of Health and Human Services published an action-planning manual targeting the mental health needs of women. This report titled *Action Steps for Improving Women's Mental Health* identified women as twice as likely as men to suffer from major depression, anxiety, and obsessive–compulsive disorder (U.S. Department for Health and Human Resources, 2009). These types of mental illness often lead to addictive behaviors and social choices contributing to the staggering cost of mental illness in the United States. Furthermore, the highest mortality rate of all mental illnesses is associated with eating disorders and women represent 90% of all these cases (Birmingham, Su, Hlynsky, Goldner, & Gao, 2005). Unfortunately, the number of studies of rural mental health services for women is limited (Thorndyke, 2005). There is a need to more adequately understand and intervene on behalf of this population of mental health consumers.

As described elsewhere in this book, definitions of rural vary greatly, and there is tremendous variation in culture, opportunity, availability of services, and distance/accessibility of services. There is no single approach that will serve women in all rural settings. Rural settings typically include women who are disproportionately poor (Eberhardt, Ingram, & Makuc, 2001) with limited opportunities to obtain paid employment. These women often experience limited social contacts, and have less access to social services and health care than their urban counterparts. Furthermore, women in rural communities are more likely to adhere to traditional gender roles, which can create barriers to education, employment, and utilization of social services (Bushy, 1998).

In 1991, The Office on Women's Health (OWH) was created within the Department of Health and Human Services with the mission to provide information needed to improve women's health. After the 1999 Surgeon General's report on mental health, the women's mental health initiative published by OWH reinforced the need to take important steps toward making changes that directly impact access, availability, and utilization of mental health care by rural women. This initiative included addressing social stigma toward individuals with mental illness, training more providers equipped to treat rural women, and combating domestic violence against women in rural settings (U.S. Department of Health and Human Services, 2009). These are all factors that contribute to the development of mental illness.

The focus of this chapter is to propose solutions for meeting the mental health and social service needs of the underserved population of rural women. Rural programs require creative, collaborative models that create trajectories of care appropriate for unique economic, social, and cultural settings. Approaches must be sufficiently generic so that they can be modeled and molded to fit the particular community needs of women in diverse settings. A holistic model for comprehensive services including assessment, intervention, and support create a foundation for conceptualizing network delivery systems. Current systems meeting other needs of this population are the focus of specific models of intervention that emphasize integration of services. Contemporary advances in technology and issues of political power move the discussion toward systemic changes that support programmatic change and financial support. In addition to direct service opportunities, mental health professionals are in a position to also serve as consultants within rural communities. Descriptions of this role are included throughout this chapter.

THE BIOPSYCHOSOCIAL MODEL

The Biopsychosocial Model, a holistic approach, is suggested as an excellent model for meeting the mental health needs of rural women. It provides a comprehensive understanding of overall health and wellness as well as psychological problems and issues related to social justice. The acceptance of the model is considered to be an important advancement in mental health counseling and therapy (Kaplan & Coogan, 2005), inclusive of a variety of professional perspectives and treatment modalities. It moves counseling away from a "one size fits all" philosophy toward a "what works best in a given situation" perspective. Historically this model was proposed in April of 1977 by George Engel, a professor of psychiatry and medicine. In his article in *Science* Engel offered the Biopsychosocial Model as a way to conceptualize human health and illness (Engel, 1977). His model reflects an understanding that, despite the value of examining the influence of distinct functional dimensions, an integrative perspective is of more value. He urged the medical community to give up the prevailing biomedical model in favor of this more comprehensive perspective. Medical schools, physicians, and particularly psychiatrists have accepted the model but in a limited way. But, when the American Psychiatric Association published its third edition of the *Diagnostic and Statistical Manual of Mental Disorders*, it added the multiaxial system which reflects an acceptance of the model in the diagnostic process.

Although the diagnostic process originates from a medical tradition, the multiaxial model of the *Diagnostic and Statistical Manual* is now widely used by psychologists for diagnosing and treating patients. Its use reflects an understanding of the influence of multiple factors on psychological disorders. A comprehensive diagnosis includes not just the mental disorder but also personality and pervasive developmental disorders, sociocultural factors, physical and biologic contributors, and current and past levels of function. Many treatment modalities, notably the multimodal approach developed by Arnold Lazarus, reflect existing theoretical and treatment approaches current within the field of psychology that incorporate this perspective and style of practice.

The Biopsychosocial Model is one that can be easily incorporated into the service delivery models for different types of professionals and provides a paradigm that can be used with female clients in a variety of rural settings. The psychologist using this approach would routinely assess and develop interventions that include physical, psychological, and sociocultural dimensions. Rather than fragment service delivery, each part is viewed in the context of the comprehensive treatment plan. For example, in many cases women seek psychological as well as medical treatment from their physician. The physician then becomes a referral source for more specialized types of psychological treatment. Likewise, knowledge of the medical as well as the psychological dimensions of care allows the psychologist to serve in a consultative position from assessment to termination. Understanding the role each plays in promoting health and wellness as well as treating mental illness and pathology equips the psychologist to communicate effectively with physicians and with female patients. Each of the three areas—biological, psychological, and social—have relevance to the work of the psychologist providing care to rural women. In a rural setting, psychologists ideally network within the system of care to comprehensively respond to female patients' mental health needs. This could include a variety of different professionals.

The "bio" part of the model includes the biology of the individual, the physical, biochemical, and genetic factors that influence mental health. The genetic history of the individual serves to mark types of vulnerability to mental disorders prevalent in the family and known to create predispositions to mental illness. For example, if grandmother and aunt had problems with depression, the likelihood the granddaughter and niece are vulnerable members of the system is well documented. Rural women who are unemployed or who have low-paying jobs suffer from poor nutrition and sanitation, substandard housing, lack of education about health-related issues, and high-risk working conditions (Rowland & Lyons, 1989). Extensive social histories help psychologists to determine the part that biology may play in mental disorders.

Psychological factors that need to be assessed include motivation, temperament, and mood. All influence mental disorders and impact on overall health. Understanding the challenges at a particular developmental level and the influence of psychopathological conditions inform treatment protocols of the practitioner. A history of relationships with female patients allows the physician to identify possible barriers to compliance with the psychological component of the treatment plan. These problems can be addressed in a preventive way and include engaging the physician in the overall plan for treatment. For example, female patients taking psychoactive prescriptive medications can be required to see the psychologist before new prescriptions are written. By networking with family and community resources, safety nets can be created for chronically ill female patients. Mood disorders are routinely treated with a combination of therapy and antidepressants. Concurrent communication between physician and psychologist, each supporting the role of the other, provides enhanced treatment. If the psychologist recognizes negative side effects from medication, feedback to the physician can avoid the consequences of dangerous or troublesome side effects. The physician can rule out alternate causes for symptomatology consistent with the diagnosis of a mood disorder helping the psychologist avoid inappropriate psychological treatment for medical disorders.

The social dimension of the Biopsychosocial Model focuses on family systems, diversity and social justice issues, and the presence or absence of social support systems. Rural women with mental health concerns are prone to suffer isolation and loneliness. Extended family, neighbors, and members of shared organizations such as churches or community groups may be the only social resources available to them. The number of social roles filled by the woman suggests the types of personal, family, and work-related stress, as well as indicating the potential for social support. If a woman is struggling with depression, works outside the home, but is also the primary caregiver of her immediate and extended family, successful treatment planning must include the identification of those who can help with her social role responsibilities.

The inclusion of social justice as a dimension of the mental health mission began in the mid-1990s with emphasis on multiculturalism and diversity (Kaplan, & Coogan, 2005). The commitment to serving ethnic minorities, the poor, and neglected leads to service delivery models and training programs that target the specific needs of the rural female population. Understanding the power of the culture in which the woman resides is a crucial aspect of mental health treatment. Rural culture values self-sufficiency, autonomy, and privacy. Therefore, provision of services must account for the ways these character-istics both help and impede access to and utilization of treatment, and therefore recovery, for female patients.

The Biopsychosocial Model provides a structure for professionals across specialties to collaboratively develop comprehensive assessment and treatment plans that encourage ongoing communication, networking, and follow-up with female patients. As proponents of this collaborative perspec-tive, mental health professionals have opportunities to serve as consultants, educating other professionals and community members about the integrative model and its usefulness within their respective helping fields. The resulting productive working alliances lead to successful patient and client outcomes. Examples of collaboration between primary care providers and psychologists, and between the church and the mental health community demonstrate how this might work.

COLLABORATION BETWEEN PRIMARY CARE PROVIDERS AND PSYCHOLOGISTS

Primary care providers have shouldered much of the burden of identification and treatment of mental disorders (Badger et al., 1999). For the physician, mental health diagnoses are sometimes confounded by poorly defined pro-blems, diffuse somatic complaints, subthreshold symptoms, and high medical comorbidity. The physician's primary treatment modality is to offer medication that ameliorates distressing and disabling mental health symptoms. Too often, medication is not coupled with counseling and may not be closely monitored to assess success or to determine timelines that allow for patients to discon-tinue medication when no longer needed (particularly in rural areas with limited available mental health services). For example, more than two-thirds of rural patients treated for depression in primary care settings still meet the criteria for depression 5 months later (Badger et al., 1999).

The Biopsychosocial Model provides a networking framework for physicians, psychologists, and adjunctive health care professionals to partner with community-based services, nonprofit organizations, and mental health programs. A psychologist or other mental health professional who understands and appreciates the necessity for integration of biological, social, and psychological needs of rural women can serve as a consultant to medical professionals, educating and encouraging the consideration of multiple aspects of a female patient's diagnosis. Consultation of this nature may occur informally during treatment team meetings or formally during in-service training sessions and continuing education seminars. Beyond educating medical professionals about the model, the mental health professional provides guidance in assessment and treatment planning and service delivery for the mental health needs of rural women considering all four dimensions, physical, social, psychological, and cultural. Those professionals and organizations dedicated to comprehensive care can provide valuable insights to each other. This holistic model is a good fit for the personality and lifestyle of the rural woman.

The opportunity for such networking can occur around a common shared experience of many women: pregnancy. Literature from the American Pregnancy Association (2011) suggests that pregnancy may be the only time many low-income women see a physician on a regular basis. The Association also provides instructive and sobering statistics highlighting the importance of addressing mental and behavioral health among rural women, as follows. There are over 6 million pregnancies annually in the United States. Over one-third of women of childbearing and childrearing age have depressive symptoms while pregnant. In all, 221,000 women use illicit drugs during pregnancy. Overall, 757,000 women drink alcohol during pregnancy, and 40% of domestic assaults begin during a pregnancy. For a woman, the biology of pregnancy includes physical changes that directly affect the mother and fetus and indirectly affect the rest of the family. The prospective mother may develop psychological problems such as changes in mood and anxiety about the birth of the child and the demands of caretaking. If married, her relationship with her husband may change. Thoughts and feelings about the new baby, and the time involved with self-care and preparation for the birth, may be threatening to the marital dyad, may bring her closer to female relatives and friends, and may complicate her ability to work. Cultural norms, values, and expectations of her community may lead to polarizing messages and beliefs about the pregnancy. Developmentally, the meaning of the pregnancy and birth differ depending on the age of the woman and the response of her social network. Depending on age and stage, she may need help learning about motherhood, balancing work and parenting, or coping with the fatigue that is part of the experience of pregnancy and motherhood. Family, friends, and the community view of her pregnancy impact on the types of help she is willing and able to receive. Women at significant risk for mental disorders who would benefit from counseling during pregnancy include women taking psychotropic medication, women with histories of mental illness, in high conflict relationships, with histories of pregnancy loss and infertility, with substance abuse problems and/or partners with substance abuse problems, very young expectant mothers, and those with socioeconomic stressors. Many of these factors are more prevalent in rural areas, emphasizing on these areas even more critical in rural care.

The Biopsychosocial Model provides a framework for physicians and psychologists to promote both physical and mental health among rural female patients. Lifestyle and behavior are assessed in multiple domains. Practitioners design developmentally appropriate intervention strategies that target healthy behavior changes and promote self-care. This collaboration among psychologists, physicians, and other health care providers is more likely to lead to healthy outcomes than the isolated operation of each provider (Stewart & Okun, 2005). Furthermore, collaboration among professionals allows more convenient opportunities for care for rural women who may lack transportation, childcare, time, and money to make multiple trips to multiple providers. Models for such integration are presented in Chapter 9.

If the mental health and medical professionals are not in the same location, they can use technological tools to collaborate. Besides the standard phone referral, professionals can fax necessary release and assessment forms. They also may use Skype or similar Internet resources to talk "face to face." They can ask for releases that allow for ongoing communication and institute formal times to staff cases. Guidelines are in place that honor HIPAA confidentiality so that communication can meet practice standards (see Chapter 10 for details).

COLLABORATION BETWEEN RELIGIOUS ORGANIZATIONS AND MENTAL HEALTH PROFESSIONALS

As discussed in Chapter 6, churches have long been a source of not only religious practices, but also social and emotional support in both urban and rural communities. Baptisms, weddings, funerals, family reunions, community meetings, and a variety of other religious and social gatherings are commonplace in neighborhood churches. In rural areas, churches have historically served as an important community center because of a lack of alternative gathering places. As part of its central role in the lives of rural women, churches have emerged as an important provider of various mental health-related services for women (Rotunda, Williamson, & Penfold, 2004).

Again, the Biopsychosocial Model is instructive. Trust, which is an essential ingredient for a successful therapeutic relationship, is naturally fostered in churches where the spiritual as well as social and emotional needs of its members are met. The perceived safety of the church, the expectation of a loving response to need, the concern of church leaders and members, and the reliance upon a spiritual philosophy contribute to the trust that women experience within a church (Welch, Sikkink, Sartain, & Bond, 2004). When needs arise, including problems in mental health, women often view the church as a natural place to turn for help. When faced with their own or the mental health needs of their children or spouses, women often turn to other women or to their religious leaders before considering seeking similar assistance from professional psychologists in the community (Kramer et al., 2007; Neergaard, Lee, Anderson, & Gengler, 2007). Women trust that the information they share will remain confidential in the spiritual community. This is especially important to rural women who find it difficult to maintain a sense of privacy in a closely knit community, but at the same time may feel emotionally and geographically isolated from mental health services that assure confidentiality.

Many churches seek to attend to the mental health needs of women through the use of lay counseling ministries. Some congregations purchase training, such as that offered through nationally marketed programs like the Stephen Ministry (http://www.stephenministeries.org/). This program is designed to provide paraprofessional training to church members who desire to mentor and assist others through difficult times. These and similar training programs require extensive study using professionally prepared training materials and result in a nonprofessional certification of training. A pastor, counseling professional, or trusted leader within the setting typically supervises the training process and supervises the helping component once the program is ready to be implemented within that given church. The ministry and the individual helpers are not referred to as "counselors" or "lay counselors" for liability purposes but may be referred to as Stephen Ministers, mentors, helpers, caregivers, or by some other similar generic term. Women naturally fall into these roles as traditional caregivers within rural communities. Stephen Ministers are trained to recognize the limits of their ability to be of help and serve for a limited period of time to reinforce the emphasis on serving people with normal developmental, nonclinical issues. Related ministry information provided to "clients" specifies the limitations of the Stephen Ministry and explains referral options. Finally, volunteers are trained to recognize the importance of assessing critical counseling-related needs and clinical issues that warrant a referral for professional assistance. Collaboration and cooperation with professional psychologists enhance the comprehensive delivery of mental health services. Stephen Ministers are unpaid, choosing to serve on a volunteer basis. This ministry can be especially beneficial for church and community members who do not necessarily require professional counseling but could benefit from a listening ear, warmth, and basic feedback related to their situation. It also is an affordable way that churches can meet some mental health needs in their communities. In these ministries women work exclusively with other women forming long lasting relationships that provide ongoing support and encouragement.

If the church is committed to providing more intense services but cannot afford to contract with professionals that require payment, they can train members to use models such as the Systemic Model for Crisis Intervention counseling (Rainer & Brown, 2007). This model has been successfully used to train paraprofessionals in third world countries and can be adapted for any type of crisis situation using approaches as simple as problem solving and stress management or more sophisticated clinical approaches such as cognitive behavioral counseling of family counseling consistent with the background and training of the paraprofessional crisis counselor. Women in the community who are seen as natural helpers can be trained with this model to be in a supportive loving relationship with other women in need. The Systemic Model has proven helpful in numerous crisis related situations that commonly affect women, such as sexual assault, family violence, and loss of a child. Professional psychologists through many avenues including medical settings, churches, and community agencies, can serve as teachers and supervisors for those who practice this model.

COLLABORATION WITH COMMUNITY-BASED PROGRAMS: CASE EXAMPLES

Medical practices and religious organizations are two valuable resources for forging partnerships that meet the needs of rural women. Other community-based programs can in a similar manner be developed to provide mental health services that support the needs of women. For example in the 1990s, a small rural community in North Carolina was fraught with unemployment, teenage pregnancy, substance abuse, violence, and school dropout. These are all problems that trouble rural women who are responsible for feeding, clothing, and protecting their children, ensuring their children are prepared for school and work, and are safe from the influence of gangs, drug abuse, and domestic violence. In this example, the mental health community was concerned about families in their geographic area, as were other community-based programs such as schools, social service agencies, public health agencies, and local industry. The solution to the problems of this community was developed by networking with the men and women in this rural area to create an infrastructure that would provide healthy community resources, forge linkages with food banks, clothing closets, and other resources, engage industrial leadership in mentoring for jobs, and enhance the sense of power the parents felt in their ability to prevent problems from occurring. The goal for establishing the local program was to develop local leadership that could continue the work begun by professionals. Two professionals were involved in creating the program, one a psychologist and one a social worker from a community-based program serving the mental health and drug abuse needs of families. The third member of the organizing committee, a minister from the local church, was personally invested in the project. His own children were in the neighborhood school system as were children from members of his congregation. The vision for a community-based program for the children and youth led to extensive community involvement and the gifting of a house from an elderly female resident to serve as a gathering place for adolescents and their families. This gift was a major component of the success of this program. This woman in this case was a respected community member. Her actions highlighted the commitment of the women and men in the community to preventing mental health problems and providing a health environment for families. Local industry provided mentors and sponsored work-related events to encourage vocational planning and job-seeking skills.

In time, the community transitioned from a high-risk neighborhood to a legally defined city that had the wherewithal to develop a wide array of services and network with existing programs to meet the diverse needs of the community. Today this community is a city with its own mayor, mailbox, and leadership. The rates of unemployment, teenage pregnancy, substance abuse, and violence are significantly lower. A key to the success of this program was the work with local leadership to effect change. To adequately serve women, communities must begin with what they have, be it personal or professional capital, community, church, and professional services. Mental health professionals serving in the roles of advocates and consultants can initiate these types of community programs by partnering with others within the community, involving influential leaders, presenting sound arguments for community mental health needs, and suggesting viable options for accomplishing desired goals. Without that type of initiative on the part of mental health professionals, rural women's mental health needs may continue to go unaddressed.

In this example, the troubled rural community had local professionals involved in all phases of the program. This may not be feasible for all programs or for some specific types of needs, but advances in technology allow people to be connected if they are in remote geographic areas. The use of cell phones as a tool for delivering psychological services has come into its own. The field of "coaching" has moved this technology from its infancy to maturity. The client of the coach negotiates a contract for service that includes when the call will be made, how long it will last, and what will be included in the content (as is increasingly being done in the broader field of psychology). Women constrained by work and family obligations may lack transportation or time, but most have phones. To travel a distance once a week to meet with a psychologist may be physically impossible. But if the therapist is willing to consult with the patient on the phone, session time can be scheduled around the work and family demands of the client. The technology of Skype, which is a free service, adds the possibility of visual contact if that is preferred. If the client has no computer, the local public library is a resource for providing a quiet confidential space for women to communicate with a therapist. Additional details on use of technology for service delivery in all rural groups can be found in Chapter 10.

In a small, rural community in Texas, a homeless shelter developed an innovative way to bring mental health treatment to the homeless (Horner, 2003). This community has no public transportation, making it difficult for patients to visit the doctor's office. The county sends caseworkers to shelters each week to evaluate needs for psychiatric help. Through a telemedicine program, a psychiatrist "sees" the residents for medication evaluation. This simulates a face-to-face meeting between the psychiatrist and patient. After the assessment, the psychiatrist faxes a prescription to a local pharmacy. Most of the clients receiving this type of care are diagnosed with a schizophrenic or bipolar disorder. In 2003, the program expanded to a shelter for women where victims of domestic violence are treated for mental health problems quickly and in the secure setting of the shelter. Funding for the program is provided through external grants and foundations.

Another example of treatment currently in place in rural areas involves in-home services. Psychologists are moving out of their offices and into the homes and community settings of their patients. This model of service delivery is identified by the term *family preservation* and is no longer limited to the work of the crisis counselor. In the homes of clients, psychologists are able to directly observe the living conditions of women and their families in relation to the natural environments and lifestyle challenges. Based on observation and assessment, the psychologist provides consultation and treatment. It may be that rural psychologists will become increasingly similar to early physicians who made house calls, rather than the present-day professional tied to an office setting. The safety of the therapist and the ability of the client to work in a private space are important considerations for the success of this model; however, it holds great potential to serve the needs of rural women who often face multiple challenges in being able to attend psychological services.

COLLABORATION WITH UNIVERSITY TRAINING PROGRAMS

Women in rural areas tend to be disproportionately without insurance coverage. Among the uninsured, approximately one-third are poor and almost a quarter live in rural areas (Rowland & Lyons, 1989). In many cases mental health services may have to be provided on a pro bono basis. Practicing psychologists may be unable or unwilling to provide these free services. However, one group of clinicians who are motivated to perform such work are interns in university psychology and counseling training programs. Insurance carriers do not routinely reimburse services provided by interns. In most cases, public and private mental health facilities that use interns do so with pro bono clients. Working in a rural setting with a student under the supervision of a seasoned supervising psychologist is a win–win for the client, for the professional, and for the psychology intern. Research suggests that most rural women respond well to theoretical approaches such as cognitive behavioral therapy (Zust, 2000). Graduate students often favor this type of treatment modality as it is associated with a relational style similar to that of a teacher and student and has enough structure to encourage confidence in therapists who are early in their professional development. It is also easier to supervise, as there are many supporting forms and homework assignments that the intern can share with the supervisor.

The Pro Bono Counseling Program in Blacksburg, Virginia (www. mhanrv.org/pro_bono), is an example of this type of approach. This program provides mental health counseling and psychiatric services to low-to-moderate-income individuals, including women who are uninsured or ineligible for other financial assistance. The program partners with 35 mental health providers and with local universities. Unlicensed graduates of masters and doctoral programs in mental health fields see four clients a week. The program pays a supervisor to provide clinical supervision once a week. Services are offered at the offices of the mental health provider or at nonprofit locations such as public libraries in the more rural area. The program coordinates medication evaluations and partners with pharmaceutical companies for inclusion in the medications for indigents drug program. Indicators of success include: an average satisfaction rating of 9 out of a high of 10; a 60% treatment completion rate by clients; a no-show rate of only 10%; and severity of symptoms and difficulties in work life and personal life were cut in half. The program has even initiated an antistigma campaign to address cultural barriers to seeking help.

The Pro Bono Counseling Program was awarded the 2000 Innovation in Programming Award by the National Mental Health Association and was a semifinalist for the American Psychiatric Association Gold Community Award. The program offers a Program Development Guide so that other areas of the country might replicate this model. This guide includes a program handbook and all the forms and documents including guidelines for grant writing so that other settings might start a pro bono counseling program.

The last, but possibly most powerful, system to engage on behalf of mental health services for rural women is the political system. This chapter began with a report from the Surgeon General on mental health services with specific references and recommendations for serving women. This same report outlined multiple interventions for improving service delivery and effectiveness of treatment. Women uniting to seek support and political change can have the twofold effect of enhancing women's sense of competence and at the same time making meaningful change possible through local, state, and federal dollars.

In 1977, a group of rural women founded Rural American Women, Inc., a nonprofit organization based in Washington, DC and focused on bringing visibility and recognition to the achievements and concerns of rural America (www.lib.lastate.edu/spcl/manuscripts/MS366.html). This group connected rural women around important issues such as vocational education and moves to cut the federal budget in ways that impacted on rural women.

Although the organization disbanded in 1982, it was part of a movement to unite women across America in ways to support mental health service delivery. Today a similar organization, the American Agri-Women (www.americanagri-women.org), serves as a national coalition of farm, ranch, and agribusiness organizations. With 53 affiliate states they have a web site, sponsor meetings and forums, and give rural women a voice in the political process. These types of organizations promote systemic change that undergirds advances in mental health delivery and theoretical models for treatment of the mental health needs of rural women.

CONCLUSION

Without creative and collaborative efforts on the part of mental health and medical professionals, rural women cannot benefit from comprehensive mental health care services. Without these services, rural women experiencing emotional crises or mental health disorders may continue suffering and face impaired functioning. Mental health and medical professionals are wise to consider the Biopsychosocial Model, a holistic framework within which they can assess, treat, and monitor rural women's mental health symptoms and disorders. As its name suggests, this model emphasizes the many unique factors that, considered together, allow for a more thorough understanding of a rural woman's mental health needs. Implementing this model requires professionals to network and utilize existing community resources such as medical offices, churches, universities, and nonprofit organizations. When working together and tapping into these natural resources, professionals can successfully assist rural women in obtaining preventive education about self-care and information about mental health referral options.

More accessible assessment and treatment services for existing or recurring mental illness are possible when professionals and community organizations collaborate. This collaboration and a holistic understanding of rural women's mental health needs are essential if professionals and communities continue to make positive strides in responding to the current lack of mental health services available to rural women in America.

REFERENCES

American Pregnancy Association. (2011). *American Pregnancy Association Statistics.* Retrieved from http://www.americanpregnancy.org/main/statistics/html

Badger, L., Robinson, H., & Farley, T. (1999). Management of mental disorders in rural primary care. *The Journal of Family Practice, 48*(10), 20–25.

Birmingham, C. L., Su, J., Hlynsky, J., Goldner, E. M., & Gao, M. (2005). The mortality rate from anorexia nervosa. *International Journal of Eating Disorders, 38*(2), 143–146.

Bushy, A. (1998). Health issues of women in rural environments: An overview. *Journal of the American Medical Women's Association, 53*(2), 53–56.

Eberhardt, M. S., Ingram, D. D., & Makuc, D. M. (2001). *Urban and rural health chartbook: Health United States 2001*. Hyattsville, MD: National Center for Health Statistics.

Engel, G. L. (1977). The need for a new medical model: A challenge for biomedicine. *Science, 196*, 129–136.

Health Resources and Service Administration. (2005). *Mental health and rural American: 1994–2005*. Rockville, MD.

Horner, K. (2003, December). Shelter residents get mental aid on screen: Innovative program brings psychiatric treatment via TV. *Dallas News*. Retrieved from http://www.dallasnews.com/archive

Kaplan, D., & Coogan, S. (2005). The next advancement in counseling: The Biopsychosocial Model. In G. Waltz, & R. Yep (Eds.), *Vistas: Compelling perspectives on counseling* (pp. 17–25). Alexandria, VA: American Counseling Association.

Kramer, T. L., Blevins, D., Miller, T. L., Phillips, M. M., Davis, V., & Burris, B. (2007). Ministers' perceptions of depression: A model to understand and improve care. *Journal of Religion and Health, 46*(1), 123–139.

Neergaard, J. A., Lee, J. W., Anderson, B., & Gengler, S. W. (2007). Women experiencing intimate partner violence: Effects of confiding in religious leaders. *Pastoral Psychology, 55*, 773–787.

Rotunda, R. J., Williamson, G., & Penfold, M. (2004). Clergy response to domestic violence: A preliminary survey of clergy members, victims and batterers. *Pastoral Psychology, 52*, 353–365.

Rainer, J., & Brown, F. (2007). *Crisis counseling and therapy*. Binghamton, NY: Haworth Press.

Rowland, D., & Lyons, B. (1989). Triple jeopardy: Rural, poor, and uninsured. *Health Services Research, 23*, 975–1004.

Stewart, B., & Okun, B. (2005). Healthy living, healthy women. In M. P. Mirkin, K. L. Suyemoto, & B. F. Okun (Eds.), *Psychotherapy with women: Exploring diverse contexts and identities* (pp. 313–334). New York, NY: Guilford Press.

Thorndyke, L. E. (2005). Rural women's health: A research agenda for the future. *Women's Health Issues, 15*, 200–203.

U.S. Department of Health and Human Services, Substance Abuse and Mental Health Services Administration, Center for Mental Health Services, National Institutes of Health. (1999). *Mental health: A report of the Surgeon General*. Rockville, MD: Author.

U.S. Department of Health and Human Services, Office on Women's Health. (2002). *A century of women's health: 1900–2000*. Rockville, MD: Author. Retrieved from: http://www.4women.gov/timecapsule/century/index.htm

U. S. Department of Health and Human Services, Office on Women's Health. (2009). *Action steps for improving women's mental health*. Rockville, MD: Author. Retrieved from: http://www.womenshealth.gov/publications/our-publications/#mentalHealth

Welch, M. R., Sikkink, D., Sartain, E., & Bond, C. (2004). Trust in God and trust in man: The ambivalent role of religion in shaping dimensions of social trust. *Journal for the Scientific Study of Religion, 43*(3), 317–343.

Zust, B. (2000). Effect of cognitive therapy on depression in rural, battered women. *Archives of Psychiatric Nursing, 14*(2), 51–63.

16

Providing Mental Health Services for Men in Rural Areas

DON GORMAN, ROBERT ELEY, AND DELWAR HOSSAIN

INTRODUCTION

*R*ural men experience more health risk factors, poorer health, and higher death rates than rural women (Ziembroski & Breiding, 2006). They also, by virtue of the fact that they live in rural areas, have less access to health services. Of particular concern are their reported poorer levels of mental health and higher rates of suicide. Issues identified by rural men as being of particular concern include isolation, stigma, lack of employment opportunities, lack of confidence in the future, few leisure activities, boredom, and limited transportation options (Quine et al., 2003). This chapter reports on the research in the literature, as well as that of the authors, focusing on the characteristics of rural men and their mental health, provision of services for this special population, considerations of best practices, and future opportunities for research and scholarly inquiry.

CHARACTERISTICS OF RURAL MEN

There are many widely accepted attitudes considered characteristic of rural men, including stoicism, self-reliance, and resilience. While these characteristics can be positive (and perhaps essential) to survival in rural communities, they can also have negative impacts on mental health. In their review of the international literature, Kosberg and Fei Sun (2010, p. 9) concluded that among rural men in different countries there were "consistent similarities in findings of the characteristics" with rural men being described as indomitable, self-reliant, and all-conquering in an environment where stoicism, rugged individualism, self-efficiency, self-reliance, and an ability to work through hard times on their own are stereotypical (McColl, 2007).

Stoic is usually the term of choice describing denial, suppression and control of emotions, and imperturbability in the face of challenges. Indeed stoic attitudes among rural men are reported as the norm, and as a result, mental illness can be considered a sign of weakness (Francis, Boyd, Aisbett, Newnham, & Newnham, 2006). This impacts not only on the psychological functioning of rural men but also on their willingness to admit to the presence of, or seek treatment for, any emerging psychological conditions. This leads to an overall avoidance of treatment which results in later stage symptom presentation when finally entering psychological treatment. An investigation of the connection between stoicism and mental health outcomes (Murray et al., 2008) found that stoicism was negatively associated with quality of life, with the relationship mediated by negative attitudes for seeking psychological help. While high stoicism scores were found in the sample of rural men, interestingly, rural women also reported having high levels of stoicism.

Overall, members of small rural communities are characterized as having a "culture of self-reliance" and community members are expected to "soldier-on" and not talk about their problems to anyone (Parr & Philo, 2003). This has led to a stereotyped portrayal of rural men in the mass media that can perpetuate images of independence and self-reliance. While this perception remains, Alston (2010) argues that the stereotype of rural men, and in particular of masculine hegemony, has changed. Women now make a major contribution to labor, income, and financial management even in rural areas, violating traditional notions of hegemonic masculinity. As a consequence, the traditional rural male position is no longer reality, thus creating tensions impacting on men's self-worth. The author concludes that for rural men "change in gender roles and relative economic contributions of women and men has destabilized men's sense of their own self-worth and undermined their stoicism and rugged individualism" (p. 4). They continue by stating "[it has] damaged men's sense of self when circumstances are beyond their control and their stoic response prevents help-seeking behaviour and reduces their ability to attend to their health needs" (p. 4).

HEALTH-RELATED BEHAVIOR

Gender and place of residence contribute to disparities in the use of mental health services (Hauenstein et al., 2006); in particular, rurality is found to reduce use of services, with rural men even less likely than rural women to use the services. Furthermore, men are generally less likely to see themselves as being at risk of illness or injury (Courtenay, 2003) and are more likely to dismiss health symptoms until they become severe or life threatening (Galdas, Cheater, & Marshall, 2005). For example, Barry, Doherty, Hope, Sixsmith, and Kelleher (2000) found that rural Irish men were more likely to conceal mental health problems than women and felt unable to talk about their problems.

When considering the underlying cause of these limits to seeking psychological help, subtle cultural differences in rural areas can act as barriers to mental health care. The culture of stoicism, resilience, and self-reliance discussed above inhibit help-seeking behaviors for social and emotional problems (de la Rue & Coulson, 2003). As O'Kane, Craig, and Sutherland (2008) stated when reporting on their Riverina district study in Australia, "Talking about health is not considered a male past-time; visiting health professionals is still seen as a last resort" (p. 70). This lack of health-mindedness is directly related to reluctance to seek help (Collins, Winefield, Ward, & Turnbull, 2009). Unfortunately, in addition to the reluctance to seek help, stigma surrounding receipt of care (particularly among men) decreases men's willingness to inform others of their treatment. Rural men are increasingly likely to limit their social interactions when under threat, fearing social opprobrium because of their sense of failure (Alston, 2010). This diminishes the positive impact of social support on mental health treatment and further complicates the treatment process for rural men.

In addition to being less likely to seek mental health treatment when needed, rural men also engage in higher levels of risk-taking behavior (Milhausen, Yarber, & Crosby, 2003). These differences are found consistently across countries; for example, the Australian Institute of Health and Welfare (2007) found that when compared with their counterparts in Major Cities, people in Inner Regional, Outer Regional and Remote/Very Remote areas of Australia exhibit far higher risk factors of smoking, risky alcohol consumption, sedentary behavior, and overweight and obesity (Australian Institute of Health and Welfare, 2010), findings that have been replicated in the United States (Gamm, Hutchison, Dabney, & Dorsey, 2003).

Young rural men have also been shown to be more likely to use alcohol than young men in metropolitan areas (Rajkumar & Hoolahan, 2004; van Gundy, 2006). Rajkumar and Hoolahan (2004) assert that early detection of concurrent alcoholism and social anxiety disorders are vital in planning effective intervention for rural men. Adolescents with comorbid psychiatric and polysubstance use disorders are challenging the mental health service system in both utilization rates and costs of services. Dependent substance users in remote areas have limited continuity of care, as service infrastructure is minimal. This creates a bleak situation in rural areas, as data show that 2.9% of young adults 18–25 use methamphetamine in areas considered the most rural. That rate is nearly double the 1.5% of young adults using meth in urban areas (Clevenger, 2010). The prevalence of illicit drug use among youth reveals an emergent trend of 14.4% in rural areas, 10.4% in counties with small metropolitan areas, and 10.4% in large metropolitan areas. More specifically, growing evidence suggests that for certain substances such as alcohol, methamphetamines, and inhalants, usage rates are higher among rural youth than urban youth (Hutchison & Blakely, 2011) and disproportionately impact male youth. The interventions for drug dependence in rural and remote areas need preventive strategies for alcohol, nicotine, cannabinoids, amphetamines, and opioids to address this growing problem, particularly among rural adolescent/young adult men. The focus for implementation should be in the community through primary care workers, with inputs from consumers and other agencies providing care and support. Additional information regarding the impact of substance use on rural populations can be found in Chapter 12.

STIGMA OF MENTAL ILLNESS

According to Corrigan (2005), there are two forms of stigma of mental illness—social stigma and self-stigma. While social stigma is imposed by the community, self-stigma is a judgment imposed on a person with mental illness by themselves, as an internalization of community attitudes. The experience of self-stigma for rural populations can be particularly profound (see Chapter 4), but the effects of mental health stigma are especially strong for rural men (Boyd et al., 2008).

All people with mental health problems are at risk of experiencing social stigma. In small rural areas, however, this experience is exacerbated by the social characteristics of rural communities (Aisbett, Boyd, Francis, Newnham, & Newnham, 2007). Rural residents are far more visible when entering mental health services, for instance. This lack of privacy combined with community perceptions of mental illness within rural communities can add to the stress experienced by men with mental health problems (Gorman et al., 2007), especially given the cultural norms that men in particular should not need external help. A man with a mental health problem in a rural area can experience feelings of rejection and isolation, ostracism or exclusion when the usual caring practices of the community are not forthcoming (Aisbett et al., 2007; Boyd et al., 2007), especially given men's already established hesitance to seek out help this stigma serves to only further complicate men's decisions to do so. Furthermore, stigmatization in rural communities serves a social distancing function; community members limit their social obligations to people with mental illness in a context where access to supportive services is already poor (Boyd et al., 2008). Members of a close-knit community typically engage in a range of caring practices if a fellow community member experiences a physical illness; however, these same caring practices may not extend to a person with a mental illness (Parr, Philo, & Burns, 2004), particularly for men.

Embarrassment and self-denial are also reported in the literature. Buckley and Lower (2002) show that rural men frequently postpone visits to health services, deny symptoms of a chronic nature, and only utilize health services when symptoms are regarded as life-threatening. Because mental health concerns are rarely recognized as being "life-threatening," rural men are very hesitant to seek treatment for any emerging mental health issues. Barriers to seeking medical attention include lack of time, dislike of waiting, and fear of knowing the true health status and are probably not uniquely rural characteristics; however, requirement for privacy is a major barrier. When coupled with a resilient and resistant attitude, this results in poor engagement with health services for rural men.

SUICIDES IN RURAL AND REMOTE COMMUNITIES

There is a well-established disparity in suicide completion between men and women, with men overall being four times as likely as women to commit suicide (Dresang, 2001). This difference is repeated in rural men both internationally and within the United States. In the United States, reported mental health deteriorates significantly as rurality increases (Hauenstein et al., 2006). More rural young men than urban young men identify symptoms of depression, a leading risk factor for suicide (Eckert, Kutek, Dunn, Air, & Goldney, 2010). Suicide rates among Australia's rural men are significantly higher than rural women, urban women, and even urban men (Alston, 2010); the Australian Bureau of Statistics (2005) data suggest that males' suicide rate is five times higher than that of women with rural–urban differences becoming even broader in recent years (Page, Morrell, Taylor, Dudley, & Carter, 2007). Sex, age, and location effects are also seen in suicide rates. For example nonmetropolitan male individuals aged 15–24 years had a 50% higher rate of suicide than their metropolitan counterparts (Wilkinson & Gunnell, 2000) and rates of suicide increase with remoteness (Australian Institute of Health and Welfare, 2007). The highest rates of male suicide occur in communities of less than 4,000 (Judd et al., 2006).

Reasons for these differences in suicide have focused on help-seeking behaviors and cultural beliefs. For example, Ní Laoire's (2001) work on rural male suicide in Ireland concluded that suicides result from a sense of entrapment and an inability to see a positive future. She argues that rural men's inability to control factors that have a major influence on their lives, such as government policy, climate, or rural restructuring, leads them to a strong sense of hopelessness. Men see their mental health as an individual failing and do not see the wider picture (e.g., drought) as being responsible. She also supports the view that changes in gender roles contribute, but recognizes these changes as one of many factors, such as agricultural rationalization, out-migration, and rural change that really are "a matter of life and death" (Ní Laoire, 2001, p. 233). Other factors contributing to suicide in rural communities include greater access to firearms, difficulty in accessing health and mental health services, a culture of reluctance to seek help for personal or health problems, perceived intolerance of difference such as same sex attraction, substance use, and limited access to educational, recreational, and employment opportunities (Patterson & Pegg, 1999; Quine et al., 2003). Further discussion on the influence of rural living on suicide can be found in Chapter 13.

PROVISION OF HEALTH SERVICES TO RURAL MEN

Rural communities tend to be small and isolated, distant from services, and affected by economies of scale and difficulties in recruiting and retaining health professionals (Gale & Deprez, 2003). Rural communities are not only different from urban communities but often from each other, requiring services tailored to their local needs (Mulder & Linkey, 2003; Sears & Evans, 2003; U.S. Department of Health and Human Services, 2006). For rural men who have access to and actually seek treatment and support, a general practitioner (GP) may be their first and only local medical contact in a rural or remote community (Caldwell et al., 2004). However, even accessing a GP can be difficult in some localities and they may vary in their level of experience with the treatment of psychological distress or mental illness. Rural residents report that although there are some good health and mental health services, there is a general perception of reduced access to GPs and other health services (Caldwell et al., 2004).

One study found lower rates of GP encounters for psychological problems in rural areas and found that GPs in remote areas prescribed mental health medications at half the rate of their counterparts in urban areas (Caldwell et al., 2004). Waiting lists, lack of treatment options, and the need to travel long distances to access health care services may result in people with mental health concerns not accessing support services, or not being seen until the condition has deteriorated significantly. This becomes particularly significant for rural men who already face personal and cultural barriers to seeking treatment; if treatment is not available when they do choose to seek it, it may decrease the likelihood of them following through and actually receiving services.

WHAT WORKS: STEPS THAT CAN BE TAKEN TO ADDRESS THE NEEDS OF RURAL MEN

Rural men participants in the current authors' research, which explores the views of rural communities into mental health issues, see the key to improving mental health for rural men as increasing information and support to community members that provide a better understanding of mental health issues. In the studies, a range of prior and novel ideas were raised to engage with the community, including free head and neck massages to help destress, and providing a support worker to visit with men to informally "work through" stressful situations. As mentioned before, there are and always will be well-acknowledged difficulties in providing professional mental health services to small, rural, and remote communities. While many different strategies are being utilized to maximize the effectiveness of these services, such as fly in fly out (health professionals visiting rural communities to provide services on a short-term basis and then leaving), traveling, and telehealth services, the area that has been least explored is that of building the capacity of communities to maximize their own mental health. Such an approach would be particularly beneficial for rural men as community action could help diminish the stigma associated with mental health services.

In one study, rural men identified factors they believed enhanced their resilience to mental illness (Gorman et al., 2007). These factors were broadly categorized into two major topics: (a) the individual and their inner strength; and (b) support strategies. The individual and inner strength were related to intrinsic factors, that is, those within the individual that helped to cope with adversity. They included positive thinking, self-awareness, self-control, focusing on the meaning of life, appreciation, and hope (Gorman et al., 2007). Focusing on the positive rather than the negative aspects in life helped to prevent negative feelings dominating and becoming disproportional (and thus reducing the ability to cope). Indeed, personality traits like optimism and pessimism can affect many areas of rural men's health and well-being. The positive thinking that typically comes with optimism is a key component of effective stress management, which is associated with many health benefits. Mayo Clinic (2011) and Seaward (2009) stated that positive thinking may provide health benefits that include increased lifespan, lower rates of depression, lower levels of distress, greater resistance to the common cold, better psychological and physical well-being, reduced risk of death from cardiovascular disease, and better coping skills during hardships and times of stress. It is also thought that positive and optimistic people tend to live a healthier lifestyle, for example, more physical activity, healthy dietary practices, and not smoking (Seaward, 2009).

Positive thinking also involves actively looking for and valuing strengths, including finding an appreciation for life and incorporating a vision of hope for the future. Rural male participants also saw importance in awareness of health, especially mental health. This self-awareness allowed them to take positive steps during particularly vulnerable times. The awareness and understanding of the factors that affect mental health and mental illness, including potential vulnerability to further episodes of illness, assisted them to engage in health-promoting and illness prevention actions (Gorman et al., 2007).

Taking ownership of the problem or situation and actively addressing it was considered important by rural men in the authors' study, that is, it gave them a sense of control. Redirecting thoughts of feeling self-pity into a proactive and outward looking focus was also seen as regaining personal control (Gorman et al., 2007). Seeking meaning in life gives a sense of purpose, something to strive for. This can include participation in religion which can be a way to explore the concept of the meaning of life. Murphy (1998) noted that by participating in religious practice or disciplined prayer and meditation, people have been shown to gain new strength and a new outlook on life and a spiritual dimension of healing. Murphy (1998) further noted that from care, people have gained some of the strength needed to cope and survive. However, having a relationship with a religious community feeds a still deeper need, one that goes further than therapy (for clients who are receptive to such an approach).

"Spirituality" has become a ubiquitous term used to encompass a variety of beliefs and behaviors (Moadel et al., 1999). For example, research has shown the following to be associated with psychosocial adjustment: religious values (Acklin, Brown, & Mauger, 1983), religious practices (Ebaugh, Richman, & Chafetz, 1984), spiritual well-being, spiritual awareness (Smith et al., 1993), and religious thoughts (Moadel et al., 1999). It is argued that spirituality or religion promotes adjustment through its ability to give meaning and hope by providing an explanation for the experience of illness and suffering (Moadel et al., 1999). In support of this theory, Mullen, Smith, and Hill (1993) found successful coping to be dependent on a sense of coherence or meaning which, in turn, was associated with higher levels of spiritual resources. Examining the importance of religion and its potential for use as an adjuvant to psychological services may be particularly important in rural areas where religiosity is typically high; further discussion of this topic can be found in Chapter 6.

The second major topic that has emerged in the mental health of rural men (Gorman et al., 2007) relates to extrinsic factors that help rural men cope with the stresses of life, and includes such things as seeking help and treatment, talking about it, life changes, being needed, support of family, and friends and distractions. Practical information about mental health can empower rural men to cope. Men often do not realize they are experiencing signs and symptoms of depression, nor that the experience is common and help is available. The benefits of acknowledging the need for professional help and seeking it are often unacknowledged. The forms of help that have been utilized include telephone support, face-to-face counseling, and support from the GP (Gorman et al., 2007).

There is evidence that men not only consult less often than women, but their method of help-seeking behavior differs. Möller-Leimkühler (2002) found that although minor emotional symptoms increase the probability of consulting a general practitioner, physical symptoms were the primary determining factor for help-seeking by men. Those men that report using pharmacological agents prescribed by their GP in their treatment regimen acknowledge the benefits of the treatment, in particular to coping with the symptoms of their illness (Gorman et al., 2007). Corney (1990) also found that men are less likely to report psychosocial problems and distress as an additional reason for consulting their physician. The fact that men and women differ in the frequency of a set of behaviors reveals little about the biological, psychological, or cultural processes responsible for any observed differences (Mechanic, 1978). However, not all men are the same, nor does it make sense to assume that individual men, especially rural men, behave similarly in all help-seeking contexts. The data show that using certain resources is not always a conscious decision, but often occurs outside of the individual's awareness. Sometimes awareness was initiated by other people, such as family and friends, with the benefits recognized later.

Talking about problems with others is another strategy reported by men. Discussion and reflection allow them to unload their burden, gain different points of view, and reflect on current position and status. The act of "talking it out" is experienced as therapeutic and is often undertaken with family and friends. The simple knowledge that there are people that care increases the benefit of the support. Relationships with others has another aspect—that of being needed. Rural men acknowledge that knowing that others depend on them provides additional strength during difficult times. It enhances a sense of obligation/purpose and boosts self-esteem (Gorman et al., 2007).

Rural men also report that consciously making life changes helps to deal with situational concerns. These changes tended not to occur until individuals recognized the reality of a particular situation, and that the situation was not likely to improve. This involved taking time out from daily life, getting away from familiar surroundings, and diverting focus from the difficult times by undertaking different activities. Taking a break is also reflected in the value of having hobbies and interests outside of daily lives. This incorporates a range of different activities with the emphasis on distraction from immediate problems (Gorman et al., 2007).

The most significant finding of the Gorman et al. (2007) study was that the men used similar strengths and strategies to overcome situations. Therefore, the resilience factors found in these men may also be found in other resilient men and may be useful as a guide for men to cope with difficult times/ mental illness. As a result of this study, a booklet was produced telling the stories of these men (Rogers-Clark & Pearce, 2004) that has proven to be a valuable resource to inform rural men about mental health.

COMMUNITY CAPACITY BUILDING

Another study with rural men (Hossain, Gorman, & Eley, 2009; Hossain, Gorman, Eley, & Coutts, 2010) showed that the provision of mental health first aid (MHFA) training to extension agents (EAs) who were staff working for various rural organizations and named variously as field officers, extension officers, catchment officers, landcare officers, financial counselors, agribusiness officers, and agricultural system officers, increased their confidence and capacity to recognize mental health issues in their rural clientele and to take appropriate action to refer to health services. Overall, following training, EAs were more competent to provide help to someone with mental health problems. This program provides an example of how building the capacity of communities to help themselves can complement the provision of professional services, which are often limited due to difficulties in recruiting, and issues related to the provision of services to small, isolated communities. Other community-based strategies such as men's groups (which encourage men to gather together for mutual support) and civic and social organizations (aimed at providing information about mental illnesses such as depression) have been shown to be beneficial.

The importance of a community approach is exemplified by McDonald and Brown (2009) who reported that independent and functional older rural men often find themselves feeling desperately lonely, socially isolated, and in a state of despair as a consequence of the lack of support and contact with peers. "Expressive support" or emotional care and support, through regular peer group participation for men living in the rural community, may reduce psychological morbidity and mortality such as depression. However, health promotion and rehabilitation programs available to address these problems for rural men are limited and knowledge about their experiences is inadequate.

CONCLUSION

In conclusion, rural men face particular challenges that exacerbate an already challenging environment for the maintenance of mental health. These challenges are the result of a combination of resource limitations, cultural values, and gender role expectations that leave rural men particularly at risk for mental and behavioral health problems. By helping rural men recognize the importance of maintaining their mental health, and that seeking help is supported and necessary, we can begin to help rural men help themselves.

REFERENCES

Acklin, M., Brown, E., & Mauger, P. (1983). The role of religious values in coping with cancer. *Journal of Religion Health*, *22*(4), 322–333.

Aisbett, D. L., Boyd, C. P., Francis, K., Newnham, K., & Newnham, K. (2007). Understanding the barriers to mental health service utilization for adolescents in rural Australia. *Rural and Remote Health*, 7, 624. Retrieved from http://www.rrh.org.au/publishedarticles/article_print_624.pdf

Alston, M. (2010). Rural male suicide in Australia. *Social Science & Medicine*. Advance online publication. doi: 10.1016/j.socscimed.2010.04.036

Australian Bureau of Statistics. (2005). *Suicides Australia catalogue* (Report No. 3309). Canberra Commonwealth of Australia: Author.

Australian Institute of Health and Welfare. (2007). *Rural, regional and remote health: A study on mortality* (2nd ed.). Canberra Commonwealth of Australia: Author.

Australian Institute of Health and Welfare. (2010). A snapshot of men's health in regional and remote Australia. *Rural health series, 11.* Canberra Commonwealth of Australia: Author.

Barry, M., Doherty, A., Hope, A., Sixsmith, J., & Kelleher, C. (2000). A community needs assessment for rural mental health promotion. *Health Education Research Theory and Practice, 15*(3), 293-304.

Boyd, C. P., Francis, K., Aisbett, D. L., Newnham, K., Sewell, J., Dawes, G. et al. (2007). Australian rural adolescents' experiences of accessing psychological help for a mental health problem. *Australian Journal of Rural Health, 15,* 196-200.

Boyd, C. P., Hayes, L., Sewell, J., Caldwell, K., Kemp, E., & Harvie, L. (2008). Mental health problems in rural contexts: A broader perspective. *Australian Psychologist, 43,* 2-6.

Buckley, D., & Lower, T. (2002). Factors influencing the utilisation of health services by rural men. *Australian Health Review, 25*(2), 11-15.

Caldwell, T. M., Jorm, A. F., Knox, S., Braddock, D., Dear, K. B. G., & Britt, H. (2004). General practice encounters for psychological problems in rural, remote and metropolitan areas in Australia. *Australian and New Zealand Journal of Psychiatry, 38,* 774-780.

Clevenger, A. (2010). Rural drug use: Deadly, and getting deadlier. *Sustained Outrage.* Retrieved from http://blogs.wvgazette.com/watchdog/2010/03/22/rural-drug-use-deadly-and-getting-deadlier/

Collins, J. E., Winefield, H., Ward, L., & Turnbull, D. (2009). Understanding help seeking for mental health in rural South Australia: Thematic analytical study. *Australian Journal of Primary Health, 15*(2), 159-165. doi:10.1071/PY09019

Corney, R. H. (1990). Sex differences in general practice attendance and help seeking for minor illness. *Journal of Psychosomatic Research, 34,* 525-534.

Corrigan, P. W. (2005). *On the stigma of mental illness.* Washington, DC: American Psychological Association.

Courtenay, W. H. (2003). Key determinants of the health and well-being of men and boys. *International Journal of Men's Health, 2*(1), 1-27.

de la Rue, M., & Coulson, I. (2003). The meaning of health and well-being: Voices from older rural women. *Rural and Remote Health, 3,* 192. Retrieved from http://www.rrh.org.au/articles/subviewnew.asp?ArticleID=192

Dresang, L. (2001). Gun deaths in rural and urban settings: Recommendations for prevention. *Guns and Violence Prevention, 14*(2), 107-115.

Ebaugh, H., Richman, K., & Chafetz, J. (1984). Life crises among the religiously committed: Do sectarian differences matter? *Journal for the Scientific Study of Religion, 23,* 19-31.

Eckert, K., Kutek, S., Dunn, K., Air, T., & Goldney, R. (2010). Changes in depression-related mental health literacy in young men from rural and urban South Australia. *Australian Journal of Rural Health, 18*(4), 153-158.

Francis, K., Boyd, C. P., Aisbett, D. L., Newnham, K., & Newnham, K. (2006). Rural adolescents' perceptions of barriers to seeking help for mental health problems. *Youth Studies Australia, 25*(4), 42-49.

Galdas, P. M., Cheater, F., & Marshall, P. (2005). Men and health help-seeking behaviour: Literature review. *Journal of Advanced Nursing, 49*(6), 616-623.

Gale, J. A., & Deprez, R. D. (2003). A public health approach to the challenges of rural mental health service integration. In B. H. Stamm (Ed.), *Rural behavioral health care: An interdisciplinary guide* (pp. 95-108). Washington, DC: American Psychological Association.

Gamm, L. D., Hutchison, L. L., Dabney, B. J., & Dorsey, A. M. (Eds.). (2003). *Rural Healthy People 2010: A companion document to Healthy People 2010 (Vol. 1).* College Station, TX: The Texas A&M University System Health Science Center, School of Rural Public Health Southwest Rural Health Research Center.

Gorman, D., Buikstra, E., Hegney, D., Pearce, S., Rogers-Clark, C., Weir, J. et al. (2007). Rural men and mental health: Their experiences and how they managed. *International Journal of Mental Health Nursing, 16*(5), 298-306.

Hauenstein, E. J., Petterson, S., Merwin, E., Rovnyak, V., Heise, B., & Wagner, D. (2006). Rurality, gender, and mental health treatment. *Community Health, 29*(3), 169-185.

Hossain, D., Gorman, D., & Eley, R. (2009). Farm advisors reflections on mental health first aid training. *The Australian e-Journal for the Advancement of Mental Health, 8*(1). Retrieved from www.auseinet.com/journal/vol8iss1/hossain.pdf

Hossain, D., Gorman, D., Eley, R., & Coutts, J. (2010). Value of mental health first aid training of advisory and extension agents in supporting farmers in rural Queensland. *Rural and Remote Health, 10*(4), 1593. Retrieved from http://www.rrh.org.au/publishedarticles/article_print_1593.pdf

Hutchison, L., & Blakely, C. (2011). Substance abuse—Trends in rural areas. In L. Gamm, L. Hutchison, B. Dabney, & A. Dorsey (Eds.), *Rural Healthy People 2010.* Retrieved from http://www.srph.tamhsc.edu/centers/rhp2010/11Volume1subabuse.htm

Judd, F., Cooper, A., Fraser, C., & Davis, J. (2006). Rural suicide—People or place effects? *Australian and New Zealand Journal of Psychiatry, 40,* 208-216.

Kosberg, J. I., & Fei Sun, M. S. (2010). Meeting the mental health needs of rural men. *Rural Mental Health, 34*(1), 5-11.

Mayo Clinic. (2011). *Positive thinking.* Retrieved from www.mayoclinic.com/health/positive-thinking/SR00009

McColl, L. (2007). The influence of bush identity on attitudes to mental health in a Queensland community. *Rural Society, 17*(2), 107-124.

McDonald, R., & Brown, P. (2009). Older people and mental health: To what extent do support groups help[Abstract]. *International Journal of Mental Health Nursing, 18,* A1-A27.

Mechanic, D. (1978). Sex, illness, illness behaviour and the use of health services. *Social Science and Medicine, 12B,* 207-214.

Milhausen, R., Yarber, W., & Crosby, R. (2003). Self-reported depression and sexual risk behaviors among a national sample of rural high school students. *Health Education Monograph Series, Special issue, 20*(2), 33-39.

Moadel, A., Morgan, C., Fatone, A., Grennan, J., Carter, J., Laruffa, G., & Dutcher, J. (1999). Seeking meaning and hope: Self-reported spiritual and existential needs among an ethnically-diverse cancer patient population. *Psychooncology, 8*(5), 378-385.

Möller-Leimkühler, A. (2002). Barriers to help seeking by men: A review of sociocultural and clinical literature with particular reference to depression. *Journal of Affective Disorders, 71,* 1-9.

Mulder, P. L., & Linkey, H. (2003). Needs assessment, identification, and mobilization of community resources, and conflict management. In B. H. Stamm (Ed.), *Rural behavioral health care: An interdisciplinary guide* (pp. 67-79). Washington, DC: American Psychological Association.

Mullen, P., Smith, R., & Hill, E. W. (1993). Sense of coherence as a mediator of stress for cancer patients and spouses. *Journal of Psychosocial Oncology, 11*(3), 23-46.

Murphy, M. A. (1998). Rejection, stigma, and hope. *Psychiatric Rehabilitation Journal, 22*(2), 185-188.

Murray, G., Judd, F., Jackson, H., Fraser, C., Komiti, A., Pattison, P., & Robins, G. (2008). Big boys don't cry: An investigation of stoicism and its mental health outcomes. *Personality and Individual Differences, 44*(6), 1369-1381. doi: 10.1016/j.paid. 2007.12.005

Ní Laoire, C. (2001). A matter of life and death? Men, masculinities, and staying 'behind' in rural Ireland. *Sociologia Ruralis, 41*(2), 220-236.

O'Kane, G., Craig, P., & Sutherland, D. (2008). Riverina men's study: An exploration of rural men's attitudes to health and body image. *Nutrition & Dietetics, 65*, 66-71.

Page, A., Morrell, S., Taylor, R., Dudley, M., & Carter, G. (2007). Further increases in rural suicide in young Australian adults: Secular trends, 1979-2003. *Social Science and Medicine, 65*(3), 442-453.

Parr, H., & Philo, C. (2003). Rural mental health and social geographies of caring. *Social and Cultural Geography, 4*, 471-488.

Parr, H., Philo, C., & Burns, N. (2004). Social geographies of rural mental health: Experiencing inclusion and exclusion. *Transactions of the Institute of British Geographers, 29*, 401-419.

Patterson, I., & Pegg, S. (1999). Nothing to do: The relationship between 'leisure boredom' and alcohol and drug addiction. Is there a link to youth suicide in rural Australia? *Youth Studies Australia, 18*, 24-29.

Quine, S., Bernard, D., Booth, M., Kang, M., Usherwood, T., & Alperstein, G. (2003). Health and access issues among Australian adolescents: A rural-urban comparison. *Rural and Remote Health, 3*, 245.

Rajkumar, S., & Hoolahan, B. (2004). Remoteness and issues in mental health care: Experience from rural Australia. *Epidemiologia e Psichiatria Sociale, 13*, 78-82.

Rogers-Clark, C., & Pearce, S. (Eds.). (2004). *Tough times: Ten rural men tell their stories on how they got through some difficult times in their lives.* Toowoomba: Centre for Rural and Remote Area Health.

Sears, S. F., & Evans, G. D. (2003). Rural social service systems as behavioral health delivery systems. In B. H. Stamm (Ed.), *Rural behavioral health care: An interdisciplinary guide* (pp. 109-120). Washington, DC: American Psychological Association.

Seaward, B. L. (2009). *Managing stress: Principles and strategies for health and wellbeing* (6th ed.). Burlington, MA: Jones & Bartlett.

Smith, E. D., Stefanek, M. E., Joseph, M. V., Verdieck, M. J., Zabora, J. R., & Fetting, J. (1993). Spiritual awareness, personal perspective on death, and psychosocial distress: An initial investigation. *Journal of Psychosocial Oncology, 11*(3), 89-103.

U.S. Department of Health and Human Services. (2006). *Mental health and rural America: 1994-2005.* Washington, DC: Health Resources and Services Administration Office of Rural Health Policy.

van Gundy, K. (2006). *Substance abuse in rural and small town America (Vol. 1)*. New Hampshire: Carsey Institute.

Wilkinson, D., & Gunnell, D. (2000). Youth suicide trends in Australian metropolitan and nonmetropolitan areas, 1988-1997. *Australian and New Zealand Journal of Psychiatry, 34*(5), 822-828.

Ziembroski, J., & Breiding, M. (2006). The cumulative effect of rural and regional residence on the health of older adults. *Journal of Aging and Health, 18*(5), 631-659. doi: 10.1177/0898264306291440.

17

Providing Mental Health Services for Children, Adolescents, and Families in Rural Areas

HEIDI LISS RADUNOVICH AND BRENDA A. WIENS

INTRODUCTION

*A*pproximately 21% of the U.S. population resides in rural areas, including a large population of children and adolescents (Gamm, Hutchison, Dabney, & Dorsey, 2003). These residents face unique challenges, as well as added risk factors impacting their mental health. This chapter outlines the need for mental health services for rural children, adolescents, and their families, challenges they face in obtaining mental health services, and strategies that may be undertaken in order to better serve the mental health needs of this population.

NEED FOR MENTAL HEALTH CARE AMONG RURAL CHILDREN, ADOLESCENTS, AND FAMILIES

While rural areas may be viewed by some as idyllic settings in which to live, many rural children and families deal with significant problems, including increased incidence of poverty, obesity and substance use, and often inferior educational, transportation, health care, and mental health care services (Welsh, Domitrovich, Bierman, & Lang, 2003). Rural children have high rates of recent and lifetime exposure to violence as victims and witnesses (Slovak & Singer, 2002). These conditions are all risk factors for rural children and families, and there is evidence that rural children may be at increased risk for various mental health and behavioral health issues (Spoth, Goldberg, Neppl, Trudeau, & Ramisetty-Mikler, 2001). Despite the presence of increased risk factors for rural children and adolescents, few are able to obtain appropriate treatment services. For example, Angold et al. (2002) reported that only 36% of rural children diagnosed with depression receive care.

Rural adolescents show a multitude of mental health issues. Most notably, incidence of depression and anxiety are high. However, unlike their urban counterparts, the literature is mixed on whether rural girls are more likely to report depression than rural boys (Peden, Reed, & Rayens, 2005; Sears, 2004). It does, however, seem that rural adolescent girls report a higher level of anxiety than boys (Puskar, Bernardo, Ren, Stark, & Lester, 2009). Substance use is also a significant problem among rural adolescents, with a report by the National Center on Addiction and Substance Abuse (CASA, 2000) at Columbia University concluding rural youth were 34% more likely to use marijuana, 29% more likely to use alcohol, and twice as likely to smoke cigarettes when compared to urban youth. Clearly there are great needs for both treatment and preventive services for children, adolescents, and their families in rural areas. However, while research on mental health needs and best practices in rural areas is lacking in general, this is especially true for the child and adolescent population (Boydell et al., 2006).

CHALLENGING ISSUES AND BARRIERS TO CARE FOR RURAL CHILDREN, ADOLESCENTS, AND FAMILIES

Providing treatment to children, adolescents, and their families is generally more involved than simply providing individual therapy services because of the need to include multiple participants in the therapy, including parents and possibly siblings. Such factors present potential complications to scheduling and transportation, as well as a need for "buy-in" from multiple family members. Children are generally dependent on parents or caregivers to initiate and provide transportation to services, as well as assistance in making any needed changes to the home environment. Without the support and involvement of parents, most children will be unable to attend or benefit from therapeutic services. While these issues are true of all children and adolescents, residing in a rural area leads to additional challenges in the ability of children to receive mental health care.

Lack of Providers

Although many children and families in rural areas are in need of evidence-based mental health services, they are particularly scarce in small communities, and specialty services such as child psychiatry are even rarer (Holzer, Goldsmith, & Ciarlo, 2000). The majority (61%) of designated Mental Health Professional Shortage Areas are in nonmetropolitan areas; it is estimated that approximately 1,200 mental health providers would be needed to alleviate this shortage (Health Resources and Services Administration, 2011). Due to shortages in mental health professionals in rural communities, some children and families turn to their primary care physicians for assistance. However, while primary care physicians are more common in rural areas than mental health professionals, there is still a shortage of these providers as well. In fact, 65% of primary medical Health Professional Shortage Areas are in nonmetro areas (Health Resources and Services Administration, 2011). It is estimated that only 10% of all physicians in America practice in rural communities (Gamm et al., 2003).

Reasons for provider shortages in rural areas are complex and discussed in detail in Chapter 1, but commonly cited reasons for shortages of rural mental health providers include: poor reimbursement for services and uncertainty of the public funding stream, higher cost of service delivery in rural areas due to low volume of patients, lack of professional support and high burnout, lack of cultural competence, and lack of financial incentives to work in rural areas (Sawyer, Gale, & Lambert, 2006). Lack of available providers in rural areas may lead to increased wait times for services, which have been shown to reduce the likelihood that children and adolescents will actually attend treatment (Sherman, Barnum, Buhman-Wiggs, & Nyberg, 2009). Due to provider shortages and the accompanying lack of psychotherapy services available, rural residents may rely on prescription medications to manage mental health needs more than their urban counterparts (Ziller, Anderson, & Coburn, 2010).

Distance

Children and families living in rural areas may need to travel long distances to access care, particularly to access child mental health or other specialty services (e.g., substance abuse treatment), which reduces the likelihood of seeking and receiving services. Furthermore, children and adolescents are generally reliant on a parent or caregiver for transportation to services. Even families who are willing and able to travel for care may experience hardships because of transportation and the associated costs, including the time needed for roundtrip travel. The availability of local community resources within short travel distances is particularly important in rural areas, which usually lack access to public transportation.

Financial Issues

Approximately 21% of rural children live in poverty (U.S. Department of Agriculture Economic Research Service, 2005). Poverty alone is a significant barrier to treatment for children. Children living in poverty are usually uninsured or underinsured, and not all providers accept state-funded sources of payment such as Medicaid. In rural areas where the primary means of employment is often agriculture and other businesses that rely on the land/nature, residents may be more likely to be self-employed or work for small businesses, and thus may not have health insurance. Even for those who are insured (public or private), there may be stringent limits on who may provide services and for how long, as well as a lack of willingness to accept service provision via tele-health models such as telephone and videoconferencing (Schopp, Demiris, & Glueckauf, 2006). In addition, natural disasters or other climate-related events that affect agricultural production profoundly affect rural economies, impact family finances, and increase familial stress.

Confidentiality and Ethical Practice Concerns

While residents in rural areas may benefit from close-knit community social networks (Pullmann, VanHooser, Hoffman, & Heflinger, 2010), these networks also present challenges for maintaining confidentiality and engaging in ethical practices in rural locations (Roberts, Johnson, Brems, & Warner, 2007; see Chapter 7 for an in-depth discussion of confidentiality and ethics in rural areas). The small number of residents makes the likelihood of dual role conflicts more likely, and preventing identification of patients to other residents can be challenging (Werth, Hastings, & Riding-Malon, 2010). These problems are amplified in service provision to children/adolescents or families simply because of the increased number of individuals involved in the therapeutic process. Questions about these issues can cause difficulties for local providers in rural areas, and potentially lead to concerns about the quality of treatment provided. They may also reduce the likelihood that children, adolescents, and their families will seek mental health treatment or remain in treatment once started (particularly as incidental encounters occur).

Stigma and Perceptions of Therapy

Attitudes toward seeking mental health services are improving. However, there are still those who harbor negative attitudes toward therapeutic services—particularly in rural areas (Starr, Campbell, & Herrick, 2002; see Chapter 4 for additional discussion). The stigma associated with seeking mental health services may be particularly problematic when partnered with the issue of reduced confidentiality in rural areas, where people may be self-conscious about "what the neighbors will think" about the need to seek mental health services. Adolescents are particularly vulnerable to stigma for mental health issues, and are developmentally more likely to be self-conscious about being viewed as different from their peers (Moses, 2010). Local attitudes, customs, and stigma regarding help-seeking in rural areas may serve as barriers to rural residents seeking mental health services from traditional mental health providers (Link & Phelan, 2006; Williams, 1996). The high value placed on self-reliance in rural areas may impede help-seeking behavior for rural residents (particularly when the family unit is involved in the therapeutic process). Research confirms that beliefs about mental health services have an impact on their utilization (Deen, Bridges, McGahan, & Andrews, 2011), which may help to explain why rural residents are less likely to use mental health services even if they are available and accessible (Petterson, Williams, Hauenstein, Rovnyak, & Merwin, 2009).

POTENTIAL SOLUTIONS FOR INCREASING SERVICE PROVISION

The key to mental health management for children, adolescents, and their families is to recognize the many systems that work together to impact child and adolescent functioning, or the "meta-system" (Kazak et al., 2010). Certainly direct assessment and treatment by mental health professionals should be provided, but this is only one piece of the larger system of care that should be considered when working with the child and adolescent population. Although not described in detail below, integration of care with primary care offices is a well-supported area of rural mental health care provision that holds much promise for rural children and families; an in-depth discussion of this topic can be found in Chapter 9.

Use of Technology for Service Provision

One part of the meta-system involves direct service provision from mental health professionals. Given the limited number of these professionals available in rural areas, efforts have been made to increase clinicians' ability to provide services in rural areas, including provision of services through primary care offices. While physical visits to these offices can be difficult for providers to make, over the last 15 years new technologies have developed that facilitate the provision of mental health services to children and adolescents at a distance (Pesämaa et al., 2004; Yellowlees, Hilty, Marks, Neufeld, & Bourgeois, 2008). In addition to the use of more traditional modalities (such as the telephone), video-conferencing and synchronous Internet-based care (i.e., telehealth) has allowed for more mental health and psychiatric providers at distant sites to provide both clinical assessment and treatment to those who would otherwise be unable to travel on a regular basis (Nelson & Bui, 2010; Schopp, Demiris, & Glueckauf, 2006). Details on the implementation of telehealth systems and evidentiary support for overall telehealth interventions can be found in Chapter 10. Research on these services suggests that these distance modalities are feasible for use with children and families, and are becoming more reliable over time (Myers et al., 2010; Myers, Valentine, & Melzer, 2008; Nelson & Bui, 2010).

There are many emerging uses of technology that might lend themselves particularly well to use by children and adolescents, such as texting, smartphone applications, videogames, asynchronous intervention approaches (such as self-guided Internet-based modules or use of podcasts), and social networking sites (Luxton, June, & Kinn, 2011). These and other technologies may be particularly important in the area of prevention in rural areas, including HIV (Juzang, Fortune, Black, Wright, & Bull, 2011), obesity (Kelders, van Gemert-Pijnen, Werkman, & Seydel, 2010; Woolford, Clark, Strecher, & Resnicow, 2010), substance use and violence prevention (Liss, 2004), and family management of children's chronic health issues such as asthma, diabetes, and epilepsy (Glueckauf et al., 2002; Hilty et al., 2006; Liss, Glueckauf, & Ecklund-Johnson, 2002). Technology has also been shown to provide support to parents and caregivers (Demiris, Oliver, Wittenberg-Lyles, & Washington, 2011; van Uden-Kraan, Drossaert, Taal, Seydel, & van de Laar, 2010).

Clients engaged in telehealth interventions, including parents and children, appear to be satisfied with the care received with distance technologies (Myers, Valentine, & Melzer, 2008; Steel, Cox, & Garry, 2011; Wagnild, Leenknecht, & Zauher, 2006). Given the complications associated with travel in rural areas, as well as concerns about confidentiality within the small local community, technology may provide an important solution to assist those who desire social support within rural areas. Not only does use of Internet-based support increase the potential support network, but the anonymity of the Internet allows support to be received without concerns over confidentiality.

School-Based Care and Coordinated Community Response

Because children spend a significant amount of time at school, educational centers can provide an excellent location for increasing outreach and providing services to underserved rural areas (Owens & Murphy, 2004; Stein et al., 2002; Weist & Evans, 2005). Schools have been identified by some as the "de facto" mental health provider for children (Burns et al., 1995). In line with this characterization, policymakers including The President's New Freedom Commission (Hogan, 2003; New Freedom Commission on Mental Health, 2003) and the former Surgeon General in his report on Children's Mental Health (United States Public Health Service, 2000) have called for schools to take an increased role in meeting children's mental health needs. While efforts to provide mental health services in and through schools are increasing (Weist et al., 2005), rural schools are less likely to provide mental health services when compared to urban schools (Slade, 2003). Increased access to students in the school system is associated with increased utilization of services (Weist, Goldstein, Morris, & Bryant, 2003); this may particularly be the case for segments of the population that are less likely to seek out mental health services. For example, Angold et al. (2002) found that even though prevalence rates for psychiatric disorders were similar between rural African American and Caucasian youth, the African American youth were less likely to use specialty mental health services. However, school-based service utilization was similar for the two groups.

There are varying models for providing mental health services through schools detailed in Chapter 11, with the most comprehensive models providing a combination of school-based and school-linked services. The term "school-based" mental health services typically refers to services provided within schools by counselors employed through the school system or outside agencies. These services can take multiple forms, including prevention services, therapy groups, individual sessions with students, teacher consultation, and family therapy provided at the school, as well as formal school-based health centers. School-linked services are provided by outside agencies that are working in collaboration with a school system to serve children and families identified by the school system to be in need of mental health or social services (Evans, Radunovich, Cornette, Wiens, & Roy, 2008). While schools provide an excellent opportunity for collaboration in rural areas, barriers to funding can still be a significant concern. In addition, many mental health services currently provided in schools range in quality, with some having little evidence of effectiveness (Hoagwood & Erwin, 1997; Rones & Hoagwood, 2000). A review by Hoagwood et al. (2007) suggests that more rigorous evaluation of school-based interventions should be conducted, but the existing literature suggests that their impact on mental health functioning is less than ideal, and that a lack of parent involvement in therapy is associated with poorer outcomes. Therefore, engaging the entire family in the therapeutic process, while more challenging to accomplish, should lead to better outcomes.

Case Example: Project CATCh

Effective collaborations with rural schools need to be tailored to the community, with consideration for the barriers, needs, and types of problems present in a particular community, and inclusion of a range of community agencies that work with children and families. Incorporation of the broad community may be particularly important when trying to provide services that will impact the entire family system; however, many existing school collaborations involve only one outside agency (Motes, Melton, Simmons, & Pumariega, 1999). An example of a school collaboration involving multiple agencies in a rural county is Project CATCh (Wack, Radunovich, & Wiens, 2009). Project CATCh's primary goals were identifying and assessing students with mental health needs, increasing linkages with community agencies to improve knowledge of and access to services, reducing stigma and barriers to services, and increasing access for ethnically diverse and low-income families. To address these goals, the district applied for and received a Safe Schools/Healthy Students grant, and later other Department of Education grants, which provided funds for project activities. The overall Project CATCh model situated the school system as the focal point for initiating referrals and handling service coordination for district students identified as having behavioral, emotional, and/or academic problems, while at the same time enhancing relationships among agencies in the community that provide services to children and families. This model allowed for children and families to be referred to more comprehensive services and tailored service referrals to help families overcome barriers to treatment (e.g., transportation, financial). Various aspects of the model have been modified over time based on family, school, and community agency feedback to enhance the fit of the model for the community. While challenging to implement, programs such as these that include multiple community agencies may result in more comprehensive service provision for children and families.

Community-Based Participatory Collaboration

In rural areas where there are fewer mental health resources, community collaborations such as those described in Project CATCh are critical in decreasing the gap between needs and services by making the most of limited community resources. In addition, working with established services or institutions that are well accepted in the rural community to provide mental health services may help reduce stigma and barriers to care (Hargrove & Breazeale, 1993). One way to do this is through Community-Based Participatory Research (CBPR). CBPR has been primarily used to engage communities to address health-related concerns and disparities. However, fewer researchers have used CBPR as an approach to address mental health concerns in communities (Stacciarini, Shattell, Madden, & Wiens, 2010), particularly in rural areas.

CBPR could be an effective approach for evaluating and addressing the mental health needs of children and families in rural communities because collaboration among community agencies that serve children, particularly schools, is important for successful implementation of mental health efforts. Utilizing CBPR approaches to address mental health disparities for children and families in rural areas could help to tailor strategies and programs to a particular community, and community collaboration would allow for the maximization of the limited resources available within communities. In addition, CBPR may be a particularly good match for addressing minority child and family mental health needs in rural areas given the presence of ethnic disparities in mental health and the fact that minority groups may be less likely to access traditional mental health services even when they are available (U.S. Public Health Service, 2000). For example, Stacciarini et al. (2011) have used CBPR to evaluate mental health needs of rural Latino immigrant mothers and children, with the goal of developing culturally appropriate interventions for this population.

Prevention-Based Focus

The literature suggests that it is much easier to prevent problems than it is to treat them once they occur; this is even more critical for children and families within rural areas where availability of treatment services is limited. Therefore, focusing efforts on increasing preventive services for children and families in rural areas may be key in improving their mental health. Prevention efforts are consistent with a public health approach to children's mental health; indeed, a number of mental and behavioral health issues faced by children (such as violence and obesity) can be conceptualized as public health problems. There are many types of preventive services targeting mental and behavioral health issues that could be beneficial for children and families. Using youth violence prevention as an example, systematic reviews and meta-analyses of universal school-based violence prevention programs have shown effectiveness in reducing violence and associated youth risk behaviors of substance use, delinquency, poor school attendance, and underachievement (Hahn et al., 2007; Wilson & Lipsey, 2007). Integrating prevention programs into schools can be an especially effective way to reach children in rural areas who might not otherwise receive mental health services. However, issues such as funding, integration and acceptance of such programs at schools, and fidelity of program implementation may limit the reach and effectiveness of such programs.

In addition to school-based prevention efforts, there are also community agencies that may serve as partners to provide or supplement preventive efforts, and to house program implementation. For example, health departments, churches, and the Cooperative Extension Service in many rural counties have served as hosts or facilitators of child and family-related prevention programming. In fact, many state Cooperative Extension Services provide low or no cost education in the areas of parenting skills, child and adolescent coping skills, nutrition education, and marriage enrichment. The Cooperative Extension Service has also served as a partner for behavioral health and mental health research, as well as assisted in the implementation of programming. An example is the Sensible Treatment of Obesity in Rural Youth (STORY) project, which involves the provision of obesity treatment through Cooperative Extension offices (Janicke et al., 2008). Additionally, the Extension Family Lifestyle Intervention Project (Janicke et al., 2011) involves the use of Cooperative Extension space in partnership with Extension agents who provide the intervention programming.

Another program associated with the Cooperative Extension Service is the 4-H youth program, which provides positive youth development programming nationally. A large-scale, longitudinal study on the impact of positive youth development programming through 4-H is currently underway, and initial results suggest that the acquisition of positive youth development skills through 4-H is associated with better outcomes related to increased positive functioning as well as reduced incidence of at-risk behaviors and depression later in life (Jelicic, Bobek, Phelps, Lerner, & Lerner, 2007). This means that programs such as 4-H could serve as a meaningful partner in providing and enhancing skill development for children and adolescents, particularly in rural areas with limited resources.

CONCLUSION

While many inroads have been made in increasing access to mental health services to the population at large, rural residents are still underserved, despite showing a greater number of risk factors. Children, adolescents, and their families' mental health needs are even more challenging to meet due to the complications associated with multiple persons involved in treatment. This is especially true in rural environments where barriers such as limited numbers of providers, stigma, negative attitudes toward therapy, confidentiality challenges, lack of public transportation, and limited finances make the likelihood of accessing or even seeking mental health services low. However, obtaining appropriate mental health and preventive services is critical in order to enhance the functioning of rural families.

In order to better meet the mental health needs of children, adolescents, and their families in rural communities, several strategies for care have been developed. Increasing the availability of direct services has been accomplished through integrated care and the provision of telehealth. These methods are promising, but as technology continues to develop rapidly, telehealth methods in particular will need to be continually assessed. There are also specific technologies that likely appeal more to children and adolescents, and continued development of programs and protocols for these technologies and research on these modes of service provision are important.

Leveraging the existing resources within a community and providing coordination of services is also of critical importance. Engaging community participants and partnering with local service agencies leads to better identification of areas of community need, as well as better care for families. Finally, given the limited resources available in rural communities and the barriers to accessing services, prevention should be a key component of rural mental health management. Recognizing the roles that local agencies such as school systems, churches, health departments, Cooperative Extension Services, and 4-H can play as providers or facilitators of prevention services, identifiers of those who need care, and locations of central service provision will help maximize the use of community resources. These strategies ensure that the entire "meta-system" involved in child and adolescent mental health care is engaged in the process.

REFERENCES

Angold, A., Erkanli, A., Farmer, E. M. Z., Fairbank, J. A., Burns, B. J., Keeler, G., & Costello, E. J. (2002). Psychiatric disorder, impairment, and service use in rural African American and white youth. *Archives of General Psychiatry, 59*, 893–901. doi: 10.1001/archpsyc.59.10.893

Boydell, K. M., Pong, R., Volpe, T., Tilleczek, K., Wilson, E., & Lemieux, S. (2006). Family perspectives on pathways to mental health care for children and youth in rural communities. *The Journal of Rural Health, 22*(2), 182–188. doi: 10.1111/ j.1748-0361.2006.00029.x

Burns, B. J., Costello, E. J., Angold, A., Tweed, D., Stangl, D., Farmer, E.M., & Erkanli, A. (1995). Children's mental health service use across service sectors. *Health Affairs, 14*(3), 147–159. doi: 10.1377/hlthaff.14.3.147

Deen, T. L., Bridges, A. J., McGahan, T. C., & Andrews, A. R. III (2011). Cognitive appraisals of specialty mental health services and their relation to mental health service utilization in the rural population. *The Journal of Rural Health, 27*(2), 1–10. doi: 10.1111/j.1748-0361.2011.00375.x

Demiris, G., Oliver, D. P., Wittenberg-Lyles, E., & Washington, K. (2011). Use of videophones to deliver a cognitive-behavioural therapy to hospice caregivers. *Journal of Telemedicine and Telecare, 17*, 142–145. doi: 10.1258/jtt.2010.100503

Evans, G. D., Radunovich, H. D., Cornette, M. M., Wiens, B. A., & Roy, A. (2008). Implementation and utilization characteristics of a rural, school-linked mental health program. *Journal of Child and Family Studies, 17*, 84–97.

Gamm, L. D., Hutchison, L. L., Dabney, B. J., & Dorsey, A. M. (Eds.). (2003). *Rural Healthy People 2010: A companion document to Healthy People 2010* (Vol. 1). College Station, TX: The Texas A&M University System Health Science Center, School of Rural Public Health, Southwest Rural Health Research Center.

Glueckauf, R. L., Fritz, S. P., Ecklund-Johnson, E. P., Liss, H.J., Dages, P., & Carney, P. (2002). Videoconferencing-based family counseling for rural teenagers with epilepsy: Phase 1 findings. *Rehabilitation Psychology, 47*(1), 49–72. doi: 10.1037// 0090-5550.47.1.49

Hahn, R., Fuqua-Whitley, D., Wethington, H., Lowy, J., Crosby, A., Fullilove, M., ... Dahlberg, L. (2007). Effectiveness of universal school-based programs to prevent violent and aggressive behavior: A systematic review. *American Journal of Preventive Medicine, 33*, S114–S129. doi: 10.1016/j.amepre.2007.04.012

Hargrove, D. S., & Breazeale, R. L. (1993). Psychologists and rural services: Addressing a new agenda. *Professional Psychology: Research and Practice, 24*, 319–324. doi: 10.1037/0735-7028.24.3.319

Health Resources and Services Administration, U.S. Department of Health & Human Services, Office of Shortage Designation, Bureau of Health Professions. (2011). *Designated health professional shortage areas statistics.* Retrieved from http:// ersrs.hrsa.gov/ReportServer?/HGDW_Reports/BCD_HPSA/BCD_HPSA_SCR50_ Smry&rs:Format=HTML3.2

Hilty, D., Yellowlees, P., Cobb, H., Bourgeois, J., Neufeld, J., & Nesbitt, T. (2006). Models of telepsychiatry-liaison service to rural primary care. *Psychosomatics, 47*(2), 152–157. doi: 10.1176/appi.psy.47.2.152

Hoagwood, K., & Erwin, H. D. (1997). Effectiveness of school-based mental health services for children: A 10-year research review. *Journal of Child and Family Studies, 6*, 435–451. doi: 10.1023/A:1025045412689

Hoagwood, K. E., Olin, S. S., Kerker, B. D., Kratochwill, T. R., Crowe, M., & Saka, N. (2007). Empirically based school interventions targeted at academic and mental health functioning. *Journal of Emotional and Behavioral Disorders, 15*(2), 66–92.

Hogan, M. F. (2003). The President's New Freedom Commission: Recommendations to transform mental health care in America. *Psychiatric Services, 54*, 1467–1474. doi: 10.1176/appi.ps.54.11.1467

Holzer, C. E., Goldsmith, H. F., & Ciarlo, J. A. (2000). The availability of health and mental health providers by population density. *Journal of the Washington Academy of Sciences, 86,* 25–33.

Janicke, D. M., Lim, C. S., Perri, M. G., Bobroff, L. B., Mathews, A. E., Brumback, B. A., . . . Silverstein, J. H. (2011). The Extension Family Lifestyle Project (E-FLIP for Kids): Design and methods. *Contemporary Clinical Trials, 32*(1), 50–58. doi: 10.1016/j.cct.2010.08.002

Janicke, D. M., Sallinen, B. J., Perri, M. G., Lutes, L. D., Silverstein, J. H., Huerta, M. G., & Guion, L. A. (2008). Sensible Treatment of Obesity in Rural Youth (STORY): Design and methods. *Contemporary Clinical Trials, 29*(2), 270–280. doi: 10.1016/j.cct.2007.05.005

Jelicic, H., Bobek, D. L., Phelps, E., Lerner, R. M., & Lerner, J. V. (2007). Using positive youth development to predict contribution and risk behaviors in early adolescence: Findings from the first two waves of the 4-H Study of Positive Youth Development. *International Journal of Behavioral Development, 31*(3), 263–273. doi: 10.1177/0165025407076439

Juzang, I., Fortune, T., Black, S., Wright, E., & Bull, S. (2011). A pilot programme using mobile phones for HIV prevention. *Journal of Telemedicine and Telecare, 17,* 150–153. doi: 10.1258/jtt.2010.091107

Kazak, A. E., Hoagwood, K., Weisz, J. R., Hood, K., Kratochwill, T. R., Vargas, L. A., & Banez, G. A. (2010). A meta-systems approach to evidence-based practice for children and adolescents. *American Psychologist, 65*(2), 85–97. doi: 10.1037/a0017784

Kelders, S. M., van Gemert-Pijnen, J. E. W. C., Werkman, A., & Seydel, E. R. (2010). Evaluation of a web-based lifestyle coach designed to maintain a healthy bodyweight. *Journal of Telemedicine and Telecare, 16,* 3–7. doi: 10.1258/jtt.2009.001003

Link, B. G., & Phelan, J. C. (2006). Stigma and its public health implications. *The Lancet, 367,* 528–529.

Liss, H. J. (2004). Telehealth/Internet services for children, adolescents and families. In R., Steele, & M., Roberts (Eds.), *Handbook of mental health services for children, adolescents, and families.* New York: Kluwer Academic Publications.

Liss, H. J., Glueckauf, R. L., & Ecklund-Johnson, E. P. (2002). Research on telehealth and chronic medical conditions: Critical review, key issues and future directions. *Rehabilitation Psychology, 47*(1), 8–30.

Luxton, D. D., June, J. D., & Kinn, J. T. (2011). Technology-based suicide prevention: Current applications and future directions. *Telemedicine and e-Health, 17*(1), 51–54. doi: 10.1089/tmj.2010.0091

Moses, T. (2010). Being treated differently: Stigma experiences with family, peers, and school staff among adolescents with mental health disorders. *Social Science & Medicine, 70,* 985–993. doi: 10.1016/j.socscimed.2009.12.022

Motes, P. S., Melton, G., Simmons, W. E. W., & Pumariega, A. (1999). Ecologically oriented school-based mental health services: Implications for service system reform. *Psychology in the Schools, 36,* 391–401. doi: 10.1002/(SICI)1520-6807(199909)36:5<391::AID-PITS3>3.0.CO;2-C

Myers, K. M., Valentine, J. M., & Melzer, S. M. (2008). Child and adolescent telepsychiatry: Utilization and satisfaction. *Telemedicine and e-Health, 14*(2), 131–137.

Myers, K. M., Vander Stoep, A., McCarty, C. A., Klein, J. B., Palmer, N. B., Geyer, J. R., & Melzer, S. M. (2010). Child and adolescent telepsychiatry: Variations in utilization, referral patterns, and practice trends. *Journal of Telemedicine and Telecare, 16*, 128–133. doi: 10.1258/jtt.2009.090712

National Center on Addiction and Substance Abuse. (2000). *No place to hide: Substance abuse in mid-size cities and rural America*. New York, NY: Author.

Nelson, E., & Bui, T. (2010). Rural telepsychology services for children and adolescents. *Journal of Clinical Psychology, 66*(5), 490–501.

New Freedom Commission on Mental Health. (2003). *Achieving the promise: Transforming mental health care in America*. Final Report (DHHS Pub. No. SMA-03-3832). Rockville, MD: Substance Abuse and Mental Health Service Administration.

Owens, J. S., & Murphy, C. E. (2004). Effectiveness research in the context of school-based mental health. *Clinical Child and Family Psychology Review, 7*, 195–209. doi: 10.1007/s10567-004-6085-x

Peden, A. R., Reed, D. B., & Rayens, M. K. (2005). Depressive symptoms in adolescents living in rural America. *The Journal of Rural Health, 21*(4), 310–316. doi: 10.1111/j.1748-0361.2005.tb00100.x

Pesämaa, L., Ebeling, H., Kuusimäki, M., Winblad, I., Isohanni, M., & Moilanen, I. (2004). Videoconferencing in child and adolescent telepsychiatry: A systematic review of the literature. *Journal of Telemedicine and Telecare, 10*, 187–192.

Petterson, S., Williams, I., Hauenstein, E., Rovnyak, V., & Merwin, E. (2009). Race and ethnicity and rural mental health treatment. *Journal of Health Care for the Poor & Underserved, 20*(3), 662–677.

Pullmann, M., VanHooser, S., Hoffman, C., & Heflinger, C. (2010). Barriers and supports to family participation in a rural system of care for children with serious emotional problems. *Community Mental Health Journal, 46*(3), 211–220. doi: 10.1007/s10597-009-9208-5

Puskar, K., Bernardo, L., Ren, D., Stark, K., & Lester, S. (2009). Sex differences in self-reported anxiety in rural adolescents. *International Journal of Mental Health Nursing, 18*(6), 417–423. doi:10.1111/j.1447-0349.2009.00622.x

Roberts, L. W., Johnson, M. E., Brems, C., & Warner, T. D. (2007). Ethical disparities: Challenges encountered by multidisciplinary providers in fulfilling ethical standards in the care of rural and minority people. *The Journal of Rural Health, 23*, 89–97. doi: 10.1111/j.1748-0361.2007.00130.x

Rones, M., & Hoagwood, K. (2000). School-based mental health services: A research review. *Clinical Child and Family Psychology Review, 3*, 223–241. doi: 10.1023/A:1026425104386

Sawyer, D., Gale, J. A., & Lambert, D. (2006). *Rural and frontier mental and behavioral health care: Barriers, effective policy strategies, best practices*. Waite Park, MN: National Association of Rural Mental Health.

Schopp, L. H., Demiris, G., & Glueckauf, R. L. (2006). Rural backwaters or front-runners? Rural telehealth in the vanguard of psychology practice. *Professional Psychology: Research and Practice, 37*(2), 165–173. doi: 10.1037/0735-7028.37.2.165

Sears, H. A. (2004). Adolescents in rural communities seeking help: Who reports problems and who sees professionals? *Journal of Child Psychology & Psychiatry, 45*(2), 396–404. doi: 10.1111/j.1469-7610.2004.00230.x

Sherman, M. L., Barnum, D. D., Buhman-Wiggs, A., & Nyberg, E. (2009). Clinical intake of child and adolescent consumers in a rural community mental health center: Does wait-time predict attendance? *Community Mental Health Journal, 45*(1), 78–84. doi: 10.1007/s10597-008-9153-8

Slade, E. P. (2003). The relationship between school characteristics and the availability of mental health and related health services in middle and high schools in the United States. *Journal of Behavioral Health Services & Research, 30*, 382–392. doi: 10.1007/BF02287426

Slovak, K., & Singer, M. I. (2002). Children and violence: Findings and implications from a rural community. *Child and Adolescent Social Work Journal, 19*, 35–56. doi: 10.1023/A:1014003306441

Spoth, R., Goldberg, C., Neppl, T., Trudeau, L., & Ramisetty-Mikler, S. (2001). Rural-urban differences in the distribution of parent-reported risk factors for substance use among young adolescents. *Journal of Substance Abuse, 13*, 609–623. doi: 10.1016/S0899-3289(01)00091-8

Stacciarini, J. R., Shattell, M. M., Madden, M. C., & Wiens, B. A. (2010). Review: Community-based participatory research approach to address mental health in minority populations. *Community Mental Health Journal.* Advance online publication. doi:10.1007/s10597-010-9319-z

Stacciarini, J. R., Wiens, B., Coady, M., Schwait, A. B., Perez, A., Locke, B., . . . Bernardi, K. (2011). CBPR: Building partnerships with Latinos in rural areas for a wellness approach to mental health. *Issues in Mental Health Nursing, 32*(8), 486–492.

Starr, S., Campbell, L. R., & Herrick, C. A. (2002). Factors affecting use of the mental health system by rural children. *Issues in Mental Health Nursing, 23*(3), 291–304. doi: 10.1080/016128402753543027

Steel, K., Cox, D., & Garry, H. (2011). Therapeutic videoconferencing interventions for the treatment of long-term conditions. *Journal of Telemedicine and Telecare, 17*, 109–117. doi: 10.1258/jtt.2010.100318

Stein, B. D., Kataoka, S., Jaycox, L. H., Wong, M., Fink, A., Escudero, P., & Zaragoza, C. (2002). Theoretical basis and program design of a school-based mental health intervention for traumatized immigrant children: A collaborative research partnership. *Journal of Behavioral Health Services & Research, 29*, 318–326. doi: 10.1007/BF02287371

U.S. Department of Agriculture Economic Research Service. (2005). *Rural children at a glance.* Retrieved from http://www.ers.usda.gov/publications/EIB1/eib1.pdf

U.S. Public Health Service (2000). *Report of the Surgeon General's conference on children's mental health: A national action agenda.* Washington, DC: Department of Health and Human Services.

van Uden-Kraan, C. F., Drossaert, C. H. C., Taal, E., Seydel, E. R., & van de Laar, M. A. F. J. (2010). Patient-initiated online support groups: motives for initiation, extent of success and success factors. *Journal of Telemedicine and Telecare, 16*, 30–34. doi: 10.1258/jtt.2009.001009

Wack, E., Radunovich, H. L., & Wiens, B. (2009). Project CATC: A model of care coordination and service delivery for children. *Journal of Rural Community Psychology, E12 (1).* Retrieved from http://www.marshall.edu/JRCP/VE12%20N1/Radunovich%20JRCP.pdf

Wagnild, G., Leenknecht, C., & Zauher, J. (2006). Psychiatrists' satisfaction with telepsychiatry. *Telemedicine and e-Health, 12*(5), 546–551.

Weist, M. D., & Evans, S. W. (2005). Expanded school mental health: Challenges and opportunities in an emerging field. *Journal of Youth and Adolescence, 34*, 3–6. doi: 10.1007/s10964-005-1330-2

Weist, M. D., Goldstein, A., Morris, L., & Bryant, T. (2003). Integrating expanded school mental health programs and school-based health centers. *Psychology in the Schools, 40*, 297–308. doi: 10.1002/pits.10089

Weist, M. D., Sander, M. A., Walrath, C., Link, B., Nabors, L., Adelsheim, S., . . . Carrillo, K. (2005). Developing principles for best practice in expanded school mental health. *Journal of Youth and Adolescence, 34*, 7–13. doi: 10.1007/s10964-005-1331-1

Welsh, J., Domitrovich, C. E., Bierman, K., & Lang, J. (2003). Promoting safe schools and healthy students in rural Pennsylvania. *Psychology in the Schools, 40*, 457–472. doi: 10.1002/pits.10103

Werth, J. L. Jr., Hastings, S. L., & Riding-Malon, R. (2010). Ethical challenges of practicing in rural areas. *Journal of Clinical Psychology, 66*(5), 537–548.

Williams, R. T. (1996). The on-going farm crisis: Extension leadership in rural communities. *Journal of Extension, 34*. Retrieved from http://www.joe.org/joe/1996february/a3.html

Wilson, S. J., & Lipsey, M. W. (2007). School-based interventions for aggressive and disruptive behavior: Update of a meta-analysis. *American Journal of Preventive Medicine, 33*, S130–S143. doi: 10.1016/j.amepre.2007.04.011

Woolford, S. J., Clark, S. J., Strecher, V. J., & Resnicow, K. (2010). Tailored mobile phone text messages as an adjunct to obesity treatment for adolescents. *Journal of Telemedicine and Telecare, 16*, 458–461. doi: 10.1258/jtt.2010.100207

Yellowlees, P., Hilty, D., Marks, S., Neufeld, J., & Bourgeois, J. (2008). A retrospective analysis of a child and adolescent e-mental health program. *Journal of the American Academy of Child & Adolescent Psychiatry, 47*(1), 103–107. doi: 10.1097/chi.0b013e31815a56a7

Ziller, E., Anderson, N., & Coburn, A. (2010). Access to rural mental health services: Service use and out of pocket costs. *Journal of Rural Health, 26*(3), 214–224. doi: 10.1111/j.1748-0361.2010.00291.x

18

Providing Mental Health Services for Older Adults and Caregivers in Rural Areas

MARTHA R. CROWTHER, FORREST SCOGIN, ERNEST WAYDE,
AND AUDREY L. AUSTIN

INTRODUCTION

Given the increasing proportion of the population of older adults and changing demographics, health professionals must be prepared to assess and treat clients who are often much older than the populations they worked with in their training. This becomes even more important in rural areas where provider shortages exacerbate existing mental health problems and conditions. Several psychotherapies have proven effective in working with older adults (Culverwell & Martin, 2000); both research and clinical experience confirm that most older adults are well suited to cognitive and behavioral therapies utilizing an approach that is collaborative, involves explicit goal setting, and acknowledges strengths. Within this approach (or any other psychotherapy), it is important for therapists to consider what adaptations might make therapy especially responsive to the concerns and style of older rural clients. Therapists would do well to utilize a biopsychosocial model in working with older rural adults, in which they plan treatment with awareness of interdisciplinary principles and resources.

This chapter describes the changing demographic profile of older adults with particular attention to rural elders. Probable adaptations of psychotherapy for the aged in rural communities are reviewed with the provision of an overview of caregiving issues for rural elders. A clinical illustration of Cognitive Behavior Therapy (CBT) for an elderly rural man is then presented. Selected references and recommended readings are included at the end of the chapter. Many of the issues discussed here have been addressed in previous work focused on elderly care across all geographic regions (Crowther & Austin, 2009; Crowther, Scogin, & Norton, 2010). This chapter expands on previous discussions to include rural caregiving.

OLDER, RURAL ADULTS

The population of the United States is growing older and becoming more ethnically diverse. According to Census Bureau projections, the number of persons aged 65 and older will increase from 35 million to 66 million by 2030 and to 82 million by 2050, a figure accounting for 20% of the entire U.S. population (U.S. Census Bureau, 2000). This "gerontological explosion" will also occur across groups of minority elders, whose respective population sizes will nearly double by 2050 (U.S. Bureau of the Census, 2000).

As discussed in Chapter 1, definitions of rurality vary; however, rural areas are commonly defined by their categorization as nonmetropolitan as opposed to metropolitan (National Advisory Committee on Rural Health and Human Services, 2008). Using this definition, 19% of the older adult population is considered to live in rural areas (Administration on Aging, 2010), whereas only 16% of the overall population resides in rural areas (U.S. Census Bureau, 2010). This suggests that the anticipated increase in the elderly population will have a greater impact on rural areas. Rural elders are increasingly becoming isolated, compounding all aspects of mental health. The proportion of older adults in rural counties is higher than in urban areas primarily as a result of younger populations moving to larger urban areas. Along with the out-migration of younger populations, there is an in-migration of retired elderly. Thus, many rural communities are aging more rapidly than urban areas (Ham, Goins, & Brown, 2003). Retirement communities, primarily in coastal regions, experienced a rate of total population increase of 28.4% from 1990 to 2000 (Johnson & Beale, 2002). There was a rapid growth of the older population moving to the rural areas of the West and Mid-Atlantic regions, mainly for retirement. However, the growth of the older population slowed or stopped in many areas in the Great Plains, Corn Belt, and lower Mississippi Delta (Whitener & McGranahan, 2003). While retiree migration does increase populations and local tax bases, studies find that it does not increase per capita income, nor contribute to increased economic stability (Ham et al., 2003).

MENTAL HEALTH AND RURAL ELDERS

Rural elders are one of the groups at greatest risk for experiencing mental health problems (Bischoff, Hollist, Smith, & Flack, 2004; Chalifoux, Neese, Buckwalter, Litwak, & Abraham, 1996). In many rural communities there are no psychosocial services to meet the needs of the elderly. Many physicians who treat elderly community-dwelling individuals have little specialized training in diagnosing or treating the most common mental health problems of older adults. Symptoms of older individuals' underlying mental health problems are often either ignored, misdiagnosed, or are simply attributed to the inevitability of the "aging process" and therefore left untreated (Butler, Lewis, & Sunderland, 1991). Where specialized services do exist, they tend to be concentrated in more densely populated cities and suburban areas. Obtaining mental health services for older people is most problematic in rural areas of the country where there is a general overall scarcity of such services for all age groups, and a lack of specialized expertise in diagnosing and treating the mental health problems of the elderly (Buckwalter, Smith, Zevenbergen, & Russell, 1991; McCulloch & Lynch, 1993). Although it is unclear exactly what characteristics of living in a rural area contribute to mental health problems, several explanations have been suggested including neighborhood or residential stability and its isolating effects, lack of community resources and health services, and diminished family and social support due to migration of younger cohorts to more populated areas.

FAMILY CAREGIVING AND RURAL ELDERS

In the discussion of issues involved in treating rural elders, caregiving is an important topic, particularly given the growth in the rural elderly population and the out-migration of rural young adults. An increasing number of older adults are family caregivers and/or the recipients of care. Family caregivers constitute the largest group of care providers in the United States, and provide primary or secondary care, full time or part time, and live with the person being cared for or live separately (Administration on Aging, 2006). Family caregivers are active in many scenarios across the lifespan, providing instrumental, therapeutic, and emotional support to care recipients (Family Caregiver Alliance, 2006). National estimates show that 44 million Americans over the age of 18 provide support to older people and adults with disabilities who live in the community and who have limited ability to carry out daily activities such as bathing, managing medications, or preparing meals.

As described above, the Administration on Aging (2007) indicates that persons 65 and older will increase 101% between 2000 and 2030. Unfortunately, over that same 30-year period the number of family members who are available to provide care for these older adults is expected to increase by only 25%, at a rate of 0.8% per year (Mack & Thompson, 2001). This difference in the rates of population increase may be even more pronounced in rural areas given the disproportionate representation of the elderly in rural areas.

Most family caregivers are women, half are employed, and most are over 50 years of age. The functional limitations of care recipients which necessitate the most assistance for the caregiver include moving around, need for help with eating, dressing, bathing, toileting, and so on, disordered learning, memory and confusion, and anxiety or depression. Caregiving is not exclusively conducted for the elderly resident; older adults are frequently caregivers themselves: approximately 4.5 million children (representing 6.3%) are living in grandparent-maintained households with no parent present (U.S. Census Bureau, 2000).

While caregiving occurs everywhere in society, rurality likely affects caregiving. Factors related to caregiving in a rural community, to some extent, are responsible for differences in the nature and outcomes of caregiving. For many rural caregivers, poverty combines with lack of health services, fewer resources, and living in an underserved area to negatively impact caregiving. Often family members, neighbors, and friends provide both direct and indirect caregiving services. However, family members may migrate to other areas seeking education, employment, and other opportunities. This often reduces the number of family members or paid caregivers available to provide care for rural elders.

Research in the area of interventions for caregivers has focused on identifying and relieving the burden of caregiving. Caregivers commonly shoulder responsibility for helping care recipients to manage multiple activities of daily living, and these responsibilities are magnified in rural areas where support resources and home health professionals are frequently unavailable. Caregivers most frequently report arranging or providing transportation, completing grocery shopping and housework, and managing finances, as well as helping the care recipient to get in and out of bed and chairs, to get dressed, and to complete personal grooming tasks (National Alliance for Caregiving & AARP, 2004). Although caregivers of varying ages and backgrounds may need to perform similar activities, living in an underserved area may influence the way rural caregivers perceive and respond to their responsibilities. Caregiver reactions, coping strategies, distress levels, acceptance of symptoms, and attitudes toward clinicians and outside help may vary considerably across different cultures ("Culture and Caregiving," 1992) and potentially within rural areas as well.

ADAPTING CBT FOR TREATING THE RURAL ELDERLY

Psychoeducation is a major component of CBT, and therapy is often framed as a "learning experience," rather than a "psychological treatment." This suggests that clients do not have to be especially "psychologically minded" to benefit. This can be an advantage to the current cohort of older adults, who were raised in an era when psychological principles were not widely disseminated, and especially for rural older adults, within whom stigma regarding psychological services is heightened (Crowther et al., 2010). However, it is noteworthy that older adults may not be as averse to psychotherapy, especially CBT, as intuition might lead one to expect. Rokke and Scogin (1995), for example, showed that older adults rated cognitive therapy as more credible and acceptable than drug therapy for depression, in direct contrast to frequently voiced expectations that older adults would prefer drug therapy and feel stigmatized when psychotherapy is recommended.

Core elements of CBT remain essential when working with older adults, even those with cognitive or physical impairments. These elements include:

1. Emphasis on a collaborative therapeutic relationship, in which the therapist and client develop a mutually responsive, goal-focused working style;
2. Recognition of the client's strengths as well as problems;
3. Focus on a small number of clearly specified goals for treatment;
4. Placing the emphasis of treatment on change, while acknowledging that understanding or insight may be an important step, but is not usually an end in itself;
5. Use of psychoeducational methods as a central treatment components, for example, sharing the treatment rationale, educating the client about techniques to be used;
6. Length of therapy established initially, or as soon as feasible, and linking length to the time expected to accomplish particular goals;
7. Setting an agenda at each meeting representing the consensus of the therapist and client about what goals have priority; and
8. Training in more effective strategies for handling problems as a frequent component of treatment (e.g., cognitive behavioral or interpersonal skills).

There are a few major content differences in therapy with older as compared to younger adults. Older adults have more health problems resulting in functional impairment and their psychological status is often related to their functional status (Zeiss, Lewinsohn, Rohde, & Seeley, 1996). In addition, older adults may face obstacles in terms of resources for supporting an adequate quality of life, such as limited financial resources, limited transportation, or the experience of loss of friends and family. The problems older adults face are not all appropriate targets for CBT, but may be important targets for the services of other health care professionals, such as geriatricians, social workers, and occupational therapists, who can work collaboratively with the CB therapist. Thus, CBT with the elderly often is part of a comprehensive, interdisciplinary treatment. Unfortunately, however, many of these services are not as readily available for rural older adults.

Because of the emphasis on learning in CBT, it is important to consider possible changes in memory and information processing with rural older adult clients and to be prepared to adapt therapy according to the specific function of each older client. Cognitive changes can be part of normal aging or can occur with more dramatic brain changes due to trauma or a dementia process. There are enormous individual differences among older adults, so the concerns briefly highlighted below are presented as *possible* cognitive changes related to aging.

Older adults, on average, show significant age decrements in performance on many kinds of memory functions, such as short-term memory, memory span, recall of lists of information, recall of paired-associate learning, and recall of prose material. Because recognition memory is generally not as impaired, older adults benefit from the possibility of reviewing lists or texts, particularly when they can set their own pace for review. Older adults generally do not show poorer ability than younger adults in strategies for making associations, imagery, or extracting main points from prose material. This finding suggests that bibliotherapy adjuncts or using imagery procedures can be as effective with older adults as with younger adults.

As a result of cognitive changes, the pace of therapy may be slower than with younger adults. More repetition of material may be necessary, and processing of new ideas may be slower. Memory aids, such as an audio tape of each session to review at home, may be helpful (particularly among rural clients who are less able to return for follow-up visits). It may help to present material in multiple ways, both because of potential sensory loss (poorer hearing or vision, for example) and because repetitions provide multiple routes to memory storage. A key phrase for therapists working with older adults is "Say it, Show it, Do it." When presenting a new idea, state it clearly, write it down, and help the client use the idea in a specific way, applying it to one's situation.

Some older adults become distracted from the main topic during a session because of memory problems and a tendency to be pulled off topic by concrete or tangential associations to words. An older person may start to tell a relevant story, for example, to provide information on a homework assignment, and then get lost in the details and become unable to return to the main point. Older people who have this problem benefit from active efforts to stay focused, including redirecting attention to the main ideas of a discussion. It can also be helpful to have the agenda clearly visible, for example, written on a white board on the wall or on a table between therapist and client.

Because older clients may have trouble processing and storing new information, they may be slow to see the relevance of ideas presented in therapy. For example, teaching an older client to be assertive with the butcher may not generalize to being assertive with a neighbor, an adult child, or the librarian. Each seems like a new situation, and the material may need to be presented in multiple contexts before the older client can be said to have developed a new "skill." This slows the pace of therapy, but is often essential to helping the client master essential points.

The changes due to cognitive deficits, strengths of the elderly, and the intrinsically interdisciplinary nature of work with older adults are summarized in the mnemonic MICKS to help therapists remember the key adaptations of CBT that should be considered with older clients, including those that are rural:

- Use **M**ultimodal teaching
- Maintain **I**nterdisciplinary awareness
- Present information more **C**learly
- Develop **K**nowledge of aging challenges and strengths
- Present therapy material more **S**lowly.

USING CBT FOR TREATING DEPRESSION IN THE RURAL ELDERLY

As a result of government initiatives, including the Surgeon General's Supplement focused on mental health (U.S. Department of Health and Human Services, 2001) and the President's New Freedom Commission on Mental Health (2003), there has been an enhanced emphasis on decreasing mental health disparities. Depression has been identified as an area in which disparities are strongly indicated by higher prevalence and/or disparity in mental health assessment, access, and treatment outcomes for minority elders. The prevalence rates of major depressive disorder range from 3% to 5% in community samples, increasing to 6% to 8% in primary care settings, and around 13% in home health care recipients (Bruce et al., 2002). Older adults have a comparable or higher prevalence of minor depression, dysthymia, or significant depressive symptoms compared with younger persons (Blazer, 2002). Data from a number of studies indicate that across the adult life span, the highest depression scores are found among younger adults and persons 75 years and older (e.g., Lewinsohn, Rohde, Seeley, & Fischer, 1991).

Why might older adults experience a high rate of symptoms without a high rate of diagnosed depression? One answer is that older adults often have comorbid chronic medical illness. Depression is often exacerbated by the presence of these comorbid conditions, in particular heart disease, stroke, diabetes mellitus, and Alzheimer's disease (Fischer Wei, Solberg, Rush, & Heinrich, 2003). Older adult patients are more likely to be widowed, have lower levels of education, have fair or poor health, and have three or more comorbid health problems than younger depressed patients. Older adults who live in rural areas typically have fewer resources and poorer mental and physical health status than do their urban counterparts (Guralnick, Kemele, Stamm, & Greving, 2003), exacerbating the effect of comorbid conditions. Mental health researchers have found that community-dwelling elderly persons with significant symptoms of depression use more general medical services and incur higher health care costs than elders who do not show such symptoms (Ganguli, Fox, Gilby, Seaberg, & Belle, 1995; Unutzer et al., 1997).

CBT is the most extensively researched psychological treatment for geriatric depression (Scogin, Welsh, Hanson, Stump, & Coates, 2005) and is one of several evidence-based treatments available for use with this population. One of the most frequently used protocols is that developed by Thompson, Gallagher-Thompson, and Dick (1995); this particular adaptation of CBT is listed in the National Registry of Evidence-Based Practices maintained by the Substance Abuse and Mental Health Services Administration. Further information on resources and training related to this protocol is available at http://oafc.standford.edu.

The use of this CBT protocol with depressed rural older adults requires consideration of several factors in addition to those mentioned with respect to older adults in general. First, many rural older adults will find twice-weekly or weekly sessions at a clinic-based office setting problematic due to mobility and transportation difficulties. Consideration of in-home or telehealth-administered sessions is suggested if such difficulties arise. Consistent contact with the therapist and application of the protocol with the use of these non-traditional means is desired above infrequent meetings in more traditional venues. A second common adaptation of CBT that occurs with depressed rural older adults is a greater emphasis on behavioral activation and a lesser emphasis on pure cognitive therapy techniques such as three and five column approaches. As illustrated in the Case Study that follows, some older adults find a focus on identification of and engagement in meaningful activities to be more consistent with their beliefs and values, as well as a better match for their educational and cognitive status. A final consideration in the use of CBT with depressed rural older adults, especially those residing in the southern parts of the United States, is the issue of religious and spiritual beliefs (Crowther, Parker, Larimore, Achenbaum, & Koenig, 2002; see Chapter 6 for a detailed discussion). Many rural older adults are deeply religious and may initially find the application of psychology to their suffering to be antithetic to their beliefs. This is most prototypically represented by clients who express that their lives are "... in God's hands." The sensitive and respectful interpretation of this belief into an action oriented approach to improvement can be a challenging task for therapists working with rural older adults. One approach taken with respect to the behavioral activation tasks of CBT is to encourage greater involvement in religious activities (e.g., prayer, listening to the Bible on tape) as a means to increase activation and begin the upper spiral to improved well-being.

CASE ILLUSTRATION

In this section, a rural older male is described who presents with depressive symptoms and family caregiving concerns. Specifically, the client is having difficulty accepting that he needs help from his children. The goal is to illustrate respect for rural elderly clients and demonstrate strategies of CBT for depression in a specific case, with attention to the unique experience of the rural client. This case illustrates some general principles in recognizing the real-life obstacles older rural clients face in understanding and utilizing mental health services along with challenges faced by rural family caregivers.

Presenting Problem and Client Description

Mr Smith was a 73-year-old African American widowed male who presented to a rural primary care clinic seeking help with back pain. Due to his symptoms of depression, the nurse practitioner referred Mr Smith to the clinical psychology graduate student psychotherapist working in the clinic. Mr Smith lived alone in rural Alabama with support from his two sons and one daughter who lived in the same county and checked on him regularly. Mr Smith had 7 years of formal education and had worked in the local manufacturing industry for most of his life. Mr Smith was raised with both his parents; he was the fifth of eight children. At the time of therapy both of his parents were deceased. He had contact with his two siblings that were still living, but did not see them as a major source of support. Mr Smith had a small, tenuous social support network, composed primarily of his children, grandchildren, and a few friends. He spent most of his time talking to his friends and playing with his grandchildren. He also attended church services on Sunday and stated that he had a strong religious belief system. Now, as a retiree, Mr Smith supported himself mostly through social security benefits and additional financial assistance from his children. Mr Smith had no previous psychotherapy experience and had very limited knowledge of psychological disorders or psychotherapy. Although prescribed an antidepressant by his primary care provider, the medication was conceptualized as a treatment for back pain, and he did not think of it as an antidepressant.

Case Formulation

During the first therapy session, Mr Smith was administered The Saint Louis Mental Status (SLUMS) as a brief cognitive screen. He scored 25 indicating that he was in the normal range and did not have cognitive impairment. He was also administered the 15-item Geriatric Depression Scale (GDS) to determine the severity of his depressive symptoms and scored a 9, indicative of moderate depression. During the initial intake interview, Mr Smith indicated that he began to feel sad about a year ago when he hurt his back and had to start using a walking cane. Mr Smith reported that his mobility became hampered and he began to require a lot more assistance from his children. He felt he was a burden to them and feared that he would only continue to become a greater burden to them as he got older. This situation was exacerbated by the death of a close friend not long after his back injury. He also reported having sleep problems and a loss of interest in all activities.

Course of Treatment

At the end of the initial one hour intake session, CBT was suggested to Mr Smith. Following the manual developed by Laidlaw, Thompson, Dick-Siskin, and Gallagher-Thompson (2003), the importance of targeting Mr Smith's maladaptive thoughts and how these related to his emotions and behaviors was explained in the context of the CBT model. He seemed unsure as to whether this would work but agreed to try it as a method of treatment. Mr Smith and the therapist agreed on five to eight sessions, some of which would be conducted over the phone due to Mr Smith's mobility and transportation issues.

During the second session, the therapist continued to gather more background information and build rapport with Mr Smith. This was an attempt to make Mr Smith feel at ease with the therapist before further treatment took place. At the beginning of session three, the issue of unhelpful thoughts was discussed. However, Mr Smith was unreceptive to the self-evaluative task of monitoring and evaluating his thoughts and behaviors for maladaptive content. Therefore, the therapist decided to move on to behavioral activation strategies with the possibility of returning to purely cognitive strategies during later sessions. Mr Smith did agree that finding and engaging in meaningful activities would help him feel better, but he was not enthusiastic about how this might be achieved considering his back pain.

In light of the fact that Mr Smith was a religious man, the therapist suggested that he start by listening to free copies of the "Bible on Tape." By starting with this activity, it would provide him with a basis of positive cognitive thoughts from which he could proceed. Mr Smith enthusiastically engaged in this activity and was even more pleased that the therapist had found a way to include his belief system. During further sessions, the therapist and Mr Smith worked collaboratively to identify other activities that Mr Smith could engage in that would provide him with pleasure. These included spending more time with his grandchildren. This had the double benefit of allowing him to play with his grandchildren, which he enjoyed, but also made him feel less of a burden to his children as he was also providing them with child care for short periods of the day.

Periodic administration of the GDS demonstrated that Mr Smith's depression scores decreased from 9 to 7 to 4 over the course of 8 treatments. The difference in his affect and behavior was also noticed by his children who had commented to him that he seemed happier. Over the course of treatment, the therapist and Mr Smith discussed ways in which his children could assist him with his care. This discussion included observation that Mr Smith and his children were entering a new phase in their relationship and addressed the reciprocal nature of the relationship. For example, Mr Smith could help with the children while they helped him. In week 6 the therapist attempted to revisit the possibility of teaching Mr Smith the self-evaluative task of monitoring and evaluating his thoughts and behaviors for maladaptive content, but Mr Smith was still unenthusiastic about this notion. Therefore, the therapist continued to focus on pleasure-inducing activities rather than belaboring the issue. During the final session, Mr Smith expressed some concern as to whether things would regress at the completion of the sessions but he was reassured when the therapist offered to check in with him for a follow-up 2 months after the end of treatment. During the follow-up, the therapist noted that Mr Smith had maintained his gains and had relatively low depression scores. He was also more accepting of the help offered from his children.

CLINICAL PRACTICES AND CONCLUSION

As evidenced in the case illustration, working with rural older adults presents some issues that are relatively unique to this population. First, limited access to specialized mental health providers is the rule rather than the exception. In Mr Smith's case, there was very little access to any mental health services, much less than those with a specialist in mental health and aging. Limited service access coupled with the stigma he felt toward such services—a view quite pervasive among rural older adults—created a circumstance in which his receipt of psychological treatment for his depressive symptoms was quite fragile. While some might view the fact that Mr Smith did not participate in all aspects of the therapeutic strategies suggested as an unsuccessful course of treatment, his engagement in many of the activities suggested was against the odds and no small feat; we believe he profited from his sessions. As illustrated by this case, access to services is one of the key barriers, if not the primary barrier, experienced by rural older adults. Providers must make efforts to reduce barriers by providing both traditional office-based services and nontraditional modalities such as home-delivered, telephone-administered, or self-administered treatments. An example of one of these alternatives in practice is the Veterans Affairs Home-Based Primary Care approach in which mental health services are provided by psychologists in the homes of mobility restricted veterans. Another issue illustrated by this case is the deviation from a strictly CBT protocol to a more eclectically-oriented, yet evidence-based, approach that included a greater focus on behavioral and reminiscence techniques. These techniques often work well with rural older adults evidencing lower literacy and diminishment of cognitive resources.

Rural older adults are unmistakably a vulnerable population. Finding ways to aid this cohort remains a challenge for those of us interested in mental health and aging. The rewards of such work are the knowledge that one has gone where few chose to tread.

REFERENCES

Administration on Aging. (2006). *A profile of older Americans: 2006*. Washington, DC: Administration on Aging (AoA), U.S. Department of Health and Human Services.

Administration on Aging. (2007). *A profile of older Americans: 2007*. Washington, DC: Administration on Aging (AoA), U.S. Department of Health and Human Services.

Administration on Aging. (2010). *A profile of older Americans: 2010*. Washington, DC: Administration on Aging (AoA), U.S. Department of Health and Human Services.

Bischoff, R. J., Hollist, C. S., Smith, C. W., & Flack, P. (2004). Addressing the mental health needs of the rural underserved: Findings from a multiple case study of a behavioral telehealth project. *Contemporary Family Therapy: An International Journal, 26*, 179–198.

Blazer, D. (2002). *Depression in late life* (3rd ed.). New York: Springer.

Buckwalter, K. C., Smith, M., Zevenbergen, P., & Russell, D. (1991). Mental health services of the rural elderly outreach program. *The Gerontologist, 31*, 408–412.

Butler, R. N., Lewis, M., & Sunderland, T. (1991). *Aging and mental health: Positive psychosocial and biomedical approaches.* New York: Macmillan.

Bruce, M., McAvay, G., Raue, P., Brown, E., Meyers, B., Keohane, D., ... Weber, C. (2002). Major depression in elderly home health care patients. *American Journal of Psychiatry, 159*, 1367–1374.

Chalifoux, Z., Neese, J., Buckwalter, K., Litwak, E., & Abraham, I. (1996). Mental health services for rural elderly: Innovative service strategies. *Community Mental Health Journal, 32*, 463–480.

Crowther, M, Scogin, F., & Norton, M (2010). Treating the aged in rural communities: The application of cognitive-behavioral therapy for depression. *Journal of Clinical Psychology: In Session, 66*(5), 1–11.

Crowther, M., & Austin, A. (2009). The cultural context on clinical work with aging caregivers. In S. Qualls, & S. Zarit (Series Eds.), *Clinical geropsychology* (pp. 45–60). Hoboken, NJ: Wiley Publishing.

Crowther, M., Parker, M., Larimore, W., Achenbaum, A., & Koenig, H. (2002). Rowe and Kahn's model of successful aging revisited: Spirituality the missing construct. *The Gerontologist, 42*(5), 613–620.

Culture and Caregiving. (1992, Winter-Spring). *Aging,* (363/364), 29–31.

Culverwell, A., & Martin, C. (2000). Psychotherapy with older people. In G. Corley (Ed.), *Older people and their needs: A multi-disciplinary perspective* (pp. 92–106). London, England: Whurr Publishers, Ltd.

Family Caregiver Alliance. (2006). *Caregiver assessment: Principles, guidelines and strategies for change.* Report from a National Consensus Development Conference (Vol. I). San Francisco: Author.

Fischer, L., Wei, F., Solberg, L., Rush, W., & Heinrich, R. (2003). Treatment of elderly and other adult patients for depression in primary care. *Journal of the American Geriatrics Society, 51*, 1554–1562.

Ganguli, M., Fox, A., Gilby, J., Seeberg, E., & Belle, S. (1995). Depressive symptoms and associated factors in a rural elderly population: The MoVIES project. *American Journal of Geriatric Psychiatry, 3*, 144–160.

Guralnick, S., Kemele, K., Stamm, B. H., & Greving, A. M. (2003). Rural geriatrics and gerontology. In B. H. Stamm (Ed.), *Rural behavioral health care: An interdisciplinary guide* (pp. 193–202). Washington, DC: American Psychological Association.

Ham, R. L., Goins, R. T., & Brown, D. K. (2003). *Best practices in service delivery to the rural elderly.* Retrieved from West Virginia University, Center on Aging: http://www.hsc.wvu.edu/coa/publications/best_practices/best-practices2003.asp

Johnson, K. M., & Beale, C. L. (2002). Non-metro recreation counties: Their identification and rapid growth. *Rural America, 17*(4), 12–19.

Laidlaw, K., Thompson, L. W., Dick-Siskin, L., & Gallagher-Thompson, D. (2003). *Cognitive behaviour therapy with older people.* New York: Wiley.

Lewinsohn, P. M., Rohde, P., Seeley, J. R., & Fischer, S. (1991). Aging and depression: Unique and shared effects. *Psychology and Aging, 6*, 247–260.

Mack, K., & Thompson, L. (2001). *Data profiles, family caregivers of older persons: Adult children.* Washington, DC: Georgetown University's The Center on an Aging Society.

McCulloch, J. B., & Lynch, M. S. (1993). Barriers to solutions: Service delivery and public policy in rural areas. *Journal of Applied Gerontology, 12*, 388–403.

National Advisory Committee on Rural Health and Human Services. (2008). *The 2008 Report to the secretary: Rural health and human services issues.* Washington, DC: Health Resources and Services Administration, U.S. Department of Health and Human Services.

National Alliance for Caregiving & AARP. (2004). *Caregiving in the US.* Washington, DC: Author.

The President's New Freedom Commission on Mental Health (2003). *Achieving the promise: Transforming mental health care in America.* Rockville, MD: Author.

Rokke, P. D., & Scogin, F. (1995). Depression treatment preferences in younger and older adults. *Journal of Clinical Geropsychology, 1*, 243–257.

Scogin, F. R., Welsh, D. L., Hanson, A. E., Stump, J., & Coates, A. (2005). Evidence-based psychotherapies for depression in older adults. *Clinical Psychology: Science and Practice, 12*(3), 222–237.

Thompson, L. W., Gallagher-Thompson, D., & Dick, L. P. (1995). *Cognitive-behavioral therapy for late life depression: A therapist manual.* Palo Alto, CA: Older Adult and Family Center, Veterans Affairs Palo Alto Health Care System.

U.S. Census Bureau. (2000). *Projections of the total resident population by 5-year age groups, race, and Hispanic origin with special age categories: Middle series, 1999–2000 and 2050–2070.* Retrieved from www.census.gov/population/projections/nation/summary/np-t4.a-g.txt

U.S. Census Bureau. (2010). *Population by Core Based Statistical Area (CBSA) and state: 2010. Statistical Abstract of the United States: 2012.* Retrieved from http://www.census.gov/compendia/statab/cats/population.html

U.S. Department of Health and Human Services. (2001). *Mental health: culture, race, and ethnicity–A supplement to mental health: A report of the Surgeon General.* Rockville, MD: U.S. Department of Health and Human Services, Substance Abuse and Mental Health Services Administration, Center for Mental Health Services.

Unutzer, J., Patrick, D. L., Simon, G., Grembowski, D., Walker, E., Rutter, C. et al. (1997). Depressive symptoms and the cost of health services in HMO patients aged 65 years and older: A 4-year prospective study. *Journal of the American Medical Association, 277*, 1618–1623.

Whitener, L. A., & McGranahan, D. A. (2003, February). Rural America: Opportunities and challenges. *Amber Waves.* Retrieved from http://www.ers.usda.gov/Amber Waves/Feb03/features/ruralamerica.htm

Zeiss, A. M., Lewinsohn, P. M., Rohde, P., & Seeley, J. R. (1996). Relationship of physical disease functional impairment to depression in older people. *Psychology and Aging, 1*, 1572–1582.

19

Providing Mental Health Services for Rural Veterans

JOHN PAUL JAMESON AND LISA CURTIN

INTRODUCTION

*R*ural residents have long been overrepresented in military service, and this is reflected in the large numbers of veterans found in rural areas today. According to the 2000 Census, rural counties feature higher concentrations of veterans than nonrural counties (Richardson & Waldrop, 2003). Evidence suggests that this trend will continue into the future; a recent report on U.S. military enlistees' demographic characteristics shows that the rural population accounts for almost 12% of recruits aged 18-24, but only 7.5% of that age group in the general population (Kane, 2006). Moreover, casualties in the conflicts in Iraq and Afghanistan are disproportionately high among soldiers from rural areas (O'Hare & Bishop, 2006), suggesting that soldiers returning to rural areas will have greater exposure to combat-related trauma than their nonrural counterparts on the whole. This may translate into greater need for mental health services among rural veterans over the coming decades, a factor that rural researchers, service providers, and policymakers should consider seriously and prepare for accordingly.

The following sections provide a brief overview of the available research, including descriptive characteristics of rural veterans and the barriers they face in accessing mental health care. Additionally, the chapter provides a clinically focused primer for providers with limited experience working with rural veterans, and concludes with recommendations for future research directions to increase our ability to serve those who have served our country.

CHARACTERISTICS OF RURAL VETERANS

Systematic investigations specific to rural veterans are sparse and often suffer from significant limitations. Available studies tend to describe retrospective data collected on health care provided in Veterans Health Administration (VA) settings prior to the year 2000, utilize inconsistent definitions of rurality, and frequently do not consider the patient as the unit of analysis (Weeks, Wallace, West, Heady, & Hawthorne, 2008). Given these limitations, it is no surprise that inconsistencies have emerged in the literature regarding differences between urban and rural veterans. A large cross-sectional survey of VA-enrolled veterans conducted in 1999 found somewhat lower rates of psychiatric disorders among rural veterans, with the exception of anxiety disorders other than posttraumatic stress disorder (PTSD), though quality of life ratings for physical and mental health were significantly lower among rural veterans (Wallace, Weeks, Wang, Lee, & Kazis, 2006). However, veterans in nonmetropolitan areas reported more days of poor mental health on average than veterans in metropolitan areas in the 2000 Behavioral Risk Factor Surveillance Survey (West & Weeks, 2006). Moreover, the West Virginia Returning Soldiers Study found a higher proportion of soldiers returning to rural West Virginia reported clinically significant symptoms of PTSD and depression (56%) than those returning to urban West Virginia (32%) or bases outside West Virginia (34%; Scotti, 2008).

Differences in physical health status and demographic factors relevant to mental health appear to exist between rural and nonrural veterans. A large-scale survey of VA enrollees indicated that rural veterans reported a higher prevalence of physical diagnoses compared to urban veterans (Weeks, Wallace, Wang, Lee, & Kazis, 2006). Although rural veterans are more likely to be older (Cully, Jameson, Phillips, Kunik, & Fortney, 2010), are less likely to be employed (Weeks et al., 2008; West & Weeks, 2006), and have lower income (Cully et al., 2010; West & Weeks, 2006) than their urban counterparts, Weeks et al. (2006) found that differences in self-reported health persisted after controlling for these demographic variables.

Despite a somewhat muddled picture of specific rural–urban differences, VA-based research that does not explicitly consider geographic status may still be cautiously applied to rural veterans, as they account for a substantial proportion of VA patients and are more likely to enroll in VA health care than nonrural veterans (West & Weeks, 2006). Based on this literature, it is clear that military veterans of past wars and current conflicts are particularly vulnerable to adjustment problems, posttraumatic stress disorder (PTSD), depression, and substance abuse regardless of whether they return to rural or urban areas (Fontana & Rosenheck, 2008; Petrakis, Rosenheck, & Desai, 2011; Wallace et al., 2006; Zatzick et al., 1997). Furthermore, many veterans meet criteria for more than one mental health diagnosis or dual diagnosis (comorbid mental illness and substance abuse; Petrakis et al., 2011; Zatzick et al., 1997). Risk of suicide increases in the context of mental illness as well (Mościcki, 2001), and a recent study found a higher rate of suicide among military veterans compared to the general population when adjusted for age and gender, although a causal link to military service has not been ascertained (McCarthy et al., 2009).

Vulnerabilities, including substance dependence, mental illness, and physical disabilities, increase the likelihood of homelessness among veterans. Although less than 1% of veterans are estimated to be homeless, veterans are overrepresented within the homeless population, and in the face of poverty, are more likely than non-veterans to become homeless (U.S. Department of Housing and Urban Development, U.S. Department of Veterans Affairs, 2009). Veterans make up approximately 8% of the total U.S. population, yet comprise approximately 12% of the homeless population. Homelessness among veterans is associated with being male, non-White, 31–50 years of age, and disabled. Though rural veterans are slightly underrepresented among the total population of homeless veterans, approximately 30% of homeless veterans are located in rural and suburban areas. Additionally, veterans tend to be most overrepresented among the total homeless population in more rural states in the South and West.

Much of the recent research has focused on veterans of Operation Iraqi Freedom (OIF) and Operation Enduring Freedom (OEF), and these studies indicate significant mental health needs among these younger veterans. Hoge, Auchterlonie, and Milliken (2006) found that 19.1% of veterans serving in Iraq, 11.3% of those serving in Afghanistan, and 8.5% of those serving elsewhere screened positively for a mental health problem postdeployment, and nearly 1% reported suicidal ideation. Of particular concern, postdeployment screenings appear to underestimate mental health needs; Milliken, Auchterlonie, and Hoge (2007) found an increase in reported mental health concerns and referrals during 3–6 month postdeployment reassessments.

Those numbers increase when examining OEF and OIF veterans in the context of VA health care. Studies indicate that approximately one-third of OEF and OIF veterans receiving VA care have a mental health or other psychosocial diagnosis (e.g., relational problem; Cohen et al., 2010; Seal et al., 2009; Seal, Bertenthal, Miner, Sen, & Marmar, 2007). For example, Seal et al. (2009) found that 21.8% of 289,328 veterans entering VA health care between 2002 and 2008 suffered from PTSD and 17.4% suffered from depression, with women veterans more likely to experience depression and men more likely to experience substance abuse. Furthermore, these veterans often present with multiple diagnoses; a study of VA-enrolled OEF and OIF veterans found that over 50% of those with a mental health diagnosis had two or more distinct disorders (Seal et al., 2007). Veterans of recent conflicts appear to experience the same psychological afflictions as veterans of past wars, most notably Vietnam (e.g., Zatzick et al., 1997), although there is some indication of lower substance abuse rates among OIF and OEF veterans (Fontana & Rosenheck, 2008). Moreover, consistent with findings among Vietnam veterans (Zatzick et al., 1997), greater exposure to combat in OIF and OEF veterans related to increased risk of PTSD (Hoge et al., 2004).

Unlike past conflicts, a significant proportion of veterans returning from OIF/OEF suffer from various levels of traumatic brain injury (TBI; Hoge et al., 2008), likely related to the use of Kevlar helmets and body armor that improve overall survival rates, as well as frequent exposure to improvised explosive devices (Long et al., 2009; Owens et al., 2008). A study of OIF combat troops estimated that nearly 15% of soldiers suffered at least one TBI during service (Hoge et al., 2008). Complicating the clinical presentation and intervention needs, TBI frequently co-occurs with PTSD, depression, and generalized anxiety disorder, and may result in cognitive dysfunction such as memory and attention impairment, difficulty with decision making, and impairment in fine motor skills (Kennedy et al., 2007). Additionally, the similarities in the symptom profiles between PTSD and persistent postconcussive symptoms (e.g., irritability, memory difficulties) can make differential diagnosis difficult (Bryant, 2001).

As more women serve in the military, rates of Military Sexual Trauma (MST) have increased. MST is defined as "sexual assault or repeated, unsolicited, threatening acts of sexual harassment that occurs during military service" (Rowe, Gradus, Pineles, Batten, & Davison, 2009; p. 388). Although men experience MST, women veterans are far more likely to report MST (Haskell et al., 2010). A large-scale exploration of over 125,000 OEF/OIF veterans seeking VA health care after service between 2001 and 2007 found 15.1% of women and 0.7% of men screened positively for MST (Kimerling et al., 2010). Similarly, a smaller study of OEF/OIF veterans seeking services between 2001 and 2007 in a single VA setting found that 14% of women and 1% of men positively screened for MST (Haskell et al., 2010). Not surprisingly, Kimerling et al. (2010) found that MST was associated with a higher likelihood of PTSD, other anxiety disorders, depression, and substance use disorders.

The mental health needs of veterans of National Guard and Reserve units who served in OEF and OIF also are particularly relevant to rural mental health care providers, as rural areas are known for high rates of service in the National Guard and Reserve units. National Guard members appear more likely than active duty returning soldiers to report mental health issues, particularly symptoms of PTSD and depression (Scotti, 2008; Milliken et al., 2007). Increased risk of mental health issues may relate to limited training, cohesion, and base-support, leaving soldiers underprepared for deployment relative to full-time, active duty military. In addition, those serving in the Reserves have less access to postdeployment military health care compared to those in active service, and the extent and duration of VA benefits are lower for Guard veterans (Milliken et al., 2007). However, the Department of Defense does not systematically track the geographic status of National Guard members, and research has yet to establish the extent to which rural National Guard and Reserve veterans represent a particularly vulnerable subgroup.

BARRIERS TO CARE FOR RURAL VETERANS

Military veterans living in rural areas experience the same barriers to care as other rural residents including decreased service availability, accessibility, and acceptability (Mohatt, Bradley, Adams, & Morris, 2005). Despite a greater likelihood to enroll in VA care (West & Weeks, 2006), studies indicate that rural veterans utilize VA health services, most notably specialty services, less often than their urban counterparts (Cully et al., 2008, 2010; Weeks, Bott, Lamkin, & Wright, 2005; Weeks et al., 2006). Decreased use of VA services likely relates to distance, as lack of transportation is frequently noted as a problem by both veterans and their family members (Weeks et al., 2008). In addition to transportation problems, an interview-based study of rural veterans utilizing VA Community-Based Outpatient Clinics found that cost and provider availability may also limit use of services (Jameson, Teal, & Blevins, 2011). Similarly, West and Weeks (2006) found that nonmetropolitan veterans between 18 and 44 years of age were less likely to access health care in the past year because of cost relative to age-matched metropolitan veterans.

Specific to access to mental health services, Cully et al. (2008) demonstrated a negative relationship between distance to a VA facility and receipt of psychotherapy, and found an average lag of 57 days between mental health diagnosis and start of psychotherapy in their sample of both rural and urban veterans. Compared to urban veterans, rural veterans with a new diagnosis of anxiety, depression, or PTSD seeking VA services were significantly less likely to have received psychotherapy during the 12 months after their initial diagnosis. This difference between urban and rural veterans persisted even after controlling for other variables related to psychotherapy use (younger age, female gender, medical illness, and distance to VA facility), and rural veterans treated with psychotherapy received fewer sessions of psychotherapy than urban veterans (Cully et al., 2010). Similarly, rural residents are more likely to use medication rather than psychotherapy for depression, and distance from the provider is associated with a reduced likelihood of receiving guideline concordant pharmacotherapy (Fortney, Harmon, Xu, & Dong, 2010; Fortney, Rost, Zhang, & Warren, 1999).

Although distance to services appears to be an important factor, it does not fully account for differences between rural and urban veterans' use of psychotherapy. Cully et al. (2010) suggest that acceptability of mental health services and stigma associated with mental illness in rural areas likely contribute to decreased receipt of psychotherapy among veterans. Rural communities typically value self-reliance and independence (Slama, 2004), which may inflate concerns about stigma related to help-seeking, especially for mental health problems which are not frequently discussed or acknowledged (Jameson et al., 2011).

Although rural–urban comparisons were not made, Hoge et al. (2004) found significant concerns related to help seeking for mental health problems in their sample of Army soldiers and Marines. Among those who screened positive for a mental illness, a minority reported seeking help from a mental health professional (low of 13% among Army soldiers prior to deployment to a high of 27% among Army soldiers after deployment to Iraq), despite 78% to 86% acknowledging a problem and 38% to 45% reporting an interest in receiving help. A majority of the participants in this study reported significant stigma-related concerns to seeking help, most notably being seen as weak, having a potentially negative impact on working relationships with leaders and peers, experiencing difficulty finding time to seek treatment, and potentially inflicting career harm. Nearly identical results were found among a sample of National Guard members and their significant others (Gorman, Blow, Ames, & Reed, 2011). Interestingly, these barriers were noted by those who screened positive for a mental illness nearly two times more frequently than those who screened negative (Gorman et al., 2011; Hoge et al., 2004).

Similarly, Ouimette et al. (2011) found that veterans diagnosed with PTSD who had not received treatment in the past 2 years reported stigma-related concerns as the most influential barrier (e.g., discomfort, social and career-related consequences) to help-seeking. Perceptions of the quality of VA care and logistical barriers such as distance were less of a concern. However, it is not known whether perceptions of stigma are more pronounced among rural veterans, though concerns regarding stigma and lack of privacy emerged as themes in interviews of rural veterans (Jameson et al., 2011) and stigma regarding mental health care is prevalent in the general rural population (see Chapter 4).

Further, the acceptability of VA care may differ among groups of veterans. Younger and White female veterans reported relatively greater concern with not fitting into the VA system, and non-White male veterans reported the greatest difficulty accessing services (e.g., transportation, not fitting in; Ouimette et al., 2011). Further, in one study, women veterans with a positive history of MST reported greater use of VA services, but relatively less satisfaction compared to women veterans without MST experiences (Kelly et al., 2008). The above findings suggest VA and other service providers need to adapt to the changing military population and consider individual differences.

WORKING WITH RURAL VETERANS: PRACTICE ISSUES

Working with rural veterans presents unique challenges to service providers, particularly those without a military background or experience in organizations that serve veteran populations (e.g., VA, Disabled American Veterans). A basic understanding of military structure, terminology, and process are often helpful in communicating with veterans and understanding their experiences. It should be noted that ranks, awards, duties, and training philosophies differ greatly between each branch of the armed forces. The complexity of organization and duties of each branch of the military prevents an exhaustive discussion of this topic. However, several online resources are available that are useful in gaining an understanding of military service.

For successful work with veterans, attention must be paid to military culture. As noted by Reger, Etherage, Reger, and Gahm (2008) military personnel (and by extension, veterans) share all of the features of a distinct cultural group, including social and behavioral norms, a belief system, rituals, a dress code, and language. Furthermore, an individual's identification with military culture may interact with one's identification with other cultural groups (e.g., Hispanic veterans; Cañive, Castillo, & Tuason, 2001). Moreover, the principles and code of conduct provided by the American Psychological Association (2002) and other professional organizations require that training, experience, supervision, or consultation be obtained when an understanding of cultural factors is imperative for the delivery of effective services. On this basis, several have argued that cultural competence is required to work effectively with military personnel and veterans (Bryan & Morrow, 2011; Hobbs, 2008; Reger et al., 2008). However, given the shortage of providers in rural areas, clinicians may often find themselves needing to learn quickly so that necessary services are not denied.

Central to the overarching military culture is the notion of the "warrior culture." Warrior culture has been described as ". . . one that values strength, resilience, courage, and personal sacrifice" (Bryan & Morrow, 2011, p. 17). Implied within these core values is the sense that one should not reveal personal weakness and the belief that physical or emotional pain is the individual's to bear. Additionally, warrior culture includes strong bonds with and responsibility to other members of the military unit. As such, seeking outside help may be viewed by the individual as a failure to live up to one's responsibilities to the unit and viewed with suspicion by other unit members. These cultural features are inherently opposed to the conceptualization of mental health issues in formal care systems (Bryan & Morrow, 2011). Though features of the warrior culture may apply most directly to active duty soldiers, such beliefs are common (to varying degrees) among veterans as well. Identification with the warrior culture may be most apparent in recently discharged veterans and less apparent in veterans who have been out of the military for longer periods of time. However, this is a generalization that does not apply to all cases, and many veterans may identify strongly with the warrior culture decades after discharge. Further, identification with warrior culture may be particularly salient when working with veterans with problems related to their service (e.g., combat-related PTSD), as such issues may activate the "warrior schema."

Though the warrior culture is likely common to veterans of all conflict eras, the experiences of veterans vary widely depending on their period of service. For example, each of the major conflicts the United States has been involved in since World War II has resulted in "signature injuries." In the Korean conflict, frostbite was rampant among combat troops; the war in

Vietnam saw a variety of physical and cognitive injuries in soldiers exposed to the herbicide Agent Orange (dioxin); during the Persian Gulf conflict, many soldiers returned with Gulf War Syndrome, a multisymptom condition that continues to be difficult to define, understand, and treat; and the recent conflicts in Iraq and Afghanistan have resulted in high rates of traumatic brain injury (TBI) among servicemen and servicewomen. Further, veterans from each of these conflicts returned to remarkably different economic and sociocultural environments at home (including access to mental health services through the VA and other care organizations), and the experiences of veterans of the smaller police actions over the past several decades (e.g., Grenada, Lebanon, and Panama in the 1980s; Somalia and Bosnia in the 1990s) are likely different from those of larger conflicts. The disparate experiences of veterans from different conflict eras can impact veterans' mental health needs and how they experience and perceive the formal treatment system.

The influence of warrior culture that is often most palpable to civilian providers working with veterans is a reluctance to enter treatment and difficulty building rapport early in treatment. A significant proportion of rural veterans may only seek treatment when mental health issues result in interpersonal conflict with family members or spouses, and may feel coerced into treatment (Jameson et al., 2011). Additionally, it is not uncommon for veterans to have reservations about working with civilian clinicians, believing that these providers will not understand their past and current experiences. veterans may also fear that clinicians will judge them for their behavior in combat situations, and therefore withhold important details regarding past experiences. These issues can appear at any time and should be monitored throughout the course of treatment, but oftentimes they become apparent immediately.

Based upon clinical experience, several recommendations are offered for engaging veterans in treatment. First, it is important to recognize and discuss any apprehension related to the clinician's background early in treatment. It is often helpful to acknowledge the differences in experiences between the veteran and the clinician and invite the veteran to teach the clinician about military culture and experiences. Asking the veteran about one's period of service, stations, Military Occupational Specialty (MOS), conditions of discharge, and other information pertinent to military service during the course of the initial interview can present a natural opportunity to have such a conversation. Simultaneously, it can be helpful to reassure the veteran that the clinician has adequate training and experience to diagnose and treat mental health issues similar (but not exactly the same) to those facing the veteran. This strategy presents the veteran the opportunity to receive needed help while building a reciprocal treatment relationship.

Second, clinicians working with veterans who reluctantly seek treatment may wish to establish concrete, reachable goals early in treatment to orient the veteran to the treatment process and help create positive expectations for treatment continuation. These goals vary from veteran to veteran, but often include improving marital or familial relationships, engaging in social activities, improving sleep, or managing anger more effectively. Establishing successes early in treatment may encourage the veteran to ultimately work on more complex issues (if longer-term treatment is available to the veteran). Strategies based on problem-solving therapy or solution-focused therapy may be particularly helpful in reaching goals early in the treatment process.

Third, providers should remain aware of the power balance in the therapeutic relationship. Many veterans, especially younger veterans and those who identify strongly with military culture, may model their relationship with their provider after one between a commanding officer and a subordinate. veterans operating under this assumption often behave very formally with their providers (e.g., standing when the provider stands, referring to the provider as sir or ma'am). This may lead to ineffective therapeutic relationships in which veterans acquiesce to the suggestions of the provider without revealing their personal needs or treatment goals. Oftentimes, veterans adhere to treatment suggestions early on, but terminate suddenly and unexpectedly when their undisclosed treatment desires and objectives do not get met. Therefore, it is suggested that providers encourage veterans to take the lead in setting the treatment agenda and provide feedback at the end of treatment sessions, especially early in treatment. These techniques are consistent with the cognitive therapy model outlined by Beck, Rush, Shaw, and Emery (1979). Additionally, creation of a less formal tone in session may counter perceptions of a power differential (e.g., suggesting the veteran refer to the provider by his or her first name, starting sessions with a brief informal conversation).

As mentioned at the beginning of this chapter, there is reason to believe that a significant number of rural veterans will use mental health services in the coming decades. We encourage providers to anticipate this influx and seek additional training to accommodate the needs of this population. Providers may consider seeking additional training in assessment and evidence-based treatments for PTSD. Three exposure-based therapies, cognitive processing therapy (CPT), eye movement desensitization and reprocessing (EMDR), and prolonged exposure (PE), have research bases demonstrating effectiveness in veteran populations (see Sharpless & Barber, 2011, for a review). Additionally, substance use disorders are often comorbid with PTSD in the veteran population. A CBT-based program called Seeking Safety is promising for the treatment of comorbid substance use disorders and PTSD. However, research to date on the effectiveness in veteran populations is encouraging but limited (e.g., Norman, Wilkins, Tapert, Lang, & Najavits, 2010).

An additional concern relevant to working with OEF and OIF veterans is the high prevalence of TBI. Limited research has demonstrated that CBT-based techniques are effective with individuals with postconcussive symptoms and depression or PTSD (Fann, Hart, & Schomer, 2009; Soo & Tate, 2007). However, it is difficult to make generalizations from such a small research base. Given the cognitive sequelae associated with TBI, more comprehensive approaches may be necessary to successfully treat individuals with TBI and psychiatric comorbidities (e.g., cognitive rehabilitation; Cicerone et al., 2000). At the least, providers should vigilantly assess for the presence of cognitive symptoms that may suggest TBI in veterans. Several self-report measures are available free of charge online to assist in TBI screenings. Positive screens may warrant referral to specialty providers. Given the difficulties rural veterans experience accessing specialty services, it is suggested that the referring practitioner facilitate the referral and follow-up with the veteran.

Further, providers should remain cognizant of issues that predominantly impact female veterans. Assessing the stability of romantic relationships, an important issue in treating all veterans, may be critical among female veterans. Marital discord is particularly common, with divorce rates two to three times higher for female service members than male service members (Karney & Crown, 2007). Additionally, practitioners should assess for MST history, especially when working with female veterans. The routinely used two-question VA MST Screen may be useful: "When you were in the military, did you ever receive uninvited or unwanted sexual attention?" and "When you were in the military did anyone ever use force or the threat of force to have sex against your will?" (Rowe et al., 2009, p. 391).

FUTURE DIRECTIONS FOR RESEARCH AND PRACTICE

There is much work to be done by both researchers and practitioners in the coming years to effectively address the mental health needs of rural veterans. Below, several areas of inquiry are demarcated that deserve particular attention. First, a more complete picture is needed of the characteristics of rural veterans. The vast majority of the extant research on rural veterans has been conducted by VA. Though much of this research is informative, utilizes large national samples, and is of the highest quality, studies focusing on rural veterans who have not enrolled in the VA system are scarce (e.g., West & Weeks, 2006). It is possible that systematic differences exist between VA-enrolled rural veterans and rural veterans not enrolled in VA in terms of demographics, health status, diagnoses, access to care, or service needs. Further, there is little understanding of why rural veterans enroll or do not enroll in VA. Barriers to access, lack of information regarding available benefits or services, or personal choice could influence enrollment, and may differ for rural and urban veterans. Such information could be used to combat barriers to VA access or design alternative service systems for veterans who are not VA-enrolled.

Second, research on the specific social, cultural, and community aspects of rural areas on veterans' willingness to seek help and general well-being is warranted. Preliminary research suggests that community factors such as the density of social relationships within the community, degree of interconnected-ness with the community, and community communication styles can influence decisions to seek treatment, and community members often serve as gate-keepers to care for veterans (Jameson et al., 2011). However, this line of inquiry is in its infancy, and more work needs to be done to understand the role of community in improving care access, creating acceptable and culturally sensitive treatments, and promoting quality of life of rural veterans.

Third, supporting rural service providers is critical if rural veterans are to have access to the best available treatments. For example, there are several effective therapies for the treatment of PTSD, but these treatments appear to be underutilized by community providers (Becker, Zayfert, & Anderson, 2004; Jameson, Chambless, & Blank, 2009). However, there is reason for opti-mism that cutting-edge treatments can be widely disseminated to rural service systems if an effective support infrastructure is developed. Becker et al. (2004) report that lack of adequate training was the most commonly cited barrier to the use of PE for PTSD among clinical psychologists. Additionally, rural provi-ders reported generally positive attitudes toward adopting evidence-based approaches and did not differ significantly from those of nonrural providers (Jameson et al., 2009). Taken together, these studies suggest that limited disse-mination of evidence-based approaches may result from a clinicians' lack of access to training, not resistance to the use of these treatments. Providing clinicians with opportunities to receive training and support for the use of evidence-based treatments may bolster the ability of existing service systems to treat the rural veteran population. However, the relative isolation and paucity of resources available to these systems will require innovation to create such an infrastructure.

Fourth, establishing and strengthening veteran-focused prevention pro-grams and informal systems of care that are functional in rural areas is critical to bolstering the effectiveness of formal care systems. The U.S. Army recently initiated the Comprehensive Soldier Fitness program, a universal prevention program to foster resilience and prevent negative outcomes during and after service among active duty members of the U.S. Army (Cornum, Matthews, & Seligman, 2011). However, the ultimate effectiveness of this program on future veterans is not yet known. Additionally, postdeployment prevention pro-grams have emerged outside of the formal mental health care system and may be particularly relevant to addressing the mental health needs of rural veterans. The Life Guard program is a 2-hour workshop based on principles of accep-tance and commitment therapy, in which National Guard members returning from deployment in Iraq or Afghanistan learn awareness, acceptance, and value-based living skills to promote resiliency and ease the transition back to civilian life (Blevins, Roca, & Spencer, 2011). Early research suggests that such programs effectively reduce postdeployment psychiatric symptoms. Empowering rural veterans to take charge of their mental health care, provide input on the delivery of services, and offer support to fellow brothers and sisters in arms will be an important component of any comprehensive effort to improve treatment. Emerging research suggests that peer education and support programs can improve veterans' sense of empowerment and well-being (Resnick & Rosenheck, 2008), and more research on the value of peer services is warranted. Adapting and disseminating such programs to the needs of rural communities and investigating their utility will be important in establishing comprehensive care systems for rural veterans.

Despite the development of prevention programs designed to address veterans' mental health, the reliable relationship between degree of combat exposure and development of PTSD as well as high rates of comorbidity between PTSD and other psychiatric conditions suggests that veterans will need tailored mental health services well into the future. Though the creation of an accessible, culturally sensitive, and high-quality care system for rural veterans presents an enormous challenge, mental health service providers can make small individual contributions to help serve veterans in need immediately. Organizations such as Give an Hour provide support and coordination for licensed clinicians willing to volunteer services to veterans locally. We encourage interested clinicians to investigate these opportunities, seek appropriate training opportunities, and support efforts to make quality services more accessible for all veterans including vulnerable rural veterans with less access to established sources of care.

REFERENCES

American Psychological Association. (2002). Ethical principles of psychologists and code of conduct. *American Psychologist, 57,* 1060–1073.

Beck, A. T., Rush, A. J., Shaw, B. F., & Emery, G. (1979). *Cognitive therapy of depression.* New York, NY: Guilford Press.

Becker, C. B., Zayfert, C., & Anderson, E. (2004). A survey of psychologists' attitudes towards and utilization of exposure therapy for PTSD. *Behaviour Research and Therapy, 42,* 277–292.

Blevins, D., Roca, J. V., & Spencer, T. (2011). Life Guard: Evaluation of an ACT-based workshop to facilitate reintegration of OIF/OEF Veterans. *Professional Psychology: Research and Practice, 42,* 32–39.

Bryan, C. J., & Morrow, C. E. (2011). Circumventing mental health stigma by embracing the warrior culture: Lessons learned from the Defender's Edge program. *Professional Psychology: Research and Practice, 42,* 16–23.

Bryant, R. A. (2001). Posttraumatic stress disorder and traumatic brain injury: Can they coexist? *Clinical Psychology Review, 21,* 931–948.

Cañive, J. M., Castillo, D. T., & Tuason, V. B. (2001). The Hispanic veteran. In W. S. Tseng, & J. Streltzer (Eds.), *Culture and psychotherapy: A guide to clinical practice* (pp. 157–172). Washington, DC: American Psychiatric Press.

Cicerone, K. D., Dahlberg, C., Kalmar, K., Langenbahn, D. M., Malec, J. F., Bergquist, T. F. et al. (2000). Evidence-based cognitive rehabilitation: Recommendations for clinical practice. *Archives of Physical Medicine and Rehabilitation, 81,* 1596–1615.

Cohen, B. E., Gima, K., Bertenthal, D., Kim, S., Marmar, C. R., & Seal, K. H. (2010). Mental health diagnoses and utilization of VA non-mental health medical services among returning Iraq and Afghanistan veterans. *Journal of General Internal Medicine, 25*, 18-24.

Cornum, R., Matthews, M. D., & Seligman, M. E. P. (2011). Comprehensive Soldier Fitness: Building resilience in a challenging institutional context. *American Psychologist, 66*, 4-9.

Cully, J. A., Jameson, J. P., Phillips, L. L., Kunik, M. E., & Fortney, J. C. (2010). Use of psychotherapy by rural and urban veterans. *The Journal of Rural Health, 26*, 225-233.

Cully, J. A., Tolpin, L., Henderson, L., Jimenez, D., Kunik, M. E., & Petersen, L A. (2008). Psychotherapy in the Veterans Health Administration: Missed opportunities? *Psychological Services, 5*, 320-331.

Fann, J. R., Hart, T., & Schomer, K. G. (2009). Treatment for depression after traumatic brain injury: A systematic review. *Journal of Neurotrauma, 26*, 2383-2402.

Fontana, A., & Rosenheck, R. (2008). Treatment-seeking veterans of Iraq and Afghanistan: Comparison with veterans of previous wars. *Journal of Nervous & Mental Disease, 196*, 513-521.

Fortney, J. C., Harmon, J. S., Xu, S., & Dong, F. (2010). The association between rural residence and the use, type and quality of depression care. *Journal of Rural Health, 26*, 205-213.

Fortney, J., Rost, K., Zhang, M., & Warren, J. (1999). The impact of geographic accessibility on the intensity and quality of depression treatment. *Medical Care, 37*, 884-893.

Gorman, L. A., Blow, A. J., Ames, B. D., & Reed, P. L. (2011). National Guard families after combat: Mental health, use of mental health services, and perceived treatment barriers. *Psychiatric Services, 62*, 28-34.

Haskell, S. G., Gordon, K. S., Mattocks, K., Duggal, M., Erdos, J., Justice, A., . . . Brandt, C. A. (2010). Gender differences in rates of depression, PTSD, pain, obesity, and military sexual trauma among Connecticut war veterans of Iraq and Afghanistan. *Journal of Women's Health, 19*, 267-271.

Hobbs, K. (2008). Reflections on the culture of veterans. *AAHON Journal, 56*, 337-341. Retrieved from http://www.ncbi.nlm.nih.gov/pubmed/18717299

Hoge, C. W., Auchterlonie, J. L., & Milliken, C. S. (2006). Mental health problems, use of mental health service, and attrition from military service after returning from deployment to Iraq or Afghanistan. *JAMA, 295*, 1023-1032.

Hoge, C. W., Castro, C. A., Messer, S. C., McGurk, D., Cotting, D. I., & Koffman, R. L. (2004). Combat duty in Iraq and Afghanistan, mental health problems, and barriers to care. *New England Journal of Medicine, 351*, 13-22.

Hoge, C. W., McGurk, D., Thomas, J. L., Cox, A. L., Engel, C. C., & Castro, C. A. (2008). Mild traumatic brain injury in U.S. soldiers returning from Iraq. *New England Journal of Medicine, 358*, 453-463.

Jameson, J. P., Chambless, D. L., & Blank, M. B. (2009). Empirically supported treatments in rural community mental health centers: A preliminary report on current utilization and attitudes toward adoption. *Community Mental Health Journal, 45*, 463-467.

Jameson, J. P., Teal, C. R., & Blevins, D. (2011, June). *The influence of community factors on perceived stigma and service utilization in rural veterans.* Paper presented at the annual convention of the National Association for Rural Mental Health, Dubuque, IA.

Kane, T. (2006). *Who are the recruits? The demographic characteristics of U.S. Military enlistment* (Report No. CDA06-09). Washington, DC: The Heritage Foundation.

Karney, B. R., & Crown, J. S. (2007). *Families under stress: An assessment of data, theory, and research on marriage and divorce in the military* (RAND Report MG599). Retrieved from the RAND Corporation website: http://www.rand.org/pubs/monographs/MG599

Kelly, M. M., Vogt, D. S., Scheideerer, E. M., Ouimette, P., Daley, J., & Wolfe, J. (2008). Effects of military trauma exposure on women veterans' use and perceptions of Veterans Health Administration care. *Journal of General Internal Medicine, 23,* 741–747.

Kennedy, J. E., Jaffee, M. S., Leskin, G. A., Stokes, J. W., Leal, F. O., & Fitzpatrick, P. J. (2007). Posttraumatic stress disorder and posttraumatic stress disorder-like symptoms in mild traumatic brain injury. *Journal of Rehabilitation Research & Development, 44,* 895–920.

Kimerling, R., Street, A. E., Pavao, J., Smith, M. W., Cronkite, R. C., Holmes, T. H. et al. (2010). Military sexual trauma among Veterans Health Administration patients returning from Afghanistan and Iraq. *American Journal of Public Health, 100,* 1409–1412.

Long, J. B., Bentley, T. L., Wessner, K. A., Cerone, C., Sweeney, S., & Bauman, R. A. (2009). Blast overpressure in rats: Recreating a battlefield injury in the laboratory. *Journal of Neurotrauma, 26,* 827–840.

McCarthy, J. F., Valenstein, M., Kim, H. M., Ilgen, M., Zivin, K., & Blow, F. C. (2009). Suicide mortality among patients receiving care in the Veterans Health Administration health system. *American Journal of Epidemiology, 169,* 1033–1038.

Milliken, C. S., Auchterlonie, J. L., & Hoge, C. W. (2007). Longitudinal assessment of mental health problems among active and reserve component soldiers returning from the Iraq war. *JAMA, 298,* 2141–2148.

Mohatt, D. F., Bradley, M. M., Adams, S. J., & Morris, C. D. (2005). *Mental health and rural America: 1994–2005.* Washington, DC: U.S. Department of Health and Human Services, Health Resources and Services Administration, Office of Rural Health Policy.

Mościcki, E. K. (2001). Epidemiology of completed and attempted suicide: Toward a framework for prevention. *Clinical Neuroscience Research, 1,* 310–323.

Norman, S. B., Wilkins, K. C., Tapert, S. F., Lang, A. J., & Najavits, L. M. (2010). A pilot study of seeking safety therapy with OEF/OIF veterans. *Journal of Psychoactive Drugs, 42,* 83–87.

O'Hare, W., & Bishop, B. (2006). *U.S. rural soldiers account for a disproportionately high share of casualties in Iraq and Afghanistan* (Fact Sheet No. 3). Retrieved from the Carsey Institute, University of New Hampshire website: http://www.carseyinstitute.unh.edu/publications/FS_ruralsoldiers_06.pdf

Ouimette, P., Vogt, D., Wade, M., Tirone, V., Greenbaum, M. A., Kimerling, R.,...Rosen, C. S. (2011). Perceived barriers to care among Veterans Health Administration patients with posttraumatic stress disorder. *Psychological Services, 8,* 212–223.

Owens, B. D., Kragh, J. F., Wenke, J. C., Macaitis, J., Wade, C. E., & Holcomb, J. B. (2008). Combat wounds in Operation Iraqi Freedom and Operation Enduring Freedom. *Journal of Trauma, 64*, 295–299.

Petrakis, I. L., Rosenheck, R., & Desai, R. (2011). Substance use comorbidity among veterans with posttraumatic stress disorder and other psychiatric illness. *The American Journal on Addictions, 20*, 185–189.

Reger, M. A., Etherage, J. R., Reger, G. M., & Gahm, G. A. (2008). Civilian psychologists in an Army culture: The ethical challenge of cultural competence. *Military Psychology, 20*, 21–35.

Resnick, S. G., & Rosenheck, R. A. (2008). Integrating peer-provided services: A quasi-experimental study of recovery orientation, confidence, and empowerment. *Psychiatric Services, 59*, 1307–1314.

Richardson, C., & Waldrop, J. (2003). *veterans: 2000* (Report No. C2KBR-22). Retrieved from United States Census Bureau website: http://www.census.gov/prod/2003pubs/c2kbr-22.pdf

Rowe, E. L., Gradus, J. L., Pineles, S. L., Batten, S. V., & Davison, E. H. (2009). Military sexual trauma in treatment-seeking women. *Military Psychology, 21*, 387–395.

Scotti, J. (2008, June). *Survey of West Virginia veterans of recent conflicts*. Paper presented at the CARE-NET Governor's Conference on West Virginia Military Members and their Families, Charleston, WV.

Seal, K. H., Bertenthal, D., Miner, C. R., Sen, S., & Marmar, C. (2007). Bringing the war back home: Mental health disorders among 103,788 US veterans returning from Iraq and Afghanistan seen at Department of Veterans Affairs facilities. *Archives of Internal Medicine, 167*, 476–482.

Seal, K. H., Metzler, T. J., Gima, K. S., Bertenthal, D., Maguen, S., & Marmar, C. R. (2009). Trends and risk factors for mental health diagnoses among Iraq and Afghanistan veterans using Department of Veterans Affairs health care, 2002–2008. *American Journal of Public Health, 99*, 1651–1658.

Sharpless, B. A., & Barber, J. P. (2011). A clinician's guide to PTSD treatments for returning veterans. *Professional Psychology: Research and Practice, 42*, 8–15.

Slama, K. (2004, January). Rural culture is a diversity issue. *Minnesota Psychologist, 53*(1), 9–12.

Soo, C., & Tate, R. (2007). Psychological treatment for anxiety in people with TBI. *Cochrane Database of Systematic Reviews, 3*, CD005239.

U.S. Department of Housing and Urban Development, U.S. Department of Veterans Affairs. (2009). *Veteran Homelessness: A Supplemental Report to the 2009 Annual Homeless Assessment Report to Congress*. Retrieved from http://www.hudhre.info/documents/2009AHARVeteransReport.pdf

U.S. Department of Veterans Affairs. (2009). *About rural veterans*. Retrieved from www.ruralhealth.va.gov/page.cfm?pg=2

Wallace, A. E., Weeks, W. B., Wang, S., Lee, A., & Kazis, L. E. (2006). Rural and urban disparities in health-related quality of life among veterans with psychiatric disorders. *Psychiatric Services, 57*, 851–856.

Weeks, W. B., Bott, D. M., Lamkin, R. P., & Wright, S. M. (2005). Veterans health administration and Medicare outpatient health care utilization by older rural and urban New England veterans. *The Journal of Rural Health, 21*, 167–171.

Weeks, W. B., Wallace, A. E., Wang, S., Lee, A., & Kazis, L. E. (2006). Rural-urban disparities in health-related quality of life within disease categories of veterans. *The Journal of Rural Health, 22*, 204–211.

Weeks, W. B., Wallace, A. E., West, A. N., Heady, H. R., & Hawthorne, K. (2008). Research on rural veterans: An analysis of the literature. *The Journal of Rural Health, 24*, 337–344.

West, A., & Weeks, W. B. (2006). Physical and mental health and access to care among nonmetropolitan veterans health administration patients younger than 65 years. *The Journal of Rural Health, 22*, 9–16.

Zatzick, D. F., Marmar, C. R., Weiss, D. S., Browner, W. S., Metzler, T. J., Golding, J. M., …Wells, K. B. (1997). Posttraumatic stress disorder and functioning and quality of life in a nationally representative sample of Vietnam veterans. *American Journal of Psychiatry, 154*, 1690–1695.

20

Working in Frontier Communities

JAEDON P. AVEY, MIMI MCFAUL, TAMARA L. DEHAY, AND DENNIS MOHATT

INTRODUCTION

*W*orking in frontier communities is qualitatively different than working in urban, suburban, and rural communities. There are numerous definitions and methods of classification for rural and frontier communities, as discussed in Chapter 1. The Office of Management and Budget (OMB), United States Department of Agriculture (USDA), United States Census Bureau, and other governmental organizations each have varying definitions of rural in the United States (see Coburn et al., 2007; Hart, Larson, & Lishner, 2005). Frontier areas have been equally cumbersome to define, as standards vary depending upon purpose (Popper, Lang, & Popper, 2000).

Four common definitions of "frontier" exist in the field of mental health. First, originating from the 1980 United States Department of Health and Human Services definition (Hewitt, 1989), frontier is used as a crude measure for a country population density less than or equal to 6 people per square mile (ppsm). Utilizing census data from the year 2000, this definition identifies 1.6% of the U.S. population as frontier. In some instances, the population density delineation has increased to 7 or 10 ppsm (Ciarlo, Wackwitz, Wagenfeld, Mohatt, & Zelarney, 1996).

Second, the Health Resources and Services Administration (HRSA) Office for the Advancement of Telehealth tasked the Center for Rural Health at the University of North Dakota (2006) to define frontier. Their expert panel recommended the following definition:

> ZIP code areas whose calculated population centers are more than
> 60 minutes or 60 miles along the fastest paved road trip to a short-term
> non federal general hospital of 75 beds or more, and are not part of a
> large rural town with a concentration of over 20,000 population. (p. 15)

Using 1998 census data this definition identifies just under 3% of the population of the United States as residing in a frontier area.

Third, under contract with HRSA's Office of Rural Health Policy, the National Center for Frontier Communities, formerly the Frontier Education Center (2007), used a consensus development methodology to create a weighted matrix definition of frontier. After six iterations among experts, the frontier definition development workgroup unanimously voted to define frontier counties based on a simple matrix consisting of population density (0–20 people per square mile), and travel distance (0–90 miles) and travel time (0–90 minutes) to a market center. The matrix establishes a point system for scoring these factors, as well as a cut off criteria for determining the designation as frontier. The matrix assigns the greatest number of points to counties with a density of less than 12 persons per square mile that are more than 90 miles and 90 minutes from the nearest market for services. Based on the matrix, less than 4% of the population of the United States as of the 2000 census resides in a frontier county.

The fourth and final definition presented herein comes from the University of Washington, Rural Health Research Center under contract with the Office of Rural Health Policy. The definition is based on the 2004 update to the Rural–Urban Commuting Areas (version 2.0). It combines census tract-based, commuting, and zip code based travel time data into definitions of functional isolation rather than objective measurements. The Rural Health Research Center does not endorse one particular definition, but the suggested categorization of frontier/remote/isolated areas indicates 4.2% of the population as of 2004 is defined as frontier. In all of the matrices, frontier areas are heavily concentrated in the Western United States and Alaska. While the various definitions of rural begin at less than 500 ppsm, each of the discussed definitions of frontier begin at a functional threshold of less than 20 ppsm (Rural Health Research Center, n.d.)

Understanding a community's sense of place, culture, and history may be more beneficial than focusing solely on technical definitions. A community may consist of as few as 10 people, or two families. Others may feel that their community is remote or frontier with thousands of residents. The community may be 50 miles from a market place or most of a day's travel to a metropolitan center. Regardless of definition, a community has a high probability of being classified as frontier if it is composed of fewer than 2,500 people, in an area of low population density, is a 2-hour drive from a "big box" store, at the end of a lengthy gravel road, or only accessible by plane. Geographic distance (isolation), economic drivers (e.g., farming/ranching, mining, manufacturing, services, recreation, government or unspecified), people (Alaska Native or American Indians, Black, White, Hispanic), or travel patterns all may characterize frontier communities (Ciarlo et al., 1996; Economic Research Service, 2004; Zelarney & Ciarlo, 2000).

When considering examples of these various types of frontier communities, two typical examples of frontier areas reliant on farming include

Forman, North Dakota, in Sargent County (population = 3,951; density = 5.1 ppsm) about 90 travel miles southwest of Fargo, and Lusk, Wyoming, in Niobrara County (population = 2,366; density = 0.9 ppsm) about 100 travel miles east of Casper. A typical frontier area, reliant on Federal or State government, is Pioche, Nevada, in Lincoln County (population = 4,794; density = 0.4 ppsm) about 180 travel miles from Las Vegas. A mining area and typical frontier "hub" community is Kotzebue, Alaska, in the Northwest Arctic Borough (population 7,444; density = 0.2 ppsm) about 440 air miles northwest of the city of Fairbanks (United States Census Bureau, 2010).

CHALLENGES AND ADAPTATIONS

As discussed throughout this book, rural mental health care delivery systems are faced with significant challenges of accessibility, availability, affordability, and acceptability for consumers of behavioral health services (Barbopoulos & Clark, 2003; Brems & Johnson, 2007). Some of these challenges are related to geographical barriers, health disparities, poverty, systemic issues, lack of trained providers, and ethical issues. Challenges intensify within increasingly frontier locations, that is, smaller and more isolated communities (Brems, Johnson, Warner, & Roberts, 2006).

Chipp et al. (2010) found that providers in Alaska and New Mexico experience mitigable challenges working in rural and frontier communities. Providers report wishing to have been primed and prepared for challenges in building relationships with the community members and professionals (e.g., differing beliefs, culture, values, broad interdisciplinary collaboration, consultation, research). They report difficulty maintaining personal or professional boundaries (due to issues around privacy, confidentiality, limited resources for diverse expansive case load, technical expertise, overlapping roles, multiple relationships, ethics), and challenges caring for personal needs and dealing with the pragmatics of rural lifestyle (e.g., travel, geography, isolation, recreation, socialization, limited services, educational and training, burnout). Other provider-level barriers that exist in addition to the lack of specific preparation and training include an expansive scope of practice, work-related stressors, and provider–patient relationship stressors (Brems & Johnson, 2007). In order to address these and many other challenges, it becomes necessary for providers to carefully adapt their practice to their setting.

Developing Relationships

Extant research has found that providers in frontier areas describe the necessity of actively working to develop an awareness or knowledge of a community's diverse resources and strengths. Providers become involved in interacting with a community in an informal capacity outside of their professional role (Chipp et al., 2010; Gifford, Koverola, & Rivkin, 2010). In the literature to date, providers in frontier areas found that participating in community activities and contacting local elders (with a focus on strengthening relationships and engaging a community) can be helpful in learning about the culture of the community, leading to a better understanding of the culture through participation, working with community resources, and increasing their ability to provide effective care. Frontier providers' relationships can further be strengthened through community workshops and by offering trainings to or participating in trainings with other providers (Chipp, Johnson, Brems, Warner, & Roberts, 2008). However, it is important to acknowledge that providers new to frontier areas must remain patient when establishing these relationships or they risk reinforcing their position as an "outsider" and thus alienating themselves (Chipp et al., 2010).

Providers have adapted to social and professional isolation common in frontier settings by purposefully establishing ties with community members and other professionals with particular expertise in consultation, supervision, program evaluation, or research. Mental health providers (psychologists in particular) may benefit from additional training to establish relationships and work with other professions, thereby increasing integration with community resources and the comprehensiveness of patient care (Jameson & Blank, 2007). Additionally, video teleconferencing has an appropriate use for training and supervision within a geographically isolated area (Stamm, 1998; Wood, Miller, & Hargrove, 2005).

Barbopoulos and Clark (2003) have suggested the formation of rural research networks to reduce professional isolation and improve the availability of rural-specific research. Researchers in frontier settings have undertaken valuable community-based participatory research (CBPR) and participatory action research (PAR) work to create useful, meaningful, influential research and interventions by honoring the spirit of community self-determination amongst indigenous peoples (Freire, 2000; Lewin, 1946; Wallerstein & Duran, 2010).

Community Self-Determination and Co-Participation

Droby (2000), a seasoned clinical psychologist working in frontier Alaska, suggests that the multifaceted, highly contextual role of frontier providers working with indigenous people should include patients and other local providers, or natural helpers, as co-participants. Providers should strive to work alongside others and develop interdependence with them, rather than working in potentially "arrogant isolation." It is beneficial for primary, secondary, and tertiary prevention strategies to honor local providers and natural helpers as co-participants. A co-participatory model stresses a decentralization of services by fostering the utilization and empowerment of natural helpers and informal supports, as well as utilizing paraprofessionals and certificate level providers to establish improved access to services. Providers collaborating by maintaining itinerant schedules or using telehealth technology must support these adjunctive individuals and the services they offer. Droby distinguishes between offering support to community members and fulfilling one's own (misplaced) agenda—Droby suggests that a professional's role should be "offering a tap on the shoulder." Frontier and indigenous peoples often have an explicit or implicit history of outsider exploitation that mental health providers should not replicate.

Boundaries and Ethics

Frontier providers may face myriad boundary issues as a result of engaging in a community and forming relationships similar to those faced by all rural providers, but to a more extreme degree. Providers that do settle in frontier areas face limited resources, an expansive scope of practice, inadequate preparation and training, work and relational stressors, and ethical issues due to overlapping roles and issues of confidentiality (Brems et al., 2006; Werth, Hastings, & Riding-Malon, 2010).

In response to boundaries of competence, providers will most likely need to expand their role through additional continuing education and self-training to meet professional responsibilities as generalists. Some literature suggests that expanding prescription privileges to psychologists may have a dramatic impact on rural and frontier regions of the United States (Jameson & Blank, 2007), and staying current on these developments and necessary continuing education is very important for providers in frontier areas.

Providers in frontier areas must seek consultation or supervision through developed professional networks to ensure the best possible patient care with limited resources and gaps in knowledge (Chipp et al., 2010). Providers that do pursue training opportunities may not have sufficient numbers of population-specific clients to benefit from an intervention, contributing to disuse (Barbopoulos & Clark, 2003). Urban models of practice, including evidence-based practices developed in urban areas, are typically not appropriate in frontier settings. Frontier providers need *clinical flexibility* in finding "creative, mobile, localized solutions" (Roufeil & Battye, 2007). Frontier providers may feel a pressure to serve consumers, as if "it's me or no one." This pressure, whether stemming from the provider's needs or the patient's, can exacerbate ethical issues of competency as well as problems with multiple relationships.

Nonsexual multiple relationships are inevitable and manageable in frontier areas (Campbell & Gordon, 2003). Accidental client encounters, overlapping roles, and multiple relationships are regular and expected occurrences. As discussed in Chapter 7, having simple protocols in place (e.g., during the informed consent process) for accidental encounters can ease the perceived risk to confidentiality for the provider and the client (Barbopoulos & Clark, 2003). In some remote communities, foregoing the exchange of greetings or pleasantries with someone can, in fact, paradoxically identify them as a client.

Schank and Skovholt (1997) conducted interviews with seasoned psychologists in rural Wisconsin and Minnesota and identified ethical dilemmas in roles and boundaries. Overlapping roles were seen in four categories: the social relationships (e.g., school, community events, volunteer activities), business or professional roles (e.g., store owners, trade labor, colleague or their family), own family network and client, (e.g., teenage children dating former clients, spouses befriending former clients), and client–client (e.g., family or friends). Schank and Skovholt (1997) suggest that these ethical risks be managed through knowledge of ethical codes of conduct, ethical training and continuing education, clear expectations and boundaries when possible, maintaining confidentiality, frequent consultation, and self-knowledge. Other literature stresses the importance of informed consent, imagining the worst case scenario, personal and professional consistency, terminating detrimental dual relationships as soon as possible, and appropriately utilizing an ethical-decision making process (Barnett, Lazarus, Vasquez, Moorehead-Slaughter, & Johnson, 2007; Campbell & Gordon, 2003; Coyle, 1999; Schank, Helbok, Haldeman, & Gallardo, 2010). To avoid unintentional breaches, a provider needs a well-developed awareness of a community's informational networks and sources. Campbell and Gordon (2003, p. 434) refer to this as "Mastering the skill of communicating in social situations with appropriate professional vagueness." Additional strategies for managing ethical risk (the importance of which is magnified in frontier settings) are discussed in Chapter 7.

RURAL LIFESTYLE AND SELF-CARE

As mentioned above, research has found that providers relocating to rural and frontier areas frequently wish that they had known more about the challenges of rural lifestyle and self-care. Providers report difficulty setting appropriate boundaries in the short-term and establishing a private-life in the long-term (Chipp et al., 2010; Droby, 2000). Rural and frontier providers experience increased rates of burnout, especially due to emotional exhaustion and low social support (Kee, Johnson, & Hunt, 2002). Vicarious trauma, also known as secondary trauma, can cause a stress reaction known as compassion fatigue (Figley, 2002; McCann & Pearlman, 1990; Sprang, Clark, & Whitt-Woosley, 2007). Figley (2002) identified that a "residue of emotional energy" produced by a provider's empathic responses and actions when attempting to relieve a client's suffering from trauma can induce compassion stress. A prolonged exposure to this stress in the absence of a sense of achievement or ability to disengage from the client's needs, and in the presence of traumatic recollections and life disruptions, can lead to compassion fatigue and burnout, which is marked by a reduction of empathy for the client. Such burnout can be more common in frontier settings, where support systems and referral options are limited (if present at all).

Vicarious trauma and compassion fatigue occur among urban, rural, and frontier providers and contribute to job burnout. Literature suggest that between 18% and 65% of behavioral health, social service, and trauma workers experience a traumatic stress response and that those in helping professions, in the public sector, and with less specialized training are at greatest risk. Among other findings, a survey of 1,100 behavioral health providers in a rural southern U.S. state revealed that limited provider experience, young age, percentage of clients with post-traumatic stress disorder (PTSD), and serving in a frontier location independently contributed to elevated burnout risk (Sprang et al., 2007). This finding is understandable in the context of high staff turnover and clients experiencing a greater acuity of symptoms seeking services later in the course of their disorder. "Limited resources, geographical isolation, few colleagues (limited peer support), and highly demanding caseloads create a 'perfect storm' of burnout risk among rural clinicians" (p. 273), which is even more amplified among frontier clinicians. Burnout and compassion fatigue have been reported to decrease one's commitment to an organization, and increase absenteeism, illness, and voluntary turnover (Maslach, Schaufeli, & Leiter, 2001). Self-care strategies that can be used to minimize burnout are discussed in Chapter 8.

The clinical caseload of a generalist in behavioral health includes greater diversity than that of a specialist, with limited options for referral due to the scarcity of providers in frontier areas. Limited referral options make a caseload less flexible and difficult to manage, partly by constricting the provider's ability to reduce exposure to traumatic stimuli. Additionally, restricted access to continuing education and training opportunities can curtail clinical diversity within a behavioral health practice. The need for providers to travel within a remote region can exacerbate imbalances in professional practice and contribute to a fragmentation of self-care practices (Brems et al., 2006). The lack of privacy and anonymity, commonly reported among providers, may reduce their likelihood of accessing specific recreational opportunities (Brems & Johnson, 2007). Though many recreational self-care opportunities that take advantage of natural amenities are available, some individuals choose to partake in more isolative in-house electronic recreational activities, dubbed "cocooning" (Barbopoulos & Clark, 2003). In the long-term, there is evidence that such escape-avoidance coping styles are associated with increased burnout (Rohland, 2000). Literature strongly recommends seeking out friends, family, and formal therapy as needed in order to improve self-care and decrease professional burnout. An intermediary option between support from friends and family and traditional therapy is found in the establishment of a relationship with a natural helper. Collegial relationships with natural helpers can often foster valuable bi-directional support, and can be a viable alternative in resource-scarce frontier areas.

WORKFORCE RECRUITMENT AND RETENTION

Recruitment, retention, and training difficulties have resulted in a stagnating frontier workforce. Two basic strategies present themselves in the literature: focus on recruiting and retaining urban professionals (trained for frontier practice) or training existing providers or natural helpers already present in frontier communities.

Dyck, Cornock, Gibson, and Carlson (2008) of the Rural and Northern Program of the Department of Health Psychology at the University of Manitoba identify a framework for providing outreach to create sustainable training and psychological practice opportunities. Their suggestions are typical of a pipelining method—plant the seeds of rural practice in the minds of students early, train psychologists in rural areas early through field practica or internships, and actively recruit these individuals. They further state that professionals should highlight the positives of frontier practice, be flexible and understanding of noncritical shortcomings, provide support, and be patient and persistent. Due to service shortages, frontier settings frequently offer providers loan repayment options that can aid in initial attraction and recruitment.

Frontier communities may require workforce training programs geared to their setting that reinforce a sense of place and connection (Roufeil & Battye, 2007). Many of these programs might describe themselves as fostering "home-grown" providers as these providers typically have much higher retention rates compared to "outsiders" (Fisher, Pearce, Statz, & Wood, 2003; Roufeil & Battye, 2007). Work-based learning models show considerable promise in providing culturally sensitive training without relocation (Roberts et al., 2011).

Once providers are recruited or trained, retention efforts should be figural. In a review of the literature, Buykx, Humphreys, Wakerman, and Pashen (2010) recommended that a comprehensive retention strategy consist of: maintaining a sufficient and stable workforce; providing realistic and competitive compensation; maintaining adequate infrastructure; encouraging effective and sustainable workplace organization; ensuring the professional environment recognizes and rewards individuals contributing to patient care; and lastly, ensuring social, family, and community support. From an administrative perspective, Buykx et al. (2010) suggest that frontier health organizations measure their desired outcome (i.e., retention) rather than the more common undesirable one (i.e., turnover).

Among long-term, primary health providers in rural Australia, strong ties to the community and adequate off-call and vacation time have been reported for their importance in finding the balance that enhances long-term retention and satisfaction (Hays, Wynd, Veitch, & Crossland, 2003). Frontier providers make decisions not only for themselves, but also for their families. As providers age, their responsibilities to their families change. They may seek to move children closer to educational opportunities, or may feel the need to move to take care of aging parents (Gifford et al., 2010).

REWARDS OF WORKING IN A FRONTIER SETTING

Despite a lack of urban amenities, health professionals in frontier settings report many fulfilling personal advantages. While there may be no running water, no indoor plumbing, no shopping malls, no restaurants, and no movie theaters (Jans, 1993), there may be fantastic natural recreational opportunities on trails for hiking, biking, skiing; ample hunting, fishing, or boating opportunities; unique community events including sports, arts, or fairs; or ample time to partake in personally meaningful activities and hobbies. Communities may have highly accessible wilderness or outdoor areas for travel or recreation. Frontier life moves at a slower pace, with fewer people, devoid of many of the headaches of urbanization (Chipp et al., 2010). If there are not many stoplights, there cannot be much traffic. Providers can succeed professionally and have time for their family (Casey, 2007). There is a certain satisfaction from providing needed services in frontier areas, which fosters a sense of accomplishment (Chipp et al., 2010; Rural Special Interest Group, 2003). Where some would cite frontier areas for lack of privacy (Brems & Johnson, 2007) or anonymity (Casey, 2007), others would note the implicit potential advantage of visibility within a community (Heyman, 1982).

Professionals in frontier areas have a chance to work flexibly outside the role of direct service provider. They can provide some services less formally, finding an increased sense of community. They have a greater chance to have meaningful collaborative relationships. They have the opportunity to use or develop innovative services that allow for the creative use of available resources (i.e., frontier mental health MacGyvers; Rural Special Interest Group, 2003).

Surveys of psychiatrists in training in rural Australia revealed that some receive much greater than the minimum number of hours of supervision. Trainees reported working with integrative supportive teams and feeling respected and accomplished for the services they provided as these rendered visible differences in the community they serve (Rural Special Interest Group, 2003). Remote communities can be professional microcosms offering both breadth and depth of clinical experience unsurpassed in urban settings (Rural Special Interest Group, 2003). This professional context offers developmental advantages for practicum students, interns, post-docs, early career psychologists, and other mental health providers. Frontier agencies can use both the physical and psychosocial environment in recruiting. The physical environment allows for lifestyle advantages whereas the psychosocial environment allows for a provider to have a visible and meaningful impact within a system (Heyman, 1982).

EXPERIENTIAL LESSONS LEARNED

The recent rise of programs offering specialized training for providing mental health services with rural and frontier populations will undoubtedly produce trainees, interns, and graduates with increased coursework and training in frontier mental health, but there is much to learn from actually being present in a frontier community. This next section highlights some lessons learned by the authors while providing services in a remote region of Alaska. It is intended for burgeoning professionals who may move to frontier regions or remote communities, and may travel itinerantly within such a region. The lessons learned consist of the logistics of rural work, presence, awareness of self and community, self-presentation, collaborations and relationships, and self-care.

Logistics

Providers working in frontier communities first realize "what they are in for" by the complexities of traveling to frontier communities—what to bring, what to wear, when to travel, whom to meet, and where to stay. Adequate and affordable housing can be exceedingly difficult to locate. Logistical problems are a complicating factor that can increase stress and anxiety in personal and professional domains. Lack of a realistic, concrete approach can transform a provider's presence from one of support to one of liability—which creates stress for those around them. Connecting with local email lists or putting an advertisement in the paper can facilitate timely acquisition of housing.

Providers may often travel to regularly scheduled services in a frontier community, known as itinerant services. Or, they may live in a frontier "hub" community, itinerating to even smaller remote communities. The novelty of itinerant travel decreases sharply over time, reducing associated excitement or anxiety. Itinerant trips require proactive planning for housing, travel, food, paperwork, and financial arrangements (e.g., adequate cash within communities where credit cards and ATMs may not be used). Often housing may be found in a local hotel, school, or clinic. Travel may be flexible; however, it should be considerate of others' schedules in small clinics. Certain food supplies can be brought, though bringing all food and water may decrease one's perceived presence and contribution to a community. Access to clinical records, paperwork, and assessment materials is vital. Advertising is also necessary; providers regularly itinerating may find it beneficial to coordinate the posting of flyers with availability of services.

Providers should prepare and dress appropriately. In the standardized human resources orientation, Norton Sound Health Corporation (2010) suggests itinerant providers traveling by plane physically carry on themselves an emergency kit consisting of "a knife, two bandages, a fire starter, clean handkerchief or triangle bandages, quick energy food, and signal mirror" and wear a full array of appropriate winter gear. Though this level of preparation may be excessive in other regions, such as those with a reliable transportation infrastructure, frontier providers need to plan and prepare trips in a self-reliant manner. Preparing vital necessities for emergencies and contingencies is advisable (e.g., vehicle emergency kits, extra clothes).

Travel difficulties can be minimized by developing a certain amount of acceptance as to what is outside of one's control combined with realism and pragmatism when scheduling services. It may be necessary to schedule blocks of time in one's schedule to act as buffers to deal with delayed travel resulting from inclement weather. There may be some days in which a provider simply cannot travel safely. Clients will understand this, colleagues will understand this, and supervisors will understand this.

Presence

The importance of presence in a frontier community cannot be understated. Community providers and residents have heard many times "they're coming soon," "they're on their way," or "next month sometime." However, community members care most about who a person is when they're actually there. In addition to physical location, one's presence can be defined by awareness of self, awareness of community, and self-presentation. All of these factors increase the provider's acceptance within the community, thus facilitating their practice.

Awareness of Self

Awareness of oneself through self-knowledge, self-monitoring, and self-assessment are imperative skills for frontier providers in particular. Beyond understanding personal motivations for becoming a helping professional, providers should recognize and identify motivations for working in a frontier community, personal and professional needs, and any possible preconceived notions or assumptions. Motivations that could be perceived as exploitive jeopardize the formation of relationships and compromise one's professional practices. Financial incentives are commonly used to attract early career providers with student debt. However, it could be said that these providers are coerced into working in frontier areas for financial reasons. Providers who relocate to receive loan repayment benefits may become ambivalent and be more likely to burnout or voluntarily seek other positions once the recognition of personal drawbacks to relocating has taken place. With the broadening of professional roles, providers should constantly assess and monitor their clinical skills and areas of personal growth. Providers who have difficulty with organization, time-management, scheduling, or coordinating with others may have additional difficulty in frontier settings. Critical and reflective practices enable providers in frontier settings to continue to develop (Lavender, 2003).

Self-assessments such as the Cross-Cultural Adaptability Inventory (CCAI) can provide individuals information about their strengths and weaknesses in adapting to other cultures before traveling and experiencing significant problems. Adaptability factors include: emotional resilience (e.g., positive attitude, tolerating intense ambiguity, and coping with stress); flexibility/openness; perceptual acuity; and personal autonomy (Kelly & Meyers, 1995). Individual questions can act as critical items indicative of potential problem areas such as potential rigidity, loneliness, sensitivity to criticism, or a need for constant approval. Self-assessments often have planning guides for addressing personal weaknesses. Planning guides allow individuals to take positive action to foster cross-cultural adaptability such as practicing slowing down, searching to find relaxation or enjoyment in solitary activities, examining their self-talk, or journaling in new ways.

Awareness of Community

Developing an awareness of community strengths and resources can positively influence the appropriateness of a provider's conduct in a community. Before traveling, new providers should do homework on the history of a community and strive to understand multiple perspectives on the historical events that have shaped the identity of a community, and the concerns, pathology, and help-seeking behavior of residents. Communities may have been defined by a combination of natural resources, industry, boom and bust cycles, colonialization, migration, religious movements, notable figures, and key historical events. Each community's self-identity may be distinct from similar communities or the region, as each has its own history, values, and culture(s). Regardless of a community's current status, formal and informal resources exist that have addressed past problems encountered by the community such as outmigration, poverty, drug and alcohol abuse, domestic violence, and suicide. These resources should be identified so that collaborative relationships can be formed.

A series of proper introductions from those with established relationships in the community is the most ideal way to establish presence. The provider should be receptive to invitations and introductions. Forming a special connection with a supportive professional mentor or cultural ambassador will aid in networking within the community, creating relationships, developing a presence, and establishing roots. Once introductions have been made, establishing a presence in a community on return trips is notably easier. Simply being visible by walking around or going to the store will cue community members to the presence of the practitioner. Until more formal relationships are formed, a mental health provider's primary method of positive contribution may be contributing to the local economy by staying at local hotels and shopping in local stores.

Intrinsic community values guide local behavior. Without an understanding of local values a provider may have little idea as to what is adaptive or normative. Local residents may value dealing with problems on one's own or seek help from familial supports, teachers, or counselors. As discussed in Chapter 6, religious practices are often a source of stability and support, but can also be a source of internal community conflict and marginalization. Awareness of local religious resources and service offerings (e.g., men's group, premarital counseling, teen group) may assist with creating referrals and with ensuring services are culturally sensitive.

Self-Presentation

Building on self-awareness and community-awareness, self-presentation strategies are vital to maintaining a relationship with a frontier community. Jameson and Blank (2007) suggested that mental health providers should avoid being as seen as "overly intellectual" (p. 292) and be careful of the manner in which they dress. Though some mental health providers believe expressing a genuine self is the most important part of their professional identity and practice, how others perceive them in a frontier community setting has a large impact on their role and work. For example, if a provider who facilitates a substance abuse treatment group which emphasizes total abstinence is seen shopping in a liquor store or frequenting a bar, clients' perceptions may be changed. Taking a walk with a client or a coworker can also raise eyebrows (especially for new providers). Before returning from such an activity, two or three friends or relatives may have already notified a significant other. Rumors spread quickly and can result in damaged relationships. Providers must monitor their associations. Meeting with an office of children's services worker or child custody investigator in a public setting may give false impressions that amplify fears and reduce client help-seeking behavior. One dinner with the wrong person or group can trap the practitioner into a troubling social network. It is best to associate with positive supportive people or with larger reputable organizations in the community.

If providers are aware of the values that exist in the community they serve, they can adapt their behavior to these values. For example, if a mental health provider is participating in a community event and happens to win a door prize of food such as a frozen turkey, the provider may choose to donate the food to a needy community member. This may align with values of responsibility to the community and respect for elders in the same way that some adolescents give away the animals caught on their first hunt.

Self-monitoring allows providers to identify their actions and make mid-course corrections based on contextual factors. For relationships to be equitable and services to be appropriate, new providers in a community should be responsive to the cultural norms and language within that community. This may constitute living in harmony with the seasons (e.g., subsistence activities) or learning to use local language (e.g., using the correct version of words such as "snowmobile," "snow go," or "snow machine"). Learning the region and how to properly pronounce place names can be an important aid in building local knowledge and rapport with clients vital for clinical work.

In a frontier community, the residents take pride in knowing everyone. Interestingly, many smaller communities' children may approach newcomers and ask, "Who are you? Are you a teacher?" since teachers are often the primary outsiders to come to the community. While in an urban community one might stop and take notice of someone familiar to them, in a frontier community, one stops and takes notice of strangers. A new provider entering a frontier community can expect to pique the interest of the local residents, and being receptive to this curiosity may help to promote their acceptance by the community.

Professional Relationships and Collaboration

Just as community awareness fosters relationship building, understanding the history of care providers in a community can provide valuable insight in building relationships with clients and coworkers. If previous providers frequently broke confidentiality, maintained poor boundaries, proselytized to those seeking services, spoke poorly about the community, or left hurriedly, clients may feel that care providers are untrustworthy, condescending, authoritarian, or do not value community members. Past provider behavior and client feelings about that behavior provide valuable insight regarding patterns of help seeking. Providers moving to frontier locations as outsiders may experience initial transference (e.g., "all outsiders are only here for the student loan repayment") or countertransference, which is important to address right away in a nonreactive, culturally responsive manner. Providers may find taking a step back to recognize role and context as helpful. Not all transference is negative. In an ethnically or socially homogenous community, victims of partner violence may identify strongly with outsiders (e.g., the logical fallacy that if men here are no good and a man is not from here, then they must be good). In some frontier communities there are notions that professionals from urban places will provide services and make things better.

Collaborating with certificate level counselors, health providers, community resources, and other agencies is imperative to providing sustainable services, working with existing services, making appropriate referrals, and seeking consultation. Local counselors may have years of localized expertise in what works, and in available resources. In many ways their place-based knowledge has more utility than academic training. However, certificate level counselors may require clinical supervision to meet their work-based training needs. Certificate level counselors should be empowered by collaborations to learn new clinical skills and to take cases that appropriately utilize new competencies. Modeling appropriate professional behavior is beneficial with regard to confidentiality, multiple relationships, scope of practice and competency, documentation, and boundaries. Providers should avoid discussing clinical issues or engaging in work-related complaining in public settings. Providers should be reflective regarding their competencies and model acknowledgment of limits in their scope of practice. Providers should model contextually appropriate boundaries with clients and providers. The professional and personal mistakes of mental health providers affect others, and providers in frontier settings especially must be able to adequately maintain relationships through an awareness of difficulties caused by their own mistakes and by repairing working relationships when needed. Those that are unaware, unapologetic, or unrelenting will have a difficult time working effectively in frontier areas.

Self-Care and Safety

Some mental health providers itinerating to small frontier communities sleep in the clinic or in the counseling office. This type of morning to night contact with clients can become physically and mentally exhausting. As indicated in the literature and discussed in Chapter 8, it is crucial to notice stress, potential impaired practice, signs of burnout, or compassion fatigue. While scales such as the Professional Quality of Life Scale can be of aid (Stamm, 2005), ongoing self-monitoring is key. If a provider continues to see clients despite feeling ill, they may be at risk of working while impaired or fostering burnout.

The pace of life and work may also be different in frontier areas. Many businesses in frontier communities are only open from 9:00 a.m. to 5:00 p.m. The provider who relocates to a frontier community may be functioning based upon the norms of city/urban time. They may feel that every second must be utilized for work purposes. They may be unable to schedule or deal with downtime. A heightened sense of self-awareness is necessary so that these individuals will not let speed of processing or sense of urgency put undue pressure on coworkers, clients, or themselves. Providers should take time away from practice to take advantage of the unique recreational opportunities available in the remote setting. Some frontier organizations offer advantageous and easily accessible leave options to allow for recreational opportunities. Enjoying the frontier setting may reduce the threat of burnout and help the provider to feel more engaged in the community.

CONCLUSION

While simplistically defined as a county population density of less than seven people per square mile, frontier areas are unique settings that offer many unique challenges and opportunities for mental health providers. Frontier providers are obligated to take the time to understand the community culture. Among the many challenges highlighted in the literature, developing relationships, maintaining boundaries, and caring for personal needs stand out as mitigable. Multiple relationships and ethical dilemmas are unavoidable, but can be managed through engaging in a consultative professional network. Involvement in a frontier community possesses the inevitable risk of creating multiple relationships and ethical dilemmas, but isolating behaviors are the main ingredients in the recipe for incompetence, compassion fatigue, and burnout. Self-care strategies should include self-monitoring, realistic thinking, process changes to work, diversification of job duties, action-oriented techniques, pleasurable activities, interpersonal support, supervision, and humor.

Frontier providers are best served by a relational, existential, developmental, competency-based approach to collaboration. If actions are not taken to sustain relationships, develop competencies, or refer to local knowledge, providers are more likely to falter in their role. The greater the differences between providers and communities, the more important increased self-awareness, awareness of the community, and self-presentation become. Mental health providers in frontier communities have the opportunity to experience a slower pace of life removed from the potential stresses of urban living, as well as to work in tight collaborative groups, expand their professional roles and competencies, and experience a distinct sense of accomplishment and fulfillment that comes from working effectively within a small community.

REFERENCES

Barbopoulos, A., & Clark, J. (2003). Practising psychology in rural settings: Issues and guidelines. *Canadian Psychology/Psychologie Canadienne*, 44(4), 410–424.

Barnett, J. E., Lazarus, A. A., Vasquez, M. J. T., Moorehead-Slaughter, O., & Johnson, W. B. (2007). Boundary issues and multiple relationships: Fantasy and reality. *Professional Psychology: Research and Practice*, 38(4), 401–410. doi: 10.1037/0735-7028.38.4.401

Brems, C., & Johnson, M. (2007). Challenges and uniqueness of rural and frontier services in the United States. *Journal of Psychological Practice, 14*, 93-122.

Brems, C., Johnson, M. E., Warner, T. D., & Roberts, L. W. (2006). Barriers to healthcare as reported by rural and urban interprofessional providers. *Journal of Interprofessional Care, 20*(2), 105-118. doi: 10.1080/13561820600622208

Buykx, P., Humphreys, J., Wakerman, J., & Pashen, D. (2010). Systematic review of effective retention incentives for health workers in rural and remote areas: Towards evidence-based policy. *Australian Journal of Rural Health, 18*(3), 102-109. doi: 10.1111/j.1440-1584.2010.01139.x

Campbell, C. D., & Gordon, M. C. (2003). Acknowledging the inevitable: Understanding multiple relationships in rural practice. *Professional Psychology: Research and Practice, 34*(4), 430-434. doi: 10.1037/0735-7028.34.4.430

Casey, C. (2007, October). Rural rewards: The career you want and the lifestyle too. *InPsych*. Retrived from Australian Psychological Society website: http://www.psychology.org.au/publications/inpsych/rural_rewards/

Center for Rural Health. (2006). *Defining the term "frontier area" for programs implemented through the Office for the Advancement of Telehealth*. Bismark, ND: University of North Dakota.

Chipp, C., Dewane, S., Brems, C., Johnson, M. E., Warner, T. D., & Roberts, L. W. (2010). If only someone had told me: Lessons from rural providers. *The Journal of Rural Health, 27*(1), 122-130. doi: 10.1111/j.1748-0361.2010.00314.x

Chipp, C., Johnson, M. E., Brems, C., Warner, T. D., & Roberts, L. W. (2008). Adaptations to health care barriers as reported by rural and urban providers. *Journal of Health Care for the Poor and Underserved, 19*(2), 532-549.

Ciarlo, J. A., Wackwitz, J. H., Wagenfeld, M. O., Mohatt, D. F., & Zelarney, P. T. (1996). *Focusing on "Frontier": Isolated rural America: Letter to the field no. 2*. Retrieved from Western Interstate Commission on Higher Education website: http://www.wiche.edu//MentalHealth/Frontier/letter2.asp

Coburn, A. F., Mackinney, A. C., McBride, T. D., Meuller, K. J., Slifkin, R. T., & Wakefield, M. K. (2007). *Choosing rural definitions:Implications for health policy* (Issue Brief No. 2). Omaha, NE: Rural Policy Research Institute Health Panel.

Coyle, B. R. (1999). Practical tools for rural psychiatric practice. *Bulletin of the Menninger Clinic, 63*(2), 202-222.

Droby, R. (2000). *With the wind and the waves: A guide for non-native mental health professionals working within Alaska native communities*. Nome, AK: Norton Sound Health Corporation.

Dyck, K. G., Cornock, B. L., Gibson, G., & Carlson, A. A. (2008). Training clinical psychologists for rural and northern practice: Transforming challenge into opportunity. *Australian Psychologist, 43*(4), 239-248. doi: 10.1080/0005006080243 8096

Economic Research Service. (2004). *Measuring rurality: 2004 County typology codes*. Retrieved from http://www.ers.usda.gov/Briefing/Rurality/Typology/

Figley, C. R. (2002). Compassion fatigue: Psychotherapists' chronic lack of self care. *Journal of Clinical Psychology, 58*(11), 1433-1441. doi: 10.1002/jclp.10090

Fisher, D. G., Pearce, F. W., Statz, D. J., & Wood, M. M. (2003). Employment retention of health care providers in frontier areas of Alaska. *International Journal of Circumpolar Health, 62*(4), 423-435.

Freire, P. (2000). *Pedagogy of the oppressed*. Trans. Myra Bergman Ramos, New York: Continuum.

Frontier Education Center. (2007). *Frontier: A new definition*. Retrieved from http://www.frontierus.org/documents/consensus_paper.htm

Gifford, V., Koverola, C., & Rivkin, I. D. (2010). Factors contributing to the long-term retention of behavioral health providers in rural Alaska. *Rural Mental Health, 34*(1), 12-22.

Hart, L. G., Larson, E. H., & Lishner, D. M. (2005). Rural definitions for health policy and research. *American Journal of Public Health, 95*(7), 1149. doi: 10.2105/AJPH. 2004.042432

Hays, R., Wynd, S., Veitch, C., & Crossland, L. (2003). Getting the balance right? GPs who choose to stay in rural practice. *Australian Journal of Rural Health, 11*(4), 193-198. doi: 10.1111/j.1440-1584.2003.tb00535.x

Hewitt, M. E. (1989). *Defining "rural" areas: Impact on health care policy and research*. Washington, DC: US Government Printing Office.

Heyman, S. R. (1982). Capitalizing on unique assets of rural areas for community interventions. *Journal of Rural Community Psychology, 3*(1), 35-48.

Jameson, J. P., & Blank, M. B. (2007). The role of clinical psychology in rural mental health services: Defining problems and developing solutions. *Clinical Psychology: Science and Practice, 14*(3), 283-298.

Jans, N. (1993). *The last light breaking: Living among Alaska's Inupiat Eskimos*. Seattle, WA: Alaska Northwest Books.

Kee, J. A., Johnson, D., & Hunt, P. (2002). Burnout and social support in rural mental health counselors. *Journal of Rural Community Psychology, 5*(1). Retrieved from http://www.marshall.edu/jrcp/sp2002/Kee.htm

Kelly, C., & Meyers, J. (1995). *Cross-cultural adaptability inventory*. Minneapolis, MN: New Computer Systems.

Lavender, T. (2003). Redressing the balance: The place, history and future of reflective practice in clinical training. *Clinical Psychology, 27*, 11-15.

Lewin, K. (1946). Action research and minority problems. *Journal of Social Issues, 2*(4), 34-46. doi: 10.1111/j.1540-4560.1946.tb02295.x

Maslach, C., Schaufeli, W. B., & Leiter, M. P. (2001). Job burnout. *Annual Review of Psychology, 52*, 397-422. doi: 10.1037/004284

McCann, I. L., & Pearlman, L. A. (1990). Vicarious traumatization: A framework for understanding the psychological effects of working with victims. *Journal of Traumatic Stress, 3*(1), 131-149. doi: 10.1007/BF00975140

Norton Sound Health Corporation. (2010). *Helpful tips for in-region (village) travel*. Nome, AK: Author.

Popper, D. E., Lang, R. E., & Popper, F. J. (2000). From maps to myth: The Census, Turner, and the idea of the frontier. *Journal of American & Comparative Cultures, 23*(1), 91-102. doi: 10.1111/j.1537-4726.2000.2301_91.x

Roberts, L., Smith, J., McFaul, M., Paris, M., Speer, N., Boeckmann, M., ... Hoge, M. A. (2011). Behavioral health workforce development in rural and frontier Alaska. *Journal of Rural Mental Health, 35*(1), 10-16.

Rohland, B. M. (2000). A survey of burnout among mental health center directors in a rural state. *Administration and Policy in Mental Health and Mental Health Services Research, 27*(4), 221-237. doi: 10.1023/a:1021361419155

Roufeil, L., & Battye, K. (2007, October). Psychology services in rural and remote Australia. *InPsych*. Retrieved from Australian Psychological Society website: http://www.psychology.org.au/publications/inpsych/rural_remote

Rural Health Research Center. (n.d.). *Travel distance and time, remote, isolated, and frontier*. Retrieved from http://depts.washington.edu/uwruca/ruca-travel-dist.php

Rural Special Interest Group. (2003). Rural special interest group news. *Australasian Psychiatry, 11*, 104–106.

Schank, J. A., Helbok, C. M., Haldeman, D. C., & Gallardo, M. E. (2010). Challenges and benefits of ethical small-community practice. *Professional Psychology: Research and Practice, 41*(6), 502–510. doi: 10.1037/a0021689

Schank, J. A., & Skovholt, T. M. (1997). Dual-relationship dilemmas of rural and small-community psychologists. *Professional Psychology Research and Practice, 28*, 44–49. doi: 10.1037//0735-7028.28.1.44

Sprang, G., Clark, J. J., & Whitt-Woosley, A. (2007). Compassion fatigue, compassion satisfaction, and burnout: Factors impacting a professional's quality of life. *Journal of Loss and Trauma, 12*(3), 259–280.

Stamm, B. (1998). Clinical applications of telehealth in mental health care. *Professional Psychology: Research and Practice, 29*(6), 536–542. doi: 10.1037/0735-7028.29.6.536

Stamm, B. (2005). The Professional Quality of Life Scale: Compassion satisfaction, burnout & compassion fatigue/secondary trauma scales. *Professional Quality of Life and Trauma Therapists, 293*. Lutherville, MD: Sidran Press.

United States Census Bureau. (2010). *State and county quickfacts*. Retrieved from http://quickfacts.census.gov/

Wallerstein, N., & Duran, B. (2010). Community-based participatory research contributions to intervention research: The intersection of science and practice to improve health equity. *American Journal of Public Health, 100*(Supplement 1), S40–S46. doi: 10.2105/AJPH.2009.184036

Werth, J. L., Hastings, S. L., & Riding-Malon, R. (2010). Ethical challenges of practicing in rural areas. *Journal of Clinical Psychology, 66*(5), 537–548. doi: 10.1002/jclp.20681

Wood, J., Miller, T., & Hargrove, D. (2005). Clinical supervision in rural settings: A telehealth model. *Professional Psychology: Research and Practice, 36*(2), 173–179. doi: 10.1037/0735-7028.36.2.173

Zelarney, P. T., & Ciarlo, J. A. (2000). *Defining and describing frontier areas in the United States: An update: Letter to the field No. 22*. Retrieved from Western Interstate Commission for Higer Education website: http://www.wiche.edu//Mental-Health/Frontier/letter22.asp

IV

Looking to the Future

21

Rural Mental Health: Future Directions and Recommendations

K. BRYANT SMALLEY AND JACOB C. WARREN

INTRODUCTION

*W*e hope that this book has provided you with insights as to the current mental health needs of rural residents and the unique strategies that have been developed to address those needs. Much of the information presented in this book portrays the status of mental health for rural residents as being somewhat dire. While it is undeniable that rural populations face unique challenges that impact on their mental health status and the outcomes of mental health conditions, there are also numerous opportunities to explore novel methods of mental health service delivery that have implications not only in rural areas, but that may innovate mental health care in urban settings as well. Finding solutions to the overwhelming need of rural areas may well lead to advances with national implications in providing cost-effective and evidence-based care in contexts with limited resources. Therefore, in addition to being a place of need, rural areas represent ideal settings for innovations in preventive efforts and mental health care delivery.

Improving the mental health status of rural America will require continued focus upon "rural" as a distinct disparity group, similar to the way in which racial and ethnic minority groups are viewed in disparity research. While the lack of a consistent definition of rural impedes this somewhat, the fact remains that rural populations are inherently *heterogeneous*, as with any other disparity group, and a definition might not be as important as many think. The daily life and contextual influences of an onion farmer in rural Southern Georgia are very different from that of a frontier Alaskan in a fishing community. "Rural" should therefore be seen as an umbrella under which multiple different types of individuals stand—united in their struggles, but complex and unique in ways of their own. A consistent definition might not be possible—what *is* important is that if decisions are being made based upon a rural definition (e.g., population size of the county), that it is not unjustly excluding areas that are in reality rural but marginally fail an arbitrary definition. Viewing rurality as a cultural issue, rather than geographic issue (as discussed previously in this book), could lead to a dramatic shift in the way rurality is viewed, and thus greatly facilitate our ability to discuss it within a somewhat consistent meaning.

The lack of an agreed-upon meaning for rural may be confusing, but repeating themes across rural areas provides distinct targets for improvement of mental health. As discussed in Chapter 1, availability, accessibility, and acceptability of mental health services are challenges faced nearly across the board in rural areas. These three factors interact with each other in such a way that addressing one without addressing the other will not improve the overall mental health status of rural populations. To truly improve mental health in rural areas, each of these factors must be addressed in concert. Some strategies that could improve these aspects are discussed below.

IMPROVING AVAILABILITY OF SERVICES

Continuing to develop new ways of attracting mental health providers to rural areas to address availability issues will be essential. In late 2011, the Health Resources and Services Administration (HRSA) estimated that it would take *more than 6,000* new mental health professionals to address all of the mental health professional shortage areas in the United States—a very tall order that currently cannot be filled. While training programs graduate thousands of clinical psychologists and therapists each year, educational training opportunities for these individuals are severely limited in rural areas, and availability of required clinical experiences (e.g., practica and internships) is even more limited. Addressing the ability of interested individuals to attend a rural-focused program *and also* have the opportunity to complete required clinical training experiences in rural settings is a vital first step in increasing the presence of mental health providers in rural areas. Increasing the availability of educational opportunities without also increasing the number of field-based clinical training opportunities will drive rural-interested practitioners into urban areas to complete their clinical training because of the lack of required training sites within rural areas. Therefore, without a functioning pipeline for rural-interested individuals to take them from the start of their training all the way through licensure within a rural setting, other efforts to increase interest in rural practice will have minimal impact. Providers will continue to be effectively forced toward urban practice because of the need for training experiences and required supervision experiences typically unavailable in rural settings.

Beyond those wishing to somewhat "specialize" in rural practice, all training programs should include discussion of rural mental health in their core curriculum. Accredited psychology training programs typically include a multicultural psychology course designed to prepare students for clinical practice with diverse clients—however, "diversity" in this context seems to focus primarily upon cultures surrounding race, ethnicity, religion, and sexual orientation. Given the fact that rural residents comprise 20% of the U.S. population, they represent one of the largest "diversity" groups and should receive associated focus in cultural training. As discussed earlier in this text, rurality *is* a diversity issue, and until this is fully recognized and integrated into training programs, practitioners will continue to be at a disadvantage when dealing with clients from rural backgrounds. Including rural-focused cultural training in psychology education programs will prepare all clinicians to work with rural clients, either within rural settings or when encountered in more urbanized catchment areas.

Another key area in increasing availability of services centers on the ongoing debate regarding scope of practice, particularly prescriptive privileges. As an example, most patients with depression (one of the most common mental health diagnoses in rural areas) receive psychoactive medication from their primary care physician rather than a psychiatrist trained in management of mental health disorders (Goldberg & Lecrubier, 1995). More often than not (73% of the time) this psychopharmacologic treatment occurs without the patient ever having being diagnosed with a mental health condition (Mojtabai & Olfson, 2011). While psychiatrists do receive in-depth training in selecting, prescribing, and monitoring psychoactive prescriptions, this training occurs mostly during the psychiatric residency, not during general medical school. Therefore, primary care physicians are not adequately trained in diagnosis of mental disorders—yet they are able to prescribe psychoactive medication. To help expand the number of individuals trained in diagnosis and treatment of mental disorders, there is a growing movement to extend prescriptive privileges to psychologists. The states of Louisiana and New Mexico (as well as the military) now allow psychologists to prescribe psychoactive medication after completing additional training in psychopharmacology. Such dual-role licensure permits a single clinician (i.e., the psychologist) to address both the therapeutic and pharmacologic treatment of mental illness. In rural settings in particular this could tremendously increase the ability of rural residents to receive psychoactive medication from individuals with intensive training in their prescription and maintenance. By allowing psychologists to gain prescriptive authority after completing an in-depth program (typically a Master's degree in psychopharmacology), rural residents will be able to receive medications from individuals additionally trained to monitor mental status. This can help make rural psychologists a "one-stop shop" of sorts, and prevent the need of having at least *two* mental health professionals in any region—a therapist and a psychiatrist. The debate is not an easy one, however, and continues to face opposition. Rural psychologists can serve an important role in bringing about this change by continuing to promote the benefits of prescriptive privileges and explaining to (often urban-based) policy makers *how much* of an impact this could have in improving rural mental health.

INCREASING ACCESSIBILITY OF CARE

As the number of practitioners (and thus their availability) increases through the methods described above, efforts must be taken to strategically allow such providers nontraditional avenues of increasing their accessibility to rural residents who need services. Dispersed populations will always be a feature of rural America; therefore, continued focus on delivery modalities that take advantage of emerging technologies (i.e., telehealth) or locations where populations already congregate (e.g., in schools) will greatly improve the ability of rural residents to access services that may be available. Tele-mental health has shown remarkable promise in addressing provider shortages; however, reimbursement regulations have not caught up to the increasing evidence base. While telemedicine (including telepsychiatry) is becoming increasingly supported and reimbursed by insurance companies and government payors such as Medicare, reimbursement for therapy services remains an ongoing challenge. Federal statutes to support reimbursement of tele-mental health services (including both psychiatric services and therapy) would go a long way toward facilitating providers establishing telehealth practices. In addition, reevaluating state-by-state licensure of mental health professionals and moving toward a nationwide licensing system or reciprocal agreement/ license portability act would remove current barriers to interstate telehealth practices (as well as increase the likelihood of convincing a practitioner to relocate to a rural area in another state). Continued expansion of the availability of mental health services in community health centers, health departments, and other free/reduced price clinics will also be important in increasing the affordability of such services. These integrations could be facilitated by telehealth as appropriate, but again such opportunities are only feasible with the reform of insurance-reimbursable services or government support of their operations for the uninsured (such as through federally qualified health centers).

IMPROVING ACCEPTABILITY OF MENTAL HEALTH SERVICES

The third part of the nexus of change is in increasing acceptability of care. While much effort has been focused on the de-stigmatization of mental health, the fact remains that rural areas still hold a considerable amount of negative perception regarding individuals with mental illnesses. This not only serves to make those with mental illnesses feel even more isolated and burdened, it also prevents rural residents from seeking mental health services at early stages of their mental illness (leading to worse outcomes and longer courses of treatment). Again, innovative approaches such as integration of care can go a long way toward decreasing stigma—by providing mental health services in the context of a "medical" setting, rural residents may begin to shift their views of mental health into being an overall *health* issue. In addition, it allows for a "safe" venue for individuals to receive mental health services—people will not be as concerned about being seen in the parking lot of their doctor's office as they would in the parking lot of the local therapist—if the therapist is colocated with the medical practice such concerns can be alleviated. Given the high comorbidity between mental and physical health conditions in rural areas and the severe transportation burden faced by rural residents, colocation of services further addresses issues of accessibility as well. Other community-based awareness efforts should be undertaken to increase the visibility of mental health needs, and to educate the rural public about how addressing these issues can improve the quality of life for their communities.

EVIDENCE-BASE FOR RURAL PRACTICE

As with many high-need areas, research has not been able to keep up with demand, and new methods of improving rural mental health develop faster than they are able to be evaluated for effectiveness. Institutions of higher learning, long regarded as the hub of research and innovation, are rarely located within rural settings. This leaves university-based researchers interested in rural mental health in a very difficult predicament—do they live within an urban area and attempt to secure research funding to travel into nearby rural settings (and in the process lose their close integration into the rural community), or do they work in a smaller university within a rural area that is much less likely to receive the types of funding given to researchers at larger, urban universities? To improve the ability of researchers to examine best practices and build an evidence base for emerging strategies for improving rural mental health, federal funders must recognize that to be maximally effective, research and innovation intended for rural areas must spring from within those rural settings. This has been recognized for other disparity groups for many years in federal agencies' attempts to recruit more minority representation into the mental health workforce and research careers, but the same emphasis has not been placed upon supporting rural research and practice. Urban universities contain many dedicated researchers who are passionate about improving rural mental health issues, but without being imbedded within their rural communities of need there are inherent barriers to generating cutting-edge, community-informed research. Without dedicated support and special consideration, university-based researchers focused on rural populations will continue to face substantial barriers in securing support for their work.

There are alternatives, however, to the traditional university-based research model. Increasingly, community-based participatory research (research in which the target community plays an active *leadership* role in setting priorities and executing research) has been viewed as an exceptional model for improving community-level mental health. Communities can and should identify and mobilize local resources able to support their own research. Rural areas without experienced researchers should be supported in pursuing connections to rural-aware assistance throughout the nation (for instance, connecting to researchers located in other rural areas via technology-mediated communication). Rural clinicians, many of whom have been trained in research methodology through their graduate education, can also facilitate community-based research by serving as a resource or leader in building capacity and community buy-in for engaging in outcome research.

THE IMPORTANCE OF ADVOCACY

Many of the preceding suggestions for the future direction of rural mental health will require either significant funding or significant policy changes. This will require long-term, data-driven advocacy to policy makers. This can only occur if rural areas unite in their efforts to convey a consistent message of need to legislators and other policy-makers. Rural practitioners can play a key role in advocating for necessary resources and policy changes needed to improve the mental health of rural areas. More information on advocating for mental health issues can be found on the websites of the National Association for Rural Mental Health (http://www.narmh.org/) and the American Psychological Association's Guide to Advocacy and Outreach (http://www.apa.org/about/gr/advocacy/).

CONCLUSION

In summary, while there is much work to be done, much work *has* been done that has led to major innovations in mental health service delivery in rural settings. Rural areas will continue to be plagued with resource issues and economic hardships, but with increased understanding of the key barriers at play, a recognition of the myriad cultural factors influencing mental health outcomes, and a fresh knowledge of the latest advancements in new models of mental health service delivery, rural mental health practitioners can truly make a difference in mental health for the one in five Americans living in rural areas.

REFERENCES

Goldberg, D., & Lecrubier, Y. (1995). Form and frequency of mental disorders across centers. In T. Ustun, & N. Sartorius (Eds.), *Mental illness in general health care: An international study* (pp. 323–334). Chichester, England: John Wiley & Sons.
Mojtabai, R., & Olfson, M. (2011). Proportion of antidepressants prescribed without a psychiatric diagnosis is growing. *Health Affairs, 30*(8), 1434–1442. doi: 10.1377/hlthaff.2010.1024

Index